D1251129

DISEASES OF THE LIVER AND BILE DUCTS

CURRENT ◊ CLINICAL ◊ PRACTICE

DISEASES OF THE LIVER AND BILE DUCTS

A PRACTICAL GUIDE TO DIAGNOSIS AND TREATMENT

Edited by

GEORGE Y. WU, MD, PHD

University of Connecticut School of Medicine, Farmington, CT

and

JONATHAN ISRAEL, MD

Hartford Hospital, Hartford, CT

Foreword by

WILLIS C. MADDREY, MD

University of Texas Southwestern Medical Center, Dallas, TX

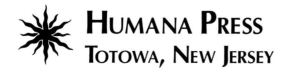

HUMANA PRESS
TOTOWA, NEW JERSEY

To my parents, my wife, Catherine, and children, Jonathan, David, and Victoria, for their patience...and to my mentors and friends: Irwin M. Arias, and Rudi Schmid for their unflagging support and guidance through the years.

George Y. Wu, MD, PhD

To my wife, Karen, and daughters, Jenna and Rebecca, and the memory of my mother, Lola Israel which continues to provide me with inspiration in all my endeavors.

Jonathan Israel, MD

© 1998 Humana Press Inc.
999 Riverview Drive, Suite 208
Totowa, New Jersey 07512

**WI
700
D6155
1998**

For additional copies, pricing for bulk purchases, and/or information about other Humana titles, contact Humana at the above address or at any of the following numbers: Tel: 973-256-1699; Fax: 973-256-8341; E-mail: humana@humanapr.com

Due diligence has been taken by the publishers, editors, and authors of this book to assure the accuracy of the information published and to describe generally accepted practices. The contributors herein have carefully checked to ensure that the drug selections and dosages set forth in this text are accurate and in accord with the standards accepted at the time of publication. Notwithstanding, as new research, changes in government regulations, and knowledge from clinical experience relating to drug therapy and drug reactions constantly occurs, the reader is advised to check the product information provided by the manufacturer of each drug for any change in dosages or for additional warnings and contraindications. This is of utmost importance when the recommended drug herein is a new or infrequently used drug. It is the responsibility of the treating physician to determine dosages and treatment strategies for individual patients. Further it is the responsibility of the health care provider to ascertain the Food and Drug Administration status of each drug or device used in their clinical practice. The publisher, editors, and authors are not responsible for errors or omissions or for any consequences from the application of the information presented in this book and make no warranty, express or implied, with respect to the contents in this publication.

Cover design by Patricia F. Cleary

This publication is printed on acid-free paper. ∞
ANSI Z39.48-1984 (American National Standards Institute) Permanence of Paper for Printed Library Materials.

Printed in the United States of America.   10 9 8 7 6 5 4 3 2 1

Library of Congress Cataloging-in-Publication Data

Diseases of the liver and bile ducts : a practical guide to diagnosis and treatment / edited by George Y. Wu and Jonathan Israel
          p.   cm.—(Current clinical practice)
     Includes index.
     ISBN 0-89603-431-1 (alk. paper)
     1. Liver—Diseases. 2. Bile ducts—Diseases. 3. Primary care (Medicine) I. Wu, George Y., 1948–   . II. Israel, Jonathan. III. Series/
     [DNLM: 1. Liver Diseases—disgnosis. 2. Liver Diseases—therapy. 3. Bile Duct Diseases—diagnosis. 4. Bile Duct Diseases—therapy. WI 700 D6155 1998.]
     RC845.D556   1998
     616.3'6—dc21
     DNLM/DLC
     for Library of Congress   98-23699
                                                                                                       CIP

FOREWORD

WILLIS C. MADDREY, MD

Executive Vice President for Clinical Affairs,
University of Texas Southwestern Medical Center, Dallas, TX

The practicing physician needs to know (and wants to know) more than ever about diseases of the liver and the biliary tract. There is surely enough emerging important information to fully warrant a well-constructed practice manual. Fortunately there is much to present, as the courses of a variety of liver diseases can now be favorably influenced. The opportunities for therapeutic intervention are exciting advancements for clinicians interested in hepatology, who heretofore were often observers with little ability to alter the natural course of acute and chronic liver diseases.

Hepatology has amply shared in the remarkable ongoing expansion of the scientific and clinical basis of medical practice. Within a quarter century, we have been given increasingly precise diagnostic tools with which to assess the liver. Developments in clinical chemistry, serology, imaging, endoscopy, and the widespread use of liver biopsy have all contributed the required tools. The ability to make secure diagnoses has been augmented. The development of liver transplantation as a successful approach to therapy has increased interest in more precise diagnosis and assessment of where the patient is in the natural history of a specific disease. The precision is of great importance in that timing for the transplantation is critical to the likelihood of success.

In this practice manual, efforts are made to provide the clinician with an understanding of the utility and limitations of the ways in which the liver is evaluated. The descriptions of tests and techniques are interwoven with outlines of the principal manifestations and the natural history of the most frequently encountered diseases of the liver. In many situations an algorithmic approach accurately presents the state of knowledge in graphic form. An algorithm based on sound observations supported by science and created by an experienced clinician is of great benefit in guiding clinical practice.

The hepatologist of today must consider a vast array of diseases. The most frequent major issues include the detection and treatment of chronic viral hepatitis B and C, assessment of drug-induced injury to the liver, diagnosis and management of the cholestatic disorders, including primary biliary cirrhosis and primary sclerosing cholangitis, evaluation of an asymptomatic or minimally symptomatic patient who is found to have an abnormality in a biochemical test or on an imaging study, and for those who have advanced disease, determining candidacy and timing for liver transplantation. The universe of recognized liver diseases continues to expand. Recent additions include nonalcoholic steatohepatitis, which is established to be a definite and quite common entity, and appreciation of the many liver diseases found in patients who are immunodeficient.

As is the case in all of medicine, our targets are ever moving. The astounding expansion of what one might know increases the focus on providing a solid base of information that one must know. Advances in virology allow precise identification of the agents that cause hepatitis A through E. Of interest has been the discovery of hepatitis G, although the importance of this virus as a cause of hepatitis remains uncertain. There has been a cascade of new information and opportunities following the discovery of the hepatitis viruses. Chronic hepatitis C and chronic hepatitis B are established major worldwide diseases affecting astounding numbers of individuals. The search for effective ways to assess the presence and extent of hepatic injury from these viruses, coupled with efforts to prevent the spread of disease, and treat those already affected, is the major activity of hepatologists. Surely the development of effective vaccines to prevent hepatitis A and B ranks among the major accomplishments of 20th century medicine. All physicians need to know when to recommend these vaccines, which thus far have been considerably underused. It may well be possible to someday add hepatitis B to the list of diseases that have been eradicated. The prevention of chronic hepatitis B is of even more importance. Patients who are long-term hepatitis B carriers have a high risk of developing chronic ongoing liver disease, cirrhosis, and hepatocellular carcinoma. The whole chain of events can be prevented through appropriate vaccination strategies. Likewise, many individuals needlessly develop hepatitis A when the use of the effective vaccine could have prevented the illness.

There is a base of knowledge about the liver and its diseases which every clinician needs to know. A few of the important issues include:

- The natural history of chronic hepatitis B and chronic hepatitis C and the potential favorable therapeutic roles of interferon and other emerging therapies.
- How to suspect, recognize, and establish the diagnosis of autoimmune disease in order to successfully intervene with immunosuppressive therapy.
- The approach to detect and treat hemochromatosis in its early stages and a plan that will achieve the most benefit from venesection for the patient and affected family members.
- When to consider Wilson's disease, recognizing that this disorder often presents with hepatic manifestations in the absence of neurological manifestations. Efforts expended in the diagnosis of Wilson's disease are amply rewarded by the often spectacular results from D-penicillamine therapy.
- When to use beta-blockers and other pharmacologic agents in patients who have bled from esophagogastric varices in order to prevent recurrent bleeding.
- The frequency with which spontaneous septicemia and bacterial peritonitis is a complication of cirrhosis and appreciation of the importance of prophylactic antibiotics in preventing recurrence of infection in a patient who has survived an initial episode.
- Appreciation of the many guises under which hepatic encephalopathy may present and how appropriate changes in diet and the use of lactulose may serve to enhance performance in these patients.
- Recognition of the opportunities afforded by the clinical development of liver transplantation and the important decisions that determine candidacy and timing.

The above list includes just a few of the important areas a clinician needs to know in caring for patients with liver diseases. This practice manual provides the clinician major blocks of sound advice in an easy-to-assimilate format. An important section of each chapter relates to interactions between the primary care physician and the specialist. Specialists often serve as educators, guides, and coaches. The primary care clinician has a vital role and needs to be fully conversant with diagnostic tests for identifying the cause of acute and chronic viral hepatitis as well as the need to promote the use of vaccines for hepatitis A and hepatitis B. When the findings are confusing, the diagnosis uncertain, and when emergency treatment or liver transplantation may be needed, the team approach is imperative. These days in hepatology there is much to do and, in fact, much more than can be done.

PREFACE

Diseases of the liver and biliary tract comprise a vast array of conditions that are often complex and bewildering. Furthermore, many recent fundamental discoveries and rapid advances in technology have led to new knowledge in the field. In this volume, we have prepared a practice manual that explains the advantages and limitations of new tests and provides algorithms for evaluation of patients and treatment of liver problems commonly encountered by the primary care physician. The first section introduces the evaluation of the patient with liver disease, aspects of the history and physical examination that can be invaluable in considering the patient with hepatobiliary disease. Nuances of serological tests for detection of viral infections of the liver are described, and radiological tests both invasive and non-invasive are presented with their application for specific circumstances. Another section covers commonly encountered specific diseases of the liver and biliary system. Treatable genetic disorders are emphasized even though many are rare because the impact of timely diagnosis and treatment is potentially great. Finally, common complications are presented with practical information on how to recognize the problems and deal with them effectively. Many experts in their fields have collaborated to produce a text that is concise, easy to understand, and definitive.

George Y. Wu, MD, PhD
Jonathan Israel, MD

ACKNOWLEDGMENTS

The expert secretarial assistance of Brenda Kawecki and Martha Schwartz is gratefully acknowledged. Research in liver diseases for GYW is supported in part by the US Public Health Service, NIH, NIDDK Grant no. DK-42182, and the Immune Response Corporation. GYW holds equity in the Immune Response Corporation.

George Y. Wu, MD, PhD

CONTENTS

CONTRIBUTORS

KHALID AZIZ, MD • *Division of GI, Veterans Administration Hospital, Newington, CT*

GABU BHARDWAJ, MD • *University of Florida College of Medicine, Gainesville, FL*

HERBERT L. BONKOVSKY, MD • *Division of Digestive Disease and Nutrition, University of Massachusetts, Worcester, MA*

SHABBIR-HUSAIN CHAIWALA, MD • *Lakewood Family Practice, Houston, TX*

HARRY CHEN, MD • *Department of Radiology, University of Connecticut Health Center, Farmington, CT*

JANNA COLLINS, MD • *Department of Pediatrics, Columbia University, New York, NY*

GARY L. DAVIS, MD • *Section of Hepatobiliary Diseases, University of Florida College of Medicine, Gainesville, FL*

THOMAS DEVERS, MD • *New Britain, CT*

MATTHEW ESTILL, MD • *Ithaca West, Ithaca, NY*

JEFF FIDLER, MD • *University of Nebraska Medical Center, Omaha, NE*

ROBERTO J. GROSZMANN, MD, FRCP • *Hepatic Hemodynamic Laboratory, Yale University School of Medicine, West Haven, CT*

MARTIN HAHN, MD • *University of Oregon Health Sciences Center, Portland, OR*

STEVEN K. HERRINE, MD • *Jefferson Medical College, Thomas Jefferson University, Philadelphia, PA*

JEFFREY HYAMS, MD • *Hartford Hospital, Hartford, CT*

YARIN ILAN, MD • *Albert Einstein College of Medicine, Bronx, NY*

JONATHAN ISRAEL, MD • *Hartford Hospital, Hartford, CT*

F. WILSON JACKSON, MD • *Thomas Jefferson University Hospital, Philadelphia, PA*

LENNOX JEFFERS, MD • *Department of Hepatology, University of Miami School of Medicine, Miami, FL*

CHRISTOPHER JUSTINICH, MD • *Hartford Hospital, Hartford, CT*

KAREN KORMIS, MD • *Pennsylvania Gastroenterology Consultants, Chapel Hill, PA*

JOHNSON LAU, MD • *University of Florida, Gainesville, FL*

THOMAS LI, MD • *DigestaCare Gastroenterology, Bridgewater, NJ*

T. JAKE LANG, MD • *NIH Liver Section NIDDK, Bethesda, MD*

ENRIQUE J. MARTINEZ • *Department of Hepatology, University of Miami School of Medicine, Miami, FL*

COLSTON A. MCEVOY, MD • *Division of Pediatric GI and Hepatology, Yale University School of Medicine, New Haven, CT*

WILLIAM H. RAMSEY, MD • *Division of GI, University of Connecticut Health Center, Farmington, CT*

CAROLINE RIELY, MD • *University of Tennessee School of Medicine, Memphis, TN*

DOUGLAS ROBERTSON, MD • *University of Connecticut Health Center, Farmington, CT*

STEVEN ROGERS, MD • *Gastrointestinal Unit, Massachusetts General Hospital, Boston, MA*

JAYANTA ROY-CHOWDHURY, MD, MRCP • *Albert Einstein College of Medicine, Bronx, NY*

NAMITA ROY-CHOWDHURY, MD, PHD • *Albert Einstein College of Medicine, Bronx, NY*

RAYMOND A. RUBIN, MD • *Atlanta Gastroenterology Associates, Piedmont Hospital, Atlanta, GA*

FRANCISCO RUIZ, MD • *University of Tennessee Medical School, Memphis, TN*

KIRAN SACHDEV, MD • *Division of GI, Middlesex Hospital, Middletown, CT*

MICHAEL SCHILSKY, MD • *Division of GI, Liver Research Center, Albert Einstein College of Medicine, Bronx, NY*

DAVID STARK, MD • *Department of Radiology, University of Nebraska Medical Center South, Omaha, NE*

IRMIN STERNLIEB, MD • *St. Luke's/Roosevelt Hospital, New York, NY*

FREDERICK SUCHY, MD • *Department of Pediatrics, The Mount Sinai Medical Center, New York, NY*

EDWARD TOFFOLON, MD • *New Britain, CT*

MARK VERSLAND, MD • *New Britain, CT*

GEORGE Y. WU, MD • *Division of GI, University of Connecticut Health Center, Farmington, CT*

MARAM ZAKKO, MD • *Hepatic Hemodynamic Laboratory, Yale University School of Medicine, West Haven, CT*

SALAM ZAKKO, MD • *Division of GI, University of Connecticut Health Center, Farmington, CT*

MARK ZERN, MD • *Jefferson Medical College, Philadelphia, PA*

I General Clinical Features of Liver Disease

1

Signs and Symptoms of Liver Disease

Khalid Aziz and Jonathan Israel

CONTENTS

1. INTRODUCTION

Liver disease is an important cause of mortality and morbidity worldwide. In third world countries, especially in Asia and Africa, viral infections are the major liver problem, whereas in the Western world, alcoholic damage is the most important cause of liver disease, accounting for up to 80% of patients with cirrhosis in some countries *(1)*. In the United States, chronic liver disease, including cirrhosis, is the fourth most frequent cause of death among individuals 30–60 yr old *(2)*. Fortunately, mortality from chronic liver disease has steadily declined in the past 10 yr in both the white and black populations *(3)*. However, it remains costly, both in terms of human morbidity and financial resources, as the course of chronic liver disease is typically characterized by recurrent complications requiring repeated hospitalizations, and often results in loss of life.

The increased use of aminotransferase assays in health surveys and screening tests has led to the incidental discovery of a large number of persons with abnormal serum liver tests. The vast majority of these people are asymptomatic. In fact, one third of patients referred to hepatologists have no complaints attributable to the hepatobiliary system *(4)*.

When symptoms are present, clinical features of the more common acute and chronic liver diseases are frequently nonspecific. As a result, use of the history and physical examination in the diagnosis and management of diseases of the liver can be challenging. Attempts to circumvent this problem with objective tests have led to a proliferation of biochemical and serologic assays, new imaging modalities, and invasive tests, such as endoscopic retrograde

From: *Diseases of the Liver and Bile Ducts: Diagnosis and Treatment*
Edited by: G. Y. Wu and J. Israel © Humana Press Inc., Totowa, NJ

cholangiopancreatography and percutaneous liver biopsy. Despite these technological advances, an accurate, organized, directed medical history is still the most important and fundamental set of data in the practice of hepatology. Accurate documentation of the precise duration of symptoms, and serum liver enzyme abnormalities, is crucial and may require scrutiny of prior medical records. Such information is essential in differentiating acute from chronic liver disease and evaluating disease progression.

2. HISTORY

As in other areas of clinical medicine, a full clinical history in patients with possible liver disease should include: chief complaint; history of present illness; past medical history; system review; family history; personal history including alcohol, substance abuse, occupational history, and foreign travel; and medications and allergies.

2.1. Chief Complaint and History of Present Illness

Patients with liver disease frequently have nonspecific symptoms such as anorexia, nausea, fatigue, malaise, and asthenia. Jaundice, generalized pruritis, right upper quadrant pain and dark urine are more suggestive of liver dysfunction. Prior symptoms such as upper abdominal pain, recent surgery, treatment with hepatotoxic drugs and history of blood or blood product administration are usually more significant. History should begin from the time the patient last felt perfectly fit and well, which may be many months or years prior to the current visit. Not infrequently, physicians have to contact the primary care provider when the patient is not able to furnish specific information about his medical history, particularly the medications, or type and details of previous surgery.

2.2. Symptoms of Liver Disease

2.2.1. FATIGUE

Nonspecific symptoms, including fatigue, malaise, listlessness, and inability to concentrate, are commonly associated with liver disease. Fatigue and malaise are the presenting features in about one third to two thirds of patients with liver disease (5). Fatigue can be the dominant, and sometimes the only, symptom in patients with chronic liver disease. A major demographic study of primary biliary cirrhosis in Canada showed that fatigue was present in 80.6% of patients and was the single most disabling symptom (6). Fatigue may be present for months or years before a diagnosis of liver disease is made. It tends to be worse during the latter part of the day. Fatigue tends to worsen as the disease progresses, and improves with improvement in liver disease, which may occur either spontaneously or in response to a specific therapy. For instance, fatigue often improves with seroconversion of hepatitis B, and treatment of autoimmune hepatitis with steroids, or after successful liver transplantation for end-stage liver disease from any cause.

The pathogenesis of fatigue is unknown. A recent study suggests that defective corticotrophin-releasing hormone-mediated neuroendocrine behavioral responses may be responsible for fatigue in this situation (7). Reports of a causal relationship between altered function of the hypothalamic-pituitary adrenal axis and abnormal behavioral state have been documented in similar animal models (8). These experimental findings may not be specific for, or applicable to, human liver disease, and further studies are necessary before their relevance in liver disease patients can be determined.

2.2.2. ANOREXIA

Anorexia is a prominent symptom in a wide variety of liver diseases and is of little specific diagnostic value. It may precede the appearance of jaundice in acute hepatitis and it may be a prominent symptom in cirrhosis and hepatobiliary malignancy. Anorexia was found to be present in almost 90% of patients with acute viral hepatitis *(9)*, and 50% with alcoholic hepatitis *(10)*. It tends to worsen with increasing severity of liver disease, and may lead to profound malnutrition with loss of muscle mass and fatty tissue. However, the total body weight may remain unchanged because of increasing edema and ascites. Worsening ascites leads to further anorexia and early satiety due to pressure on the stomach. The etiology of anorexia in liver disease is not well elucidated, but changes in the palatability of food or changes in the level of circulating hormones such as glucagon, somatostatin, cholecystokinin, gastrin, and bombesin or various nutrients such as glucose, free fatty acids, or amino acids may all be involved *(11)*.

2.2.3. DISORDERED TASTE AND SMELL

Disturbances of taste and smell are common in patients with liver disease. A recent study evaluated chemosensory function, food preferences and appetite in patients with liver disease, including hepatitis, cirrhosis, primary biliary cirrhosis, and sclerosing cho-langitis. Recent changes in taste and smell were reported by 40 and 27%, respectively in patients with liver disease, compared to only 6% of healthy age- and gender-matched controls. Compared to controls, a greater proportion of patients with liver disease reported food cravings (47–17%) and food aversions (33–13%). Foods with a predominantly bitter taste were less preferred in patients with liver disease. Patients were also more likely to report poor to fair appetite than controls (37 vs 5%) *(12)*. Altered taste probably explains aversion to smoking in acute viral hepatitis and other liver diseases. In another study, decreased subjective taste acuity and increased use of salt and sugar was noted in 84% of patients with liver disease, whereas 74% of patients with acute viral hepatitis complained of obnoxious taste and smell for fried foods and 90% to meat *(9)*. In another study, the taste threshold was elevated for salt, sugar, hydrochloric acid, and urea *(13)*. Although the mechanisms are not clear, zinc and vitamin E supplementation have been shown to improve taste sensation in patients with alcoholic cirrhosis *(14)*.

2.2.4. NAUSEA AND VOMITING

Nausea and vomiting are common complaints in patients with liver disease. They may occur independently of each other, but are more often seen concurrently, and are presumed to be mediated by related neuropathways. Nausea and vomiting are often striking features of acute biliary obstruction due to gallstones and hepatic tumors in patients with viral and drug-induced hepatitis, as well as other parenchymal liver diseases. Metoclopramide has been shown to suppress nausea and vomiting in patients with advanced cirrhosis, but can cause worsening of edema and ascites due to enhanced secretion of aldosterone *(15)*.

2.2.5. ALTERATION IN BODY WEIGHT

Unintentional weight loss is commonly seen in patients with chronic liver diseases. Mechanisms include anorexia, early satiety due to pressure of ascites on the stomach, and accelerated metabolism. Precipitous weight loss in patients with chronic liver disease may suggest development of complications such as malignancy or infection. Gradual weight loss accompanies end-stage liver disease secondary to loss of muscle mass and adipose tissue from a hypercatabolic state due to an infectious or other metabolic disorder.

Weight gain or stability in patients with late, chronic liver disease is usually due to noncompliance with low salt diet or, secondarily, to deterioration in liver disease resulting in worsening ascites. In these patients, significant malnutrition may occur without changes in body weight. Conversely, in patients with early liver disease, weight gain may be due to simple obesity.

2.2.6. ABDOMINAL PAIN

Abdominal pain is common in hepatobiliary disease. Pain may be pleuritic in nature, especially in patients with inflammatory diseases of the gallbladder. It may be located in the right upper quadrant or may be felt in the right shoulder, especially if the diaphragm is involved. Pain or discomfort along with tenderness on palpation may occur due to rapid or gross enlargement of the liver or spleen. Acute biliary colic may be localized in the right upper quadrant, epigastrium or retrosternal area. Massive accumulation of ascites may be associated with generalized abdominal pain.

2.2.7. JAUNDICE

Jaundice, or icterus, refers to the yellow pigmentation of the skin or sclera caused by deposition of bilirubin. It may be noted by the patient himself or pointed out by friends or family members. It is important to determine whether it is predominantly due to unconjugated or conjugated hyperbilirubinemia. A simple clue in this regard is whether bilirubin is present in the urine. Its absence in the urine suggests unconjugated hyperbilirubinemia, because conjugated bilirubin is filtered by the glomerulus and unconjugated bilirubin is not. Patients should be asked about pruritus, clay colored stools, and abdominal pain as clues to the presence of biliary obstruction.

2.2.8. ALTERATION IN BOWEL FUNCTION

Patients should be queried about the frequency, color, and consistency of stools. Stools may be pale or clay colored in patients with bile duct obstruction or intrahepatic cholestasis. Pancreatic steatorrhea may also result in pale gray stools. Black stools may be due to melena, or excessive oral iron intake. Greenish-black stools can be caused by bismuth therapy.

A moderate increase in stool frequency is common in many liver diseases, but particularly in alcoholics and acute viral hepatitis *(16)*. Biliary obstruction is associated with steatorrhea due to fat malabsorption, and is particularly common if the pancreatic duct is blocked. For unclear reasons, diarrhea may occur in patients with hepatocellular carcinoma. Diarrhea may be caused by a disease which is secondarily associated with liver involvement. For instance, sclerosing cholangitis is often associated with ulcerative colitis, and hepatic metastases can occur in patients with carcinoid syndrome.

2.2.9. EDEMA AND ASCITES

Ascites and edema may be caused by liver, heart, renal diseases, malnutrition, and protein-losing states. It is important to remember that abdominal distention may be due to causes other than ascites, such as enlargement of abdominal viscera, gaseous distention or, more commonly, obesity. Mild ascites may be difficult to diagnose clinically, but moderate to severe ascites is easily detectable. Severe ascites may be associated with abdominal discomfort, presumably due to increased intra-abdominal pressure and stretching of visceral peritoneum. Massive ascites is also associated with the appearance and enlargement of hernias, early satiety, dyspnea, and occasional numbness on the lateral aspect of the thigh due to pressure on the lateral cutaneous nerve.

2.2.10. PRURITUS

Pruritus is associated with intra- or extrahepatic cholestasis from causes such as primary biliary cirrhosis, sclerosing cholangitis, cholestasis of pregnancy, and common bile duct obstruction due to strictures, stones, or malignancy. It can also be a feature of acute hepatitis A and, more rarely, alcoholic hepatitis when cholestasis is present in those conditions. Pruritus is usually more severe on the extremities, and milder or absent on the trunk. It rarely affects the neck, face, or genitals and is frequently worse after a hot shower, at night, and in warm weather. The mechanism of pruritis has been postulated to be related to interaction between the nerve endings and one or more substances (bile acids) that are retained in the body as a result of cholestasis *(17)*. Antihistamines, cholestyramine, ursodeoxycholic acid, and naloxone have shown a variable degree of efficacy in treating pruritus. Occasionally, patients with primary biliary cirrhosis develop severe pruritus unresponsive to traditional management and require liver transplantation for relief.

2.2.11. BLEEDING

Patients with acute or chronic liver disease may complain of spontaneous bleeding from the gums or nose or of easy cutaneous bruising. The severity of the complaint is related to the degree of hepatic compensation.

Thrombocytopenia related to portal hypertension and splenomegaly, as well as prolonged prothrombin time from diminished clotting factors, are likely contributing factors.

2.2.12. FEVER

Fever is common in liver disease and is associated with its infective complications, such as acute cholangitis or spontaneous bacterial peritonitis. It may be associated with chills. Elevated body temperatures are also seen in acute viral, alcoholic, and drug-induced hepatitis. Fever may also be a presenting feature of hepatocellular carcinoma.

2.2.13. MENTAL CONFUSION AND SLEEP DISTURBANCE

Patients with advanced liver disease often have somnolence during the day, and insomnia at night. This occurs in early hepatic encephalopathy. Mental confusion, slow response to various stimuli, stupor, and eventually coma occurs with increasing severity of encephalopathy. With early hepatic encephalopathy, there is intellectual deterioration, short attention span, inability to solve mental problems, memory loss and, finally, inability to communicate effectively. Patients may develop personality disorders with euphoria, depression, irritability, anxiety, or apathetic state. Hepatic encephalopathy and its implications are discussed in greater detail in Chapter 28.

2.2.14. SEXUAL DYSFUNCTION

Impotence is common in patients with cirrhosis from any cause, especially alcoholism. In alcoholics, impotence is present for a longer period of time, is more severe, and appears earlier in the course of disease as compared to nonalcoholic cirrhotics *(18)*. Sexual behavior is also altered in women with a variety of liver diseases. In one study, reduced sexual desire occurred in 33% of patients, difficulty with arousal in 18%, lack of orgasm in 25%, and dyspareunia in 21% *(19)*.

2.2.15. MUSCLE CRAMPS

Cramps affecting the calf muscles are more frequent in cirrhotic patients than controls (72 vs 40%). Twenty-three percent of cirrhotics vs 9% of controls reported more than three cramp crises a week. Cirrhotics with cramps had more severe disease than those without cramps *(20)*. Three variables independently predicted cramping in cirrhotics: the presence of ascites, low value of mean arterial pressure, and increased plasma renin activity. These factors suggest that a decreased plasma volume may cause cramping in cirrhotics. Consistent with this theory, albumin infusion significantly improved plasma renin activity, and decreased the frequency of cramping in a subgroup of cirrhotic patients with frequent severe muscle cramping *(10)*. Quinidine sulfate has proven effective in some patients with this problem *(21)*.

3. PAST MEDICAL HISTORY

A history of transfusion of blood or blood products raises the possibility of cirrhosis from hepatitis B, D, or C. Previous surgery for cancer is important, because liver abnormalities may represent metastatic disease. Jaundice in a patient with a previous cholecystectomy may be due to either retained gallstones or a postoperative stricture.

4. FAMILY HISTORY

Investigation of family history in patients with liver disease is important in uncovering genetic liver diseases. Because penetrance of affected genes can be variable, the proband may be many generations apart from the index case. A family history is not only important in cases of genetically determined diseases, such as Wilson's disease, hemochromatosis, and alpha-1-antitrypsin deficiency, but also infectious liver diseases such as hepatitis B, in which the most common route of spread is transmission from mother to child.

5. MEDICATION HISTORY

Medications are an important cause of liver disease. One of the initial steps in the investigation of abnormal serum liver enzymes is to review all prescribed, and illicit drugs used by the patient. Specific inquiry should also be made regarding over-the-counter, herbal medications, and megadose vitamins. Drug-induced hepatotoxicity is discussed in greater depth in Chapter 13.

6. PERSONAL HISTORY

Inquiry into the patient's occupational history and exposures, alcohol use, intravenous drug abuse, and sexual preference must be made. Patients notoriously underestimate their alcohol consumption, and more accurate estimation can often be obtained from the patient's spouse or other close family members. Prior travel history and ethnic background may also give clues to liver disease. For example, acute viral hepatitis is more likely after travel to an endemic area. Cirrhosis may occur in patients who have emigrated even 20 yr earlier from these same areas. Similarly, patients who have lived in endemic areas can develop portal hypertension from schistosomiasis years later. Certain organic solvents have been associated with liver dysfunction. Possible exposures should be investigated with respect to previous reported cases of liver disease associated with that substance.

7. PHYSICAL EXAMINATION

Physical examination is the cornerstone of clinical evaluation of patients with liver disease. Some signs are relatively specific, such as the Kayser-Fleisher rings of Wilson's disease or a large gallbladder in patients with carcinoma of the pancreas (Courvoisier's gallbladder). Others, such as asterixis and hepatic encephalopathy or abdominal collaterals in portal hypertension, although not specific for the type of liver disease, strongly suggests its presence. Physical examination in patients with liver disease should include a general physical examination and a detailed examination of the abdomen. Examination of other systems is pursued as appropriate.

7.1. General Physical Examination

The physical examination begins with a general examination to assess the overall condition. The body build is important, as loss of muscle bulk is a sign of relatively advanced liver disease or cancer, and is particularly common in cirrhosis. Obesity may cause abnormal liver function tests because of fatty liver. Xanthalasma suggests chronic cholestasis, which is commonly seen in primary biliary cirrhosis. Parotid enlargement is sometimes seen in patients with alcohol abuse, primary biliary cirrhosis with sicca syndrome, as well as malnutrition, and is usually painless.

Vital signs, including pulse, blood pressure, and temperature, should be noted. Patients with advanced liver disease and ascites are predisposed to spontaneous bacterial peritonitis. Fever may also be due to a variety of infectious diseases in which the liver is secondarily involved, such as leptospirosis, Epstein-Barr virus, and cytomegalovirus. It is also frequently seen in patients with AIDS. Patients with established liver disease may present with fever for which no cause is found despite extensive work up. Fever is common in patients with alcoholic cirrhosis who drink heavily, have a poor diet, and have advanced clinical and biochemical signs of liver disease and alcoholic hepatitis (22). Fever is also an important sign of primary or metastatic liver disease.

Conjunctival examination may show pallor of anemia due to blood loss from portal gastropathy, varices, or anemia due to hypersplenism. Kayser-Fleischer rings are highly suggestive of Wilson's disease, and, if prominent, can be seen by the naked eye. A slit lamp examination is required in questionable cases.

Patients may have tachypnea that is multifactorial. Massive ascites with restriction of diaphragmatic excursion, pleural effusion, or massive abdominal organomegaly all may contribute to this sign.

Icterus, with few exceptions, is a hallmark of liver disease. Jaundice is usually noticeable when serum bilirubin level exceeds 2 mg/dL. Patients with obstructive jaundice have dark urine due to bilirubinuria. However, patients with hemolytic anemia and jaundice do not usually develop dark urine.

Diffuse hyperpigmentation, due to increased melanin pigmentation in the skin, is common in patients with various forms of liver disease. These disorders include primary biliary cirrhosis, various forms of biliary obstruction, hemochromatosis, and porphyria cutanea tarda. A cutaneous examination should include a search for tattoos, skin popping scars, sclerotic veins, excoriations, and xanthalasma. In addition, the skin should be examined very carefully for stigmata of chronic liver disease. Spider nevi, palmar erythema, petechial hemorrhages, and easy bruisability are important clues to the presence of chronic liver disease. Palmar erythema can be hereditary and be unrelated to liver disease. Therefore, recent onset, or lack of palmar erythema in the past, is suggestive of the development of chronic liver disease. Gynecomastia is present in some patients with chronic liver disease, but is also seen in patients who use spironolactone as well as in patients with certain other medical disorders. It is diagnosed when there is a palpable enlargement of glandular tissue under the areola. The glandular tissue may be exquisitely tender and necessitate discontinuation of medications causing it.

Patients with advanced hepatic failure may have a fishy odor (fetor hepaticus) on their breath.

Patients with alcoholic liver disease may have Dupuytren's contractures. This phenomenon has been attributed to liver damage, but in one study the prevalence was similar in alcoholic cirrhotics, nonalcoholics, and in alcoholics without liver disease (23). Various abnormalities affecting the nails have been described in liver disease. These include shiny nails due to scratching, and transverse white lines when serum albumin falls below 2.2 gm/L (24). These changes may be found in other conditions associated with low serum albumin, such as nephrotic syndrome or protein-losing enteropathy. Mild clubbing is common with end-stage liver disease, especially in patients with primary biliary cirrhosis.

7.2. Examination of the Abdomen

Inspection of the abdomen may reveal distention, which could be diffuse, due to ascites, obesity, or massive organomegaly from the liver, spleen, gallbladder, or hernias. Specifically, bulging flanks and eversion of umbilicus suggest free intraperitoneal fluid. Prominent umbilical veins (Caput Medusae) may be seen in patients with severe portal hypertension. The sudden development of abdominal wall collaterals in patients with cirrhosis may indicate acute hepatic vein thrombosis (Budd-Chiari syndrome). Dilated veins on the abdominal wall should be evaluated for direction of filling (centrifugal vs centripetal).

Palpation should be performed to look for tenderness or to detect organomegaly from the spleen or liver. Signs of peritonitis with rebound tenderness and guarding raises concern about a perforated viscus or bacterial peritonitis, although it has been documented that the latter, in the majority of cases, have no abdominal tenderness.

Percussion should be performed to look for shifting dullness or fluid wave to diagnose ascites and to define spleen and liver size. Small amounts of ascites can be detected by a "puddle sign." Auscultation may reveal arterial bruits which are common with atherosclerotic involvement of various abdominal vessels. A splenic artery bruit may be heard in the epigastrium in patients with pancreatic tumors. Vascular tumors such as hepatocellular carcinoma and cholangiocarcinoma, or arteriovenous malformation, may be associated with bruit on the surface of the liver. A transient bruit lasting a day or so may be heard after liver biopsy due to temporary arteriovenous fistula. Similarly, a bruit in the left upper quadrant may be heard in patients with an aneurysm of the splenic artery, splenic arteriovenous fistula, or splenomegaly due to any cause. A friction rub is a scratchy sound which is heard over the liver if there is hepatic infarction, abscess, or a tumor invading the visceral pleura. It can also be heard in the Fitz-Hugh Curtis syndrome (gonococcal or chlamydial perihepatitis). Splenic infarction or inflammation causes a similar rub over the splenic area.

7.3. Physical Signs and Other Symptoms

A flapping tremor (asterixis) is a brief flexion of all the fingers when both arms are stretched in front of the patient and suggests hepatic encephalopathy. Percussion of the patient's back may reveal a pleural effusion, usually right-sided, and may be seen in patients with cirrhosis and ascites. Hemorrhoids are often evident in patients with portal hypertension from liver disease.

8. PRESENTATIONS OF LIVER DISEASE

Clinical presentations of liver disease may range from asymptomatic liver serum test abnormalities to fulminant hepatic failure with encephalopathy and coma. As mentioned earlier, an apparently healthy adult with an unexpected elevation on routine liver function tests poses a common problem. In fact, one third of the patients referred to hepatologists have no complaints attributable to the hepatobiliary system *(4)*. The original complaints or reasons for performing the blood tests may identify subtle clues relevant to underlying hepatobiliary disease. However, the majority of patients are discovered on routine blood tests for annual physical examination or Red Cross screening at the time of blood donation. Tests commonly called liver function tests do not actually determine liver function. These should instead be referred to as serum liver tests. These liver tests can be classified according to the pathophysiological processes they reflect.

The first step in the evaluation of abnormal liver tests is to determine if they are hepatitic (necroinflammatory) or cholestatic (*see* Fig. 1). Hepatitic markers include the aminotransferases AST (SGOT) and ALT (SGPT). Cholestatic markers include alkaline phosphatase, gamma glutamyl transpeptidase, 5' nucleotidase, and bilirubin. Twofold or greater elevations in aminotransferases with normal or less than twofold increases in alkaline phosphatase or gamma glutamyl transpeptidase would suggest a hepatitic process. Conversely, twofold increases in alkaline phosphatase or gamma glutamyl transpeptidase with normal or less than twofold increases in aminotransferases suggest a cholestatic process. Whereas hepatitic and cholestatic serum markers generally reflect their respective type of liver injury when enzyme levels are high, they are less specific when their levels are low, and crossover can be seen when

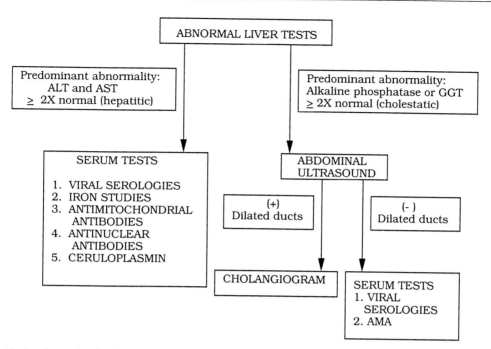

Fig. 1. A schematic plan for the evaluation of abnormal serum liver tests.

mixed effects are present. The evaluation of elevated liver serum tests proceeds as outlined in algorithm *(1)*.

8.1. AST and ALT Elevations

The serum aminotransferases include aspartate amino-transferase (AST), and alanine amino transferase (ALT), and are primarily used as markers for hepatic inflammation and necrosis. AST elevation is not specific for liver disease. It may be elevated in other conditions affecting heart, skeletal muscle, or kidneys. However, ALT is specific for hepatocellular injury. The magnitude of elevation of aminotransferases does not relate to prognosis. A patient with hepatitis A and an AST of 2000 IU/L does not necessarily have a worse prognosis than another patient with hepatitis A and an AST level of 1000 IU/L. However, absolute and relative values of AST and ALT are helpful in the differential diagnosis. Very high levels, exceeding 1000 IU/L, are seen in viral hepatitis, shock liver, toxic liver damage, a flare-up of autoimmune hepatitis, and early acute common bile duct obstruction. In contrast, alcoholic liver disease and chronic active hepatitis cause only modest elevations. The diseases that cause massive elevation of aminotransferases such as acute viral hepatitis, shock liver, and toxic hepatic injury are usually symptomatic, but diseases causing less than 10-fold elevation are usually asymptomatic. Evaluation of patients with chronically elevated hepatitic liver enzymes should include detailed history for possible drug or toxin ingestion, alcohol and substance abuse, exposure to patients with hepatitis, and previous history of serum liver test abnormality. In these patients, viral serology and tests for metabolic liver disease (iron and copper studies, autoimmune markers) should be performed (*see* Table 1).

8.2. Cholestatic Abnormalities

Alkaline phosphatase, gamma glutamyl transpeptidase (GGT), 5'-nucleotidase, and bilirubin are used as indicators of cholestasis. However, these do not differentiate intrahepatic from extrahepatic cholestasis. GGT and alkaline phosphatase are found in several tissues including

Table 1

Some Diseases that more Commonly Present with a Hepatitic (Necroinflammatory) Pattern

Viral hepatitis
Autoimmune hepatitis
Metabolic liver disease
Alcoholic liver disease
Hemochromatosis
Wilson's disease
Alpha-1-antitrypsin disease
Congestive heart failure
Drug/toxin exposure

bone, intestine, and placenta. Fortunately, combined elevation of alkaline phosphatase, 5'-nucleotidase, and GGT is highly suggestive of liver disease. GGT is inducible, and is elevated in individuals consuming drugs such as phenobarbital, phenytoin, and alcohol. Increase in serum alkaline phosphatase is due to stimulation of hepatic synthesis of this enzyme. Imaging studies such as ultrasound or CAT scan should be employed to distinguish between intra- and extrahepatic cholestasis. Table 2 lists common causes of cholestatic liver enzymes.

8.3. Isolated Hyperbilirubinemia

Unconjugated bilirubin originates mainly from the breakdown of RBC hemoglobin, which is transported to liver cells bound to plasma albumin. In the liver, it is conjugated mainly with glucuronic acid and excreted through the biliary system. The bilirubin level is a reflection of the balance between bilirubin production and clearance. The bilirubin production rate is directly related to red blood cell survival time. In hemolytic disorders, the bilirubin level rises in direct proportion to decreasing red cell survival time. Hemolytic anemia causes elevation of unconjugated serum bilirubin (indirect bilirubinemia). Gilbert's syndrome, resolving hematoma and some medications are other common causes of unconjugated hyperbilirubinemia.

9. INDICATIONS FOR CONSULTING A SPECIALIST

A specialist should be sought when specialized diagnostic or therapeutic measures are required. Patients who require a liver biopsy, endoscopic cholangiography, or endoscopic hemostasis should be referred to a specialist. In addition, patients developing fulminant hepatic failure will also require special care. Tertiary care facilities are essential in the proper management of these patients. As chronic liver disease progresses, transfer to a facility that has liver transplantation capability is important if the patient is an appropriate candidate. As a general rule, even for relatively stable chronic liver disease patients, referral to a transplant center for evaluation early is always preferable. Specific treatments and appropriate points for referral are discussed in subsequent chapters on specific diseases.

10. CONCLUSIONS

Liver disease is an important cause of morbidity and mortality worldwide and in the United States. In the United States, the majority of patients with liver disease are asymptomatic and come to the medical attention of the primary care physician when serum liver test abnormalities are noted. A complete and thorough history and physical is the essential first step in the evaluation. Categorization of the abnormalities into cholestatic or hepatitic disease is the next step. Complications of chronic liver disease resulting in decompensation, or poor response to medical management, will generally require a specialist *(25)*.

Table 2

Some Diseases that Commonly Present with a Cholestatic Pattern of Serum Liver Enzymes

Primary biliary cirrhosis
Primary sclerosing cholangitis
Malignancies (pancreatic, gall bladder, bile duct)
Granulatous diseases (tuberculosis, sarcoid)
Bile duct stricture
Bile duct stones

SUMMARY

Patients with liver disease are frequently asymptomatic.

Most cases of liver disease in the United States are discovered by finding abnormalities in screening blood tests.

Early symptoms of liver disease are nonspecific and include anorexia and easy fatigability.

Imaging studies are required to distinguish between intra- and extrahepatic cholestasis.

Abnormal liver blood tests can be divided into predominantly hepatitic (necro-inflammatory) or cholestatic, each requiring different diagnostic evaluation.

REFERENCES

1. Saunders JB, Latt, N. Epidemiology of alcoholic liver disease. Bailliere's Clin Gastro 1993;7:555–579.
2. Deaths and hospitalizations from chronic liver disease and cirrhosis–United States, 1980–1989. MMWR 52&53, 1993;4:969–973.
3. Age adjusted death rate for selected causes of death according to sex and race–United States, selected years 1950–1992. Health United States 1994: pp. 97,98.
4. Tamburro CH. Clinical evaluation of liver status. In: Gitnick G, ed. Diagnosis of liver and biliary disease. Mosby, St. Louis, MO, 1992: 95–135.
5. McIntyre N. Symptom and signs of liver disease. In: McIntyre N, Benhamon J, Bircher J, Rizzetto M, Rodes J, eds. Oxford textbook clin hepatol. Oxford University Press, Oxford, UK, 1991: pp. 273–290.
6. Witt-Sullivan H, Heathcote J, Cauch K, Blandis L, Ghent C, Katz A, Milner R, Pappas C, Rankin J, Wanless R. The demography of primary biliary cirrhosis in Ontario, Canada. Hepatology 1990;12:98–105.
7. Swain MG, Maric M. Defective corticotropin-releasing hormone mediated neuroendocrine and behavioral responses in cholestatic rats: Implications for cholestatic liver disease-related sickness behaviors. Hepatology 1995;5:1560–1564.
8. Swain MG, Patchev V, Vergalla J, Chrousos G, Jones EA. Suppression of hypothalamic-pituitary-adrenal axis responsiveness to stress in a rat model of acute cholestasis. J Clin Invest 1993;91:1903–1908.
9. Henkin RI, Smit FR. Hyposmia in acute viral hepatitis. Lancet 1971;1:823–826.
10. Mendenhall CL. Alcoholic hepatitis. Clin Gastroenterology 1981;10:417–441.
11. Nicholl CG, Polack JM, Bloom SR. The hormonal regulation of food intake, digestion and absorption. Ann Rev Nutr 1985;5:213–239.
12. Deems RO, Friedman MI, Friedman LS, Munoz SJ, Maddrey WC. Chemosensory function, food preferences and appetite in human liver disease. Appetite 1993;3:209–216.
13. Smith FR, Henkin IH, Dell RB. Disordered gustatory acuity in liver disease. Gastroenterology 1976;70:568–571.
14. Garrett-Laster M, Russell RM, Jacques PF. Impairment of taste and olfaction in patients with cirrhosis: the role of vitamin A. Hum Nutr-Clin Nutr 1984;3:203–214.
15. Uribe M, Briones A, Ramos GG. Successful administration of metoclopramide for the treatment of nausea in patients with advanced liver disease. Gastroenterology 1985;88:757–762.
16. Mezey E. Intestinal function in chronic alcoholism. Ann NY Acad Sci 1975;252:215–227.
17. Jones EA, Bergasa NV. The pruritis of cholestasis: from bile acids to opiate agonists. Hepatology 1990;11:884–887.
18. Cornely CM, Schade RR, Van Thiel D, Gavaler JS. Chronic advanced liver disease and impotence: cause and effect? Hepatology 1984;4:1227–1230.
19. Bach N, Schaffner F, Kapelman B. Sexual behavior in women with nonalcoholic liver disease. Hepatology 1989;9:698–703.

20. Angeli P, Albino G, Carraro P, Dalla Pria M, Merkel C, Caregaro L, DeBei E, Bortoluzzi A, Plebani M,Gatha A. Cirrhosis and muscle cramps: evidence of a causal relationship. Hepatology 1996;23:264–273.

21. Lee FY, Lee SD, Tsai YT, Lai KH, Chao Y, Lin HC, Wang SS, Lo KJ. A randomized controlled trial of quinidine in the treatment of cirrhotic patients with muscle cramps. J Hepatol 1991;2:236–240.

22. Podolsky DK, Isselbacher KJ. Cirrhosis of the liver. In: Wilson JD, Braunwald E, Isselbacher KJ, eds. Harrison's principles of internal medicine. McGraw Hill, New York, 1991: pp. 1340–1350.

23. Attali P, Ink O, Pelletier G, Vernier G, Jean F, Moulton L, Etienne JP. Dupuytren's contracture, alcohol consumption and chronic liver disease. Arch Int Med 1987;147:1065–1067.

24. Muehrcke RC. The finger-nails in chronic hypoalbuminemia. BMJ 1956;1:1327–1328.

25. Munoz SJ, Maddrey WC. Major complications of acute and chronic liver disease. Gastroenterol Clin North Am 1988;17:265–287.

II   Approach to Screening for Liver Disease

2

Routine Screening Blood Tests for Liver Disease

Shabbir Chaiwala and George Y. Wu

1. INTRODUCTION

This chapter describes biochemical or enzymatic tests commonly used to screen for the presence of hepatobiliary diseases. In general, these tests provide substantial sensitivity, but do not provide great specificity.

2. SERUM AMINOTRANSFERASES (TRANSAMINASES)

2.1. Principles

Alanine aminotransferase (ALT) and aspartate aminotransferase (AST) are enzymes involved in gluconeogenesis by converting amino acids to the corresponding alpha keto acids. AST is present in mitochondria and cytoplasm of cells in a wide variety of tissues such as heart, skeletal muscle, kidneys, and brain in addition to the liver. ALT is limited to the cytoplasm, and appears to be localized primarily in the liver. It is, therefore, more specific for hepatic disease *(1)*.

2.2. The Assays

The enzymatic assay for ALT and AST involves coupled enzymatic reactions. In the ALT assay, alanine and alpha ketoglutarate react in the presence of the enzyme ALT to form pyruvate and glutamate. Subsequently, pyruvate is reduced to form lactic acid in the presence of enzyme lactate dehydrogenase, and NADH is oxidized to NAD. This reaction leads to a change

From: *Diseases of the Liver and Bile Ducts: Diagnosis and Treatment*
Edited by: G. Y. Wu and J. Israel © Humana Press Inc., Totowa, NJ

in absorbance at a specific wavelength. The change in the absorbance is directly proportional to ALT activity in the tested sample *(2)*.

In the AST assay, aspartate and alpha ketoglutarate react in the presence of the enzyme AST to form oxaloacetate and glutamate. Subsequently, oxaloacetate is reduced to form malic acid in the presence of enzyme malate dehydrogenase, and NADH is oxidized to NAD. This reaction leads to a change absorbance at a specific wavelength that is directly proportional to the enzymatic activity in the tested sample *(2)*.

2.3. Clinical Significance

Both ALT and AST are normally present in low concentrations in the serum, ranging from 30–40 IU/L. Although these hepatitic serum liver tests are frequently called "liver function tests," they do not provide measures of functional or metabolic capacity of the liver *(1)*.

These enzymes generally indicate the presence of hepatocellular damage *(3)*.

1. Mild elevations (50–400 IU/L) in aminotransferases are seen in certain conditions such as drug- or ethanol-induced liver injury, parenteral nutrition, fatty liver of pregnancy, chronic viral or autoimmune liver disease, intrahepatic malignant tumor, passive hepatic congestion, or extrahepatic biliary obstruction *(3)*.
2. Moderate elevation (400–2000 IU/L) in aminotransferases are associated with conditions such as acute biliary obstruction, acute viral hepatitis, autoimmune hepatitis, toxin exposure, and ischemia associated with left ventricular failure or shock *(3)*.
3. Very high elevations in aminotransferases (2000–30,000 IU/L) are associated with severe hepatocellular necrosis such as in acute acetaminophen toxicity, mushroom poisoning, fulminant hepatitis, or shock liver *(3)*. Generally, high levels of aminotransferases indicate a high likelihood of severe hepatic injury. However, severe hepatic damage can occur with minimal or even normal aminotransferase elevations. Therefore, the absence of aminotransferase elevations does not exclude the possibility of hepatic injury.
4. After acute hepatocellular injury, a decline in AST and ALT in the serum may be a sign of recovery. However, with severe damage such a decline can be indicative of a poor prognosis *(1)*.
5. During the resolution phase of viral hepatitis, serum ALT levels are often higher than AST levels, because ALT has a longer half-life than AST *(3)*.
6. It is uncommon for aminotransferases to rise above 300 IU/L in simple alcoholic liver disease.
7. A ratio of AST to ALT levels of greater than 2:1 is considered highly suggestive of alcoholic liver disease, although the majority of patients with alcoholic liver disease do not have this ratio. The cause of this reversed ratio in alcoholics is due to a deficiency of pyridoxal 5-phosphate, which causes a decrease in the level of ALT without affecting the level of AST *(3)*. It should be noted that a ratio of AST to ALT of greater than two, when ALT levels are high (>200 IU/L), is not characteristic of alcoholic liver disease.
8. AST and ALT will often be elevated in biliary obstruction with levels of AST and ALT >300 IU/L in the majority of the patients. The rise in the aminotransferases can be up to 1000 IU/L with AST rising more than ALT.

2.4. Advantages

1. These tests are easy to perform, are reproducible, and are widely available as part of automated serum screening tests.
2. The tests are helpful in determining whether there is ongoing hepatocellular damage *(1)*.
3. Relative cost: $.

2.5. Limitations

1. Aminotransferase elevations, and especially AST, are not specific for liver diseases.
2. Normal enzyme levels do not exclude the presence of hepatocellular damage *(1)*.

3. Aminotransferase levels may be falsely diminished in patients with uremia or those patients who are on long-term hemodialysis. This effect has been attributed either to the loss of the enzymes through dialysis or deficiency of pyridoxine *(1)*.

3. ALKALINE PHOSPHATASE

3.1. Principles

Alkaline phosphatase (ALP) has been identified in the liver, bone, intestine, placenta, kidney, and leukocytes *(1)*. In the liver, alkaline phosphatase is a membrane-bound enzyme localized at the bile canalicular pole of hepatocytes *(3)*. Measurement of this enzyme in serum is useful in suspected biliary obstruction because, in that condition, synthesis of alkaline phosphatase is induced in hepatocytes *(1)*. When this occurs, some of the enzyme is released into the circulation from the sinusoidal surface of the hepatocytes due to a combination of misguided intracellular routing of newly synthesized proteins, and paracellular escape of the enzymes from bile canaliculi directly into the bloodstream *(3,4)*.

3.2. The Assay

The serum ALP activity can be determined by a variety of methodologies. Most are two-point techniques. However, a continuous monitoring technique, based on a method devised by Bowers and McComb, allows calculation of ALP activity based on molar absorptivity of p-nitrophenol. In this assay, p-nitrophenyl phosphate (a colorless compound) is hydrolyzed to p-nitrophenol (a yellow-colored compound) leading to an increase in absorbance at a specific wavelength. That increase is directly proportional to ALP activity in the sample *(2)*.

Alkaline phosphatase arising from bone is unstable at 56°C ("bone burns"), whereas alkaline phosphatase of hepatic origin is stable at this temperature ("liver lives") *(3)*. However, most automated clinical laboratory assays do not distinguish between the two.

3.3. Clinical Significance

1. A rise in serum alkaline phosphatase of hepatic origin is associated with cholestasis (extrahepatic or intrahepatic). Because the enzyme is present in other tissues, the hepatic origin of an elevation in alkaline phosphatase levels should be confirmed by measuring GGT or 5'-nucleotidase levels *(3)* (*see* Sections 4 and 5).
2. Although the degree of elevation of alkaline phosphatase cannot be used to distinguish between various etiologies, it sometimes can be helpful in suggesting the presence of certain clinical conditions *(3)*.
   a. High elevations (>750 IU/L) in alkaline phosphatase are commonly present in primary biliary cirrhosis, primary sclerosing cholangitis, hepatic lymphoma, sarcoidosis, candidiasis, and HIV cholangiopathy *(3)*.
   b. Moderate elevations (250–750 IU/L) in alkaline phosphatase are seen in hepatitis (viral, autoimmune, and alcoholic), intrahepatic malignant tumors, extrahepatic obstruction (tumor, stone, stricture), and primary biliary cirrhosis *(3,4)*.
3. Complete obstruction of the bile duct (e.g., stone or stricture) results in a rise in alkaline phosphatase after a rise in aminotransferases *(5)*.
4. A rise in alkaline phosphatase activity, unaccompanied by a corresponding serum bilirubin elevation, suggests space-occupying lesions, or partial bile ductal obstruction *(5)*.
5. A low level of serum alkaline phosphatase can be seen in Wilson's disease, hypothyroidism, pernicious anemia, congenital hypophosphatasia, and zinc deficiency *(1)*.

3.4. Advantages

1. The assay for alkaline phosphatase is easy to perform and widely available.
2. The assay has reasonably good sensitivity for the detection of cholestasis, especially if hepatic origin of the alkaline phosphatase is confirmed with an elevation of GGT or 5'-nucleotidase (*see* Sections 4 and 5).

3. Elevations in alkaline phosphatase may be seen before the appearance of clinical manifestations of cholestasis. It also rises in cases of focal cholestasis *(5)*.
4. Relative cost: $.

3.5. Limitations

1. Alkaline phosphatase is not specific for hepatobiliary diseases, as it can be elevated in bone diseases such as Paget's disease, bone fractures, and bony tumors (primary and secondary).
2. Alkaline phosphatase rises physiologically during pregnancy, but peak levels are no more than two times the normal level in the third trimester.
3. There are age, sex, and genetic variations in serum alkaline phosphatase levels. The level is high in young children, and in children near puberty, plateauing in middle age, and increasing again in old age *(1)*.
4. The level of alkaline phosphatase activity may not reflect the degree of cholestasis, and can vary 10-fold or more in individuals having the same condition *(5)*.
5. After resolution of cholestasis, the activity of alkaline phosphatase drops slowly because of its long half-life, and may remain abnormal for months. In this way, the enzyme activity does not truly correlate with recovery from the disease process *(4,5)*.

4. GAMMA GLUTAMYL TRANSPEPTIDASE

4.1. Principles

Gamma glutamyl transpeptidase (GGT) is another screening test for hepatobiliary disease. The enzyme is responsible for the transfer of a gamma glutamyl group from peptides like glutathione to other amino acids. This property of GGT is used in measuring its enzyme activity in the serum *(1)*. GGT is present in biliary epithelial cells, and its synthesis is increased in the acute phase of cholestasis *(1)*.

4.2. The Assay

The GGT assay involves use of gamma-glutamyl-p-nitroanilide as a substrate. The reaction involves transfer of a gamma-glutamyl group to glycylglycine and release of p-nitroaniline, resulting in a change in the absorbance of the tested sample. This change varies directly with enzymatic activity *(2)*.

4.3. Clinical Significance

1. GGT assay is helpful in confirming that an elevation of alkaline phosphatase is of hepatic origin. Because GGT is not found in bone, it should be elevated if the source of alkaline phosphatase is liver, but not if it is from bone *(1)*. Elevation of GGT along with alkaline phosphatase is the most sensitive indicator of biliary tract disease *(1)*.
2. GGT activity in the serum rises in parallel to alkaline phosphatase. However, it can be elevated alone by certain drugs that cause induction of this enzyme such as alcohol, acetaminophen, and phenytoin *(5)*. Some investigators have used GGT for detection of surreptitious alcohol intake in patients with a history of alcoholism because GGT is strongly induced by alcohol *(1)*.
3. The degree of GGT elevation is also helpful in certain clinical situations *(3)*:
   a. High elevations (>1000 IU/L) may be seen in patients with primary biliary cirrhosis, hepatic lymphoma, sarcoidosis, and candidiasis *(3)*.
   b. Moderate elevations (500–1000 IU/L) can be seen in patients with alcoholic hepatitis, intrahepatic malignant tumors, extrahepatic biliary obstruction, and primary biliary cirrhosis *(3)*.
   c. Mild elevations (250–500 IU/L) may be seen in patients with acute and chronic alcohol ingestion, drugs, and very early primary biliary cirrhosis *(3)*.

4.4. Advantages

1. Serum GGT is among the most sensitive tests for detecting hepatobiliary disease.
2. GGT carries an excellent negative predictive value. A normal test result strongly favors a lack of hepatobiliary disease *(1)*.
3. GGT is elevated very early in primary biliary cirrhosis, even with a normal level of alkaline phosphatase *(3)*.
4. Relative cost: $.

4.5. Limitations

1. The serum GGT is not a specific test for hepatobiliary diseases, as it can be found elevated in nonhepatobiliary diseases such as myocardial infarction, renal failure, chronic obstructive pulmonary diseases, diabetes mellitus, pancreatic diseases, and chronic alcoholism.
2. Because GGT is induced by drugs such as alcohol, barbiturates, and phenytoin, the test may not be helpful in assessing the hepatobiliary status in patients who are taking these drugs.
3. Because of the lack of specificity of GGT assay, it is less useful than 5′-nucleotidase.
4. There is an age and sex variability in the enzyme levels. Reference values are greater for men than for women and they increase with age in adults. Neonates may have values five to eight times greater than those for adults.

5. 5′-NUCLEOTIDASE

5.1. Principles

5′-Nucleotidase is an enzyme that causes hydrolysis of nucleotides by releasing inorganic phosphates from the 5′-position of the pentose ring. Besides liver, it is present in other tissues such as the intestine, blood vessels, endocrine pancreas, brain, and heart. The enzyme is associated with canalicular and sinusoidal plasma membranes of the hepatocytes *(1)*.

5.2. The Assay

The enzyme activity in serum can be assayed by either measuring the released phosphate or by assaying adenosine released from adenosine 5′-monophosphate by adenosine deaminase *(1)*.

5.3. Clinical Significance

1. In spite of its widespread tissue distribution, elevation of serum 5′-nucleotidase is always considered to be of hepatobiliary origin *(1)*.
2. Because serum 5′-nucleotidase is very specific for the liver, it can be used to confirm the hepatic origin of alkaline phosphatase.
3. 5′-Nucleotidase is also helpful in diagnosing liver disease in children and in pregnant women, because alkaline phosphatase, as mentioned earlier, can be elevated physiologically in children and in pregnant women. 5′-Nucleotidase is not elevated physiologically in either of these two disease-free populations *(1)*.
4. Measuring serial levels of 5′-nucleotidase in the serum can be helpful in following the progression or regression of hepatic metastases.

5.4. Advantages

1. Assays for 5′-nucleotidase are much more specific than GGT and alkaline phosphatase assays.
2. It has a higher predictive value and has a lower false positivity than GGT and alkaline phosphatase in diagnosing hepatobiliary diseases *(1)*.
3. It is a useful screening test for metastatic liver diseases *(1)*.
4. It has reasonably good sensitivity and it is widely available in most laboratories.
5. Relative cost: $.

5.5. Limitations

It is not usually included in automated serum screening tests.

6. BILIRUBIN

6.1. Principles

Serum bilirubin represents the breakdown product of heme and heme-containing compounds (cytochromes) in the body. In a normal person, 70–80% of the serum bilirubin is derived from the degradation of hemoglobin, and the rest comes from the degradation of other nonhemoglobin heme protein (cytochromes and catalase). An average person produces about 4 mg/kg of bilirubin per day. The process of erythrocyte destruction takes place in reticuloendothelial cells of spleen, liver, and bone marrow. Heme, a degradation product of hemoglobin, is converted to biliverdin by heme oxygenase. Biliverdin is rapidly converted to bilirubin by biliverdin reductase and does not appear in plasma. Bilirubin circulates in plasma, binds to albumin and is taken up to hepatocytes by a carrier-mediated process. Bilirubin in the hepatocytes is conjugated to bilirubin monoglucuronide and bilirubin diglucuronide (BMG, BDG). Conjugated bilirubin is excreted via the bile canaliculi into the bile. There is about 5% reflux of total conjugated bilirubin into the plasma to account for the normal concentration of conjugated bilirubin in the plasma. Conjugated bilirubin is water soluble and can be excreted via the kidneys, whereas unconjugated bilirubin cannot. Bilirubin, which is excreted via bile into the intestine, is deconjugated by intestinal bacteria to be excreted in stool in the form of a brown colored compound stercobilin. Approximately 20% of the intestinal deconjugated bilirubin is absorbed back into the plasma as urobilinogen, a colorless compound. Much of the reabsorbed urobilinogen is re-excreted in bile and the remainder appears in urine *(6)*.

6.2. The Assay

Bilirubin is routinely detected by a test called the Van den Bergh reaction. This reaction involves a diazo color reaction. In this reaction, bilirubin reacts with a reagent, diazotized sulfanilic acid, to form a colored compound that is read spectrophotometrically.

Bilirubin that is detected by this reaction in the absence of agents that dissociate bilirubin from serum proteins, urea, or ethanol, is called direct or conjugated bilirubin, whereas the detection of bilirubin in the presence of ethanol or urea is called indirect or unconjugated bilirubin *(7)*. Indirect or unconjugated bilirubin is assessed by the difference of total bilirubin and direct bilirubin. The elevation of serum bilirubin is observed in the form of jaundice when the total bilirubin level is >3 mg/dL *(7)*. Sometimes the combination of conjugated and unconjugated bilirubin does not equal the total bilirubin, and that difference is due to the presence of delta bilirubin. Delta bilirubin is irreversibly bound to albumin and has a longer half life than the conjugated bilirubin. Delta bilirubin can be present for a longer time after an acute icteric illness *(3)*.

Serum bilirubin is found to be elevated, either because of the increased production or decreased clearance from the liver *(7)*.

6.3. Clinical Significance

1. Total levels of serum bilirubin in disease-free individuals range from 0.3–1.0 mg/dL or 5.1–17 mmole/L. Levels of direct reacting bilirubin range from 0.1–0.3 mg/dL, and indirect reacting levels from 0.2–0.7 mg/dL. A ratio of conjugated to total bilirubin level of >30% suggests conjugated hyperbilirubinemia. Because bilirubin is a component of bile, cessation of bile flow or cholestasis can be accompanied by hyperbi-

lirubinemia. However, the presence of hyperbilirubinemia does not always indicate cholestasis.

2. Because conjugation is required for water solubility, bilirubin in the urine indicates the presence of conjugated bilirubin.
3. Isolated unconjugated hyperbilirubinemia in the absence of liver dysfunction often arises from an increased degradation of red blood cells such as in patients with hemolysis, ineffective erythropoiesis, blood transfusions or resorption of hematomas.
4. Isolated unconjugated hyperbilirubinemia can also be found in patients with decreased hepatic uptake or conjugation of bilirubin in conditions such as Gilbert's, Criggler-Najjar Type I and II. These are covered in more detail in Chapter 23. Rifampin, novobiocin, flavaspidic acid, and some radiographic dyes can also cause this type of unconjugated hyperbilirubinemia. The level of bilirubin elevation in these patients is usually low, 1.3–4 mg/dL *(3)*.
5. Isolated conjugated hyperbilirubinemia in the presence of normal liver function tests can be found in patients with Dubin-Johnson syndrome and Rotor syndrome. These patients are found to have decreased bilirubin secretion into the bile canaliculus *(7)*.
6. Elevations of both conjugated and unconjugated hyperbilirubinemia in the presence of abnormal aminotransferases are usually due to hepatocellular injury *(7)*, especially if the values are high. This can occur in acute hepatocellular injury as with viral hepatitis, ethanol, hepatotoxins, ischemia, and drugs. Chronic hepatocellular injury can be due to viral hepatitis, autoimmune diseases, alpha-1 antitrypsin deficiency, Wilson's disease, or Vitamin A toxicity.
7. Elevation of serum bilirubin and alkaline phosphatase with relatively normal aminotransferases can be seen in various infiltrative diseases of the liver. Examples include granulomatous diseases of the liver (tuberculosis, leprosy, fungal infections, mycobacterium avium infection, and Weggener's granulomatosis), lymphomas, and metastatic malignancies *(7)*. In these conditions there is impairment of regional bile flow with preservation of liver function and patency of the extrahepatic bile ducts.
8. Hyperbilirubinemia (levels of conjugated higher than unconjugated) with relatively higher alkaline phosphatase, compared to aminotransferases, are seen in biliary duct obstruction. Biliary duct obstruction can be intrahepatic or extrahepatic and be due to inflammation, neoplasm, or mechanical obstruction *(7)*.
9. Hyperbilirubinemia due to hepatic disease alone generally does not exceed 30 mg/dL. Levels above this suggest additional disorders such as renal disease impairing excretion of conjugated bilirubin, or hemolysis.

6.4. Advantages

1. Bilirubin assays are inexpensive, easy to perform, and widely available in automated clinical screening kits.
2. The discrimination between direct and indirect bilirubin is sometimes useful in determining the cause of hyperbilirubinemia in terms of its hepatic vs nonhepatic origin. Unconjugated hyperbilirubinemia is more commonly associated with nonhepatic causes *(7)*.
3. Severity of injury and prognosis can be correlated to the degree of rise in the serum bilirubin in the phase of acute hepatocellular damage. Progressive rise in the bilirubin is generally due to ongoing liver cell injury.
4. In the absence of increased bilirubin production, bilirubin level can be used as a liver function test, as it reflects the hepatic capacity to take up, process, and secrete bilirubin into the bile.
5. Relative cost: $ (if direct and total bilirubin are ordered together).

6.5. Limitations

1. Bilirubin assay is not very sensitive or specific for the reasons mentioned above.
2. In chronic liver diseases, the level of bilirubin cannot be correlated to the prognosis and severity of liver disease.
3. Bilirubin level can be normal in early primary biliary cirrhosis, primary sclerosing cholangitis, and patients with less than 24 h of biliary obstruction *(3)*.
4. Many substances interfere with the diazo assay: ascorbic acid, heme, high serum lipids, and drugs such as propranolol *(8)*.
5. When bilirubin levels are low, the differentiation between direct and indirect reacting fractions is unreliable. A small, but constant proportion of unconjugated bilirubin reacts directly, resulting in overestimates of this form *(8)*.

7. AMMONIA

7.1. Principles

Hyperammonemia is frequently associated with liver disease. A major source of ammonia is bacterial production in the large intestine. Bacteria in the large intestine produces a free ammonium ion from proteins, amino acids, and urea. Ammonia is absorbed by the splanchnic circulation and carried to the liver where it is converted into urea by the urea cycle. A defect in the detoxification process of ammonia can occur in patients with liver disease. Patients with advanced liver disease and portal systemic shunting are frequently found to have elevated serum ammonia levels. Ammonia is also removed peripherally by skeletal muscle. In skeletal muscle, ammonia is converted to glutamine by its condensation with glutamate. Patients with advanced liver disease are found to have low muscle mass, which further impairs ammonia detoxification *(9)*.

7.2. The Assay

Ammonia in the sample is measured by a one-stage automated assay. In this assay, ammonium ion reacts with oxoglutarate in the presence of NADPH and glutamate dehydrogenase to form glutamate and NADP. The change results in an increase in absorbance at a specific wavelength which can be measured, and is directly proportional to the amount of ammonia present *(10)*.

7.3. Clinical Significance

1. Hyperammonemia is associated with advanced liver disease and hepatic encephalopathy. However, it does not seem to be the agent solely responsible in causing neurotoxicity in patients with hepatic encephalopathy *(9)*.
2. Hyperammonemia is also seen in patients with Reye's syndrome and urea cycle enzyme deficiency. These patients can also have neurological manifestations of encephalopathy *(9)*.

7.4. Advantages

1. The test is automated, and available in most laboratories.
2. Relative cost: $.

7.5. Limitations

1. The test is not specific for liver disease and there is poor correlation between blood ammonia level and the presence or stage of hepatic encephalopathy *(9)*.
2. Hyperammonemia has been described as a complication of valproic acid therapy, asparaginase therapy, ureterosigmoidostomy, hemodialysis, and neurogenic bladder infections (9).
3. Transient elevation in the serum ammonia level is also seen in patients receiving treatment for leukemia *(9)*.

SUMMARY

Aminotransferases are only markers of cellular injury, not measures of functional or metabolic capacity of the liver.

Alkaline phosphatase is a marker of cholestasis. Hepatic origin should be confirmed by measuring gamma glutamyl transpeptidase or 5′-nucleotidase levels.

Gamma glutamyl transpeptidase is the most sensitive indicator of biliary tract disease; however, it lacks the specificity as it can be induced by alcohol, acetaminophen, and phenytoin.

5′-Nucleotidase is very specific for hepatobiliary disease.

Bilirubin assay is not very sensitive or specific for liver disease, although it is considered to be one of the true liver function tests.

Ammonia elevation in serum is considered neither sensitive nor specific for the diagnosis or severity of liver disease or hepatic encephalopathy.

REFERENCES

1. Stolz A, Kaplowitz N. Biochemical tests for liver disease. In: Zakim D, Boyer TD, eds. Hepatology: A textbook of liver disease, 2nd ed. Saunders, New York, 1990, pp. 637–667.
2. Hutruk BL, Krefetz RG. Enzymes. In: Bishop M, Duben-Engelkirk JL, Fody EP, eds. Clinical chemistry, principles, procedures, correlations, 2nd ed. Lippincott, Philadelphia, 1992, p. 230.
3. Neuschwander-Tetri, BA. Common blood tests for liver disease. Postgraduate Med 1995;98:49–63.
4. Kaplan MM. Laboratory tests. In: Schiff L, Schiff ER, eds. Diseases of the liver, vol. 1, 7th ed. Lippincott, Philadelphia, 1993, pp. 108–144.
5. Schaffner F. Cholestasis. In: Haubrich WS, Schaffner F, Berk JE, eds. Bockus gastroenterology, vol. 3, 5th ed. Saunders, New York, 1995, pp. 1931–1954.
6. Scharschmidt BF. Bilirubin metabolism, bile formation, and gallbladder and bile duct function. In: Sleisenger MH, Fordtran JS, eds. Gastrointestinal disease, pathophysiology/diagnosis/management, vol. 2, Saunders, New York, 1993, p. 1730.
7. Lidofsky SD. Jaundice. In: Sleisenger MH, Fordtran JS, eds. Gastrointestinal disease, pathophysiology/diagnosis/management, vol. 2, Saunders, New York, 1993, pp. 1931–1954.
8. Blanckaert N, Fevery J. Physiology and pathophysiology of bilirubin metabolism. In: Zakim D, Boyer TD, eds. Hepatology: a textbook of liver disease, 1st ed. Saunders, New York, 1990, pp. 254–302.
9. Schafer DF, Jones EA. Hepatic encephalopathy. In: Zakim D, Boyer TD, eds. Hepatology: a textbook of liver disease, 1st ed. Saunders, New York, 1990, pp. 447–460.
10. Balistreri WF, Shaw LM. Liver Function. In: Tietz NW, ed. Textbook of clinical chemistry. Saunders, New York, 1986, pp. 1373–1433.

3 Specific Diagnostic Blood Tests

Shabbir Chaiwala and George Y. Wu

CONTENTS

INTRODUCTION
SEROLOGICAL TESTS FOR VIRAL HEPATITIS
MOLECULAR DIAGNOSTIC TECHNIQUES OF VIRAL HEPATITIS
REFERENCES

1. INTRODUCTION

This chapter describes blood tests for the serological and molecular diagnosis of hepatitis.

2. SEROLOGICAL TESTS FOR VIRAL HEPATITIS

This section discusses the serological diagnostic techniques for hepatitis viruses A, B, C, D, E, G, Epstein-Barr virus, and cytomegalovirus.

2.1. Hepatitis A Virus

2.1.1. PRINCIPLES

2.1.1.1. Antibodies. The host immune response to hepatitis A viral infection results in development of IgM and IgG antibodies against the HAV capsid *(1)*. These antibodies are easily detected and form the basis of the most commonly used tests for detection of exposure to the virus.

2.1.1.2. Time Course of Host Serological Response. Diagnosis of acute HAV infection is confirmed by detection of IgM anti-HAV. IgM anti-HAV begins to appear 2–6 wk after exposure to HAV. The incubation period for HAV is 21–42 d *(2)*. As IgM antibody levels increase, viremia decreases. Then IgG anti-HAV levels begin to rise, reaching a peak in 3–12 mo after the onset of illness *(3)*. IgM antibodies against HAV can be detected in the serum at the time of the onset of symptoms, and low levels of IgM antibodies can continue to be detected for more than 200 d after the acute phase of illness in about 13% of patients *(3)*. The duration of IgM HAV positivity is shorter in asymptomatic patients than the symptomatic patient *(see* Fig. 1).

2.1.2. THE ASSAYS

These are competitive binding assays in which anti-HAV from a patient competes with radio-labeled-labeled (RIA) or horseradish peroxidase conjugated (ELISA) human anti-HAV for binding to HAV-antigen attached to polystyrene beads. The presence of anti-HAV is detected by gamma counter or by a change in the color of the media in RIA and ELISA, respectively *(3)*.

From: *Diseases of the Liver and Bile Ducts: Diagnosis and Treatment*
Edited by: G. Y. Wu and J. Israel © Humana Press Inc., Totowa, NJ

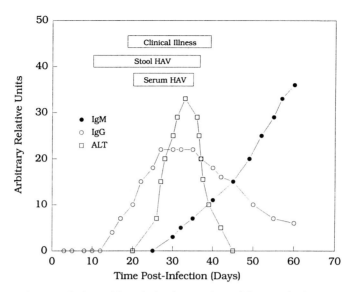

Fig. 1. Time course of events in hepatitis A infection. (Adapted from ref. *1*.)

2.1.3. Clinical Significance

1. Elevation of IgM anti-HAV helps to confirm the diagnosis of HAV in patients with clinical evidence of acute hepatitis and elevations of aminotransferases.
2. IgG anti-HAV appears a little later than IgM antibodies, persists indefinitely, and is indicative of past exposure to the virus. In addition, the antibody is protective, and indicates an immune state *(3)*.
3. Negative HAV serological tests indicate a patient has not been exposed, or is in an early phase of infection.
4. Chronic disease does not occur with Hepatitis A infection, so that the presence of IgM indicates a recent exposure to the virus.

2.1.4. Advantages

1. HAV serological assays are simple and widely available.
2. IgM HAV assays are positive in 97% of the patients who have symptoms. There is no window period in most cases, and the diagnosis can be made immediately as soon as symptoms start appearing.
3. Relative cost: $.

2.1.5. Limitations

1. IgM HAV assays can be negative in up to 3% of patients tested within 3 or 4 d after the onset of symptoms. However, they can become positive in the first two weeks of the illness.
2. HAV serological assays are less often positive during the incubation period of the illness *(1)*.

2.2. Hepatitis B Virus

2.2.1. Principles

The diagnosis of HBV infection can be made using serologic and molecular diagnostic techniques. Serological diagnosis involves assays to detect viral antigens and immunological responses of the host against viral proteins.

2.2.1.1. Viral Antigens.

1. Hepatitis B surface antigen (HBsAg) is the major antigen on the viral envelope.
2. Hepatitis B core antigen (HBcAg) is associated with inner nucleocapsid or the core of HBV *(3)*. Even though it is present in liver and serum, routine clinical laboratory tests cannot detect it.

3. Hepatitis Be antigen (HBeAg) is a soluble antigen that is immunologically distinct from HBcAg and HBsAg. It is a form of core of HBV, and is synthesized from the same precursor polypeptide *(3)*.

2.2.1.2. Host Antibodies.

1. Anti-hepatitis B surface antibody (HBsAb) is directed against the surface determinants of HBV, and small spherical and tubular forms that are not viral particles *(3)*.
2. Anti-hepatitis B core antibody (HBcAb) is directed against the core antigen of HBV *(3)*.
3. Anti-hepatitis Be antibody (HBeAb) is directed against the hepatitis Be antigen *(3)*.

2.2.1.3. Time Course of Serological Events.

Acute hepatitis B infection has an incubation period (40–150 d), a preicteric phase (3–7 d), an icteric phase (when present, lasting a few days to several months), and convalescence phase (weeks to months; *see* Fig. 2). During the incubation period, the patient may be positive only for HBsAg, whereas all other serological markers for HBV are usually negative *(2)*. In an acute HBV infection, HBsAg is the first viral marker to rise, usually beginning in the first month, and reaches a peak between 3 and 4 mo after exposure. HBeAg is detectable usually 1–2 wk after HBsAg. Both HBsAg and HBeAg appear before aminotransferase levels rise, beginning 2–3 mo after exposure. Host immune response to acute HBV infection begins with the appearance of HBcAb in the serum followed by HBeAb and HBsAb. The first HBcAb antibody is an IgM that appears shortly before the onset of symptoms, or at the time of elevation of aminotransferases, and prior to the development of IgG HBcAb. HBeAb can appear as early as the fourth week after the onset of HBV infection and after HBcAb. Unlike HBcAb and HBeAb, HBsAb, is a neutralizing and protective antibody. It starts appearing during the late convalescent phase, typically weeks to months after the disappearance of HBsAg, and four or more months after the onset of acute illness. This antibody is synthesized early in acute HBV infection. However, it is frequently not detectable in the serum when levels are low because it forms complexes with HBsAg. Three forms of HBsAb are synthesized: IgM, IgG, and IgA. IgM disappears quickly whereas IgG persists for a long period *(4)*.

In chronic HBV infection, HBsAg and HBeAg usually persist, although levels can be quite variable. The HBcAb can be frequently detected when HBsAb is not detectable (*see* Fig. 3).

2.2.2. HEPATITIS B SURFACE ANTIGEN (HBSAG)

2.2.2.1. The Assays.

HBsAg is measured by radioimmunoassay (RIA) or ELISA. The RIA is a sandwich assay in which test sample is added to beads coated with anti-HBs. After incubation, beads are washed and allowed to incubate a second time with radiolabeled anti-HBs IgG. After incubation and washing, beads are counted in a gamma counter for captured HBsAg from the test sample *(5)*.

The principles of the ELISA are identical to those of RIA, except that the second antibody is conjugated to horseradish peroxidase or alkaline phosphatase. These enzymes are reacted in an additional step with a specific substrate resulting in change in the color of the sample, which can be measured *(5)*.

2.2.2.2. Clinical Significance.

1. The level of HBsAg does not correlate with the severity of clinical disease *(6)*.
2. In resolving acute infection, antigen levels may become undetectable as antibody levels rise in the "window period."
3. Persistence of HBsAg for more than 6 mo, in most cases, is considered a marker of chronicity, because antigenemia disappears in 80–90% of cases within 6 mo of onset of disease *(3,7)*.
4. The hepatitis B vaccines induce host production of only HBsAb. The presence of HBcAb or HBeAb indicates an exposure to virus, not vaccine.

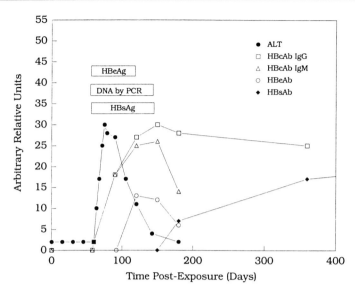

Fig. 2. Time course of events in acute hepatitis B infection. (Adapted from Hoofnagle JH, Di Bisceglie AM. Antiviral therapy of viral hepatitis. In: Galasso GJ, Whitley RJ, Merigan TC, eds. Antiviral agents and viral diseases of man. 3rd ed. Raven Press, New York, 1990; pp. 415–459.)

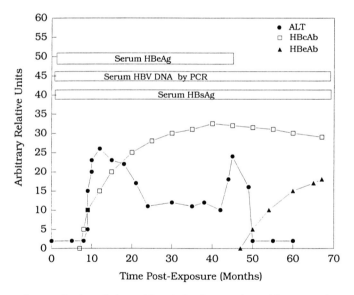

Fig. 3. Time course of events in chronic hepatitis B infection. (Adapted from Hoofnagle JH, Di Bisceglie AM. Antiviral therapy of viral hepatitis. In: Galasso GJ, Whitley RJ, Merigan TC, eds. Antiviral agents and viral diseases of man. 3rd ed. Raven Press, New York, 1990; pp. 415–459.)

2.2.2.3. Advantages. HBsAg is good for the screening of HBV in patients with clinical and biochemical evidence of acute hepatitis. This test has a very high sensitivity with an antigen detection limit between 0.02 and 1 ng/mL *(3)*.

2.2.2.4. Limitations.

1. The presence of HBsAg alone can not be used to differentiate between the acute and chronic HBV infection.
2. The test may be falsely negative during the incubation phase of infection or, in chronic infection, when levels of secreted HBsAg are below the limits of detection *(2)*. In such instances,

HBcAb is usually positive. The presence of HBV infection can be determined by detection of viral DNA (*see* Section 3.1 discussed below).

3. Relative cost: $$.

2.2.3. HEPATITIS BE ANTIGEN (HBEAG)

2.2.3.1. The Assays. The assays used for detecting HBeAg are RIA and ELISA, and utilize the same principles as described earlier with HBsAg and HBcAb.

2.2.3.2. Clinical Significance.

1. The presence of HBeAg indicates the presence of viral particles in the serum, and generally correlates with the infectivity the serum and replication of the HBV. The presence of HBeAg suggests high viremia ($>10^5$ genomes/mL of serum) *(2)*.
2. In immunocompetent individuals, the level of viremia generally correlates with the degree of liver disease *(2)*.

2.2.3.3. Advantages.

1. The assay is useful in following the course of the HBV infection. Persistence of HBeAg for more than 6 mo after the onset of the disease suggests chronic liver disease *(2,8)*.
2. HBeAg and HBeAb are surrogate markers for HBV DNA. These assays can be useful in monitoring the outcome of HBV infection when assays for HBV DNA are not available *(2)*.
3. Relative cost: $.

2.2.3.4. Limitations.

1. Detection of HBeAg is not absolutely reliable as a screening test for HBV infection. HBeAg can be negative in rare cases of mutations in the precore region of HBV.
2. False positive HBeAg in the absence of HBsAg can rarely occur *(2)*.

2.2.4. HEPATITIS B CORE ANTIBODY (HBCAB)

2.2.4.1. The Assays. The assays for HBcAb are RIA and ELISA. Antibodies in the test sample and adsorbed HBcAb compete for a standardized amount of HBcAg added to the reaction before the addition of labeled HBcAb. As with other competitive assays, the proportion of radioactive antibodies or enzyme-labeled antibodies bound to the HBcAg are inversely proportional to the concentration of unlabeled antibodies in test sample *(5)*.

2.2.4.2. Clinical Significance.

1. HBcAb assay is positive in active and resolved HBV infection. It is an indicator of HBV exposure.
2. HBcAb IgM is present in recent or chronic hepatitis B infection. It cannot be used alone to distinguish between the two *(2)*. The presence of HBcAb IgM and lack of IgG suggests an early infection, because the former becomes positive 2–8 wk prior to the onset of symptoms or biochemical evidence of liver disease and usually disappears 6 mo after exposure in individuals who recover from the infection (*see* Fig. 2).
3. A lack of IgM HBcAb suggests that an episode of acute hepatitis is caused by an agent other than HBV *(2)*.
4. HBcAb is not protective against HBV re-exposure.

2.2.4.3. Advantages.

1. HBcAb assay is useful in screening for HBV infection, especially during suspected acute infection in the "window period" when both HBsAg and HBsAb are negative *(2)*.
2. In an acute hepatitis, HBcAb IgM is the most reliable and specific serological marker for diagnosis of HBV infection. All symptomatic patients with clinical evidence of acute HBV will have an IgM HBcAb in the serum, except in immunocompromised patients.
3. As a marker of previous HBV infection, determination of HBcAb is superior to HBsAb, because HBcAb lasts longer in convalescent sera *(2)*.

4. Because HBcAb is not induced by vaccination with standard surface antigen vaccines, it can be used to distinguish HBsAb from infection versus immunization.

2.2.4.2. LIMITATIONS

1. This assay is not useful in immunocompromised patients because the test can be negative in spite of active viral replication *(2)*.
2. HBcAb can become negative, in some cases, after several decades of infection *(2)*.
3. Because IgM HBcAb persists for a long time after the acute phase of HBV infection, qualitative assays can not differentiate between chronic and acute HBV infection *(2)*.
4. Relative cost: $.

2.2.5. HEPATITIS BE ANTIBODY (HBEAB)

2.2.5.1. The Assays. The assays used for HBeAb are RIA and ELISA, with basic principles similar to those for HBcAb. Antibodies in the test sample and adsorbed HBeAb compete for a standardized amount of HBeAg added to the reaction well before the addition of labeled HBeAb. As with other competitive assays, the proportion of radioactive antibodies or enzyme-labeled antibodies bound to the HBeAg are inversely proportional to the concentration of unlabeled antibodies in test sample *(5)*.

2.2.5.2. Clinical Significance.

1. In a manner similar to HBcAb, HBeAb can be useful in the "window period" of acute infection when HBsAg and HBsAb are both negative.
2. The presence of HBeAb signifies developing immunity against HBeAg and HBV. Positive assays often, but not always, indicate declining viremia.
3. HBeAb is not protective against re-exposure to HBV.

2.2.5.3. Advantages.

1. The assays are widely available
2. Relative cost: $.

2.2.5.4. Limitations.

1. In approx 30% of the patients with negative HBeAb, viremia may be high ($> 10^5$ genomes/mL of serum). These patients may have HBcAg (precore) mutations that prevent secretion of HBeAg into the serum.
2. HBeAb does not persist for long after resolution of HBV infection *(2)*.

2.2.6. HEPATITIS B SURFACE ANTIBODY (HBsAB)

2.2.6.1. The Assays. The assays used for HBsAb are RIA and ELISA, in which the sample is incubated with fixed HBsAg. Antibody, if present, combines with fixed HBsAg and the captured antibodies are detected by adding labeled antibodies *(5)*.

2.2.6.2. Clinical Significance.

1. The HBsAb assay is useful for assessing the convalescence in patients with HBV infection, and for monitoring the success of the HBV vaccination.
2. A positive HBsAb assay suggests a previous HBV infection, HBV active vaccination, or passive immunization with the HB immunoglobulin.
3. HBsAb and HBsAg can be positive simultaneously in cases of hepatitis B infection when antigen and antibody levels are similar, and usually low *(6)*.

2.2.6.3. Advantages.

1. The assays are widely available.
2. Relative cost: $.

2.2.6.4. Limitations.

1. HBsAb is not a very sensitive assay; it can be negative in 1–5% of acute infections *(6)* and in about 20% of patients who recover from HBV infection *(2)*.
2. This assay can also become negative because of loss of antibodies in about 20% of people within a few years after HBV convalescence, and hepatitis B vaccination *(2)*.
3. In spite of good specificity, this assay can still be falsely positive in about 1% of normal subjects who have no other markers for HBV infection and have never had a hepatitis B vaccination *(2)*.
4. Conversion to detectable HBsAb takes several weeks to months after the loss of the HBsAg.
5. The presence of HBsAb does not imply the complete eradication of the HBV DNA. Extremely low levels of HBsAb can sometimes be detected in serum and liver by molecular amplification techniques *(2)*. The clinical significance of low levels of DNA has not been determined.

2.3. Hepatitis C Virus

2.3.1. ENZYME IMMUNOASSAY

2.3.1.1. Principles. Serological assays for the hepatitis C virus (HCV) include enzyme immunoassays (EIA) and recombinant immunoblot assays (RIBA). Many HCV polypeptides are used as antigens to identify corresponding circulating antibodies in serum *(8–11)*.

2.3.1.2. The Assays. In enzyme-linked immunosorbent assays (ELISA), the serum is tested for the presence of IgG antibodies against C200 (C100-3 + C33c) or C22 antigens (only the C100-3 antigen in EIA-I). The serum of the patient is added to the ELISA plate coated with recombinant C200 and C22 antigens and then washed with monoclonal antihuman IgG antibodies coupled to horseradish peroxidase. If the serum contains antibodies against these antigens, then the assays lead to the development of color, the intensity of which is measured *(11)*.

2.3.1.3. Clinical Significance.

1. EIA II is a useful screening test for HCV in low prevalence groups such as United States blood donors. If the HCV antibody test is positive in these groups, it should be confirmed by RIBA II *(11)*.
2. The presence of HCV antibody in high prevalence groups, such as patients in hospital and liver clinics, almost always confirms the diagnosis of HCV infection. RIBA is not required in high prevalence groups with clinical evidence of hepatitis along with elevation in ALT (*see* Fig. 4).
3. A positive HCV antibody assay may suggest either acute HCV infection, resolved HCV infection or, in rare circumstances, a false-positive result. When in doubt, a false-positive EIA should be confirmed by RIBA II.

2.3.1.4. Advantages.

1. The assays are widely available.
2. Later generation assays are more sensitive and specific, compared to the first generation EIA.
3. There is an earlier seroconversion for C22 and C33c antigens. Therefore, the period for seroconversion to anti-HCV tends to be shorter (i.e., time from exposure to development of detectable antibody is shorter).
4. Elimination of false positives in first generation assays due to superoxide dismutase (SOD) has resulted in lower false positivity with second generation assays.

2.3.1.5. Limitations.

1. Because of delayed seroconversion, the assay can be falsely negative in early-acute HCV infection. After acute HCV infection, the mean seroconversion period is 15 wk. However, it can require as long as 1 yr *(11)*.
2. The tests can be falsely positive in patients with rheumatoid arthritis, hypergamma-globulinemia, autoimmune disease, and paraproteinemia.

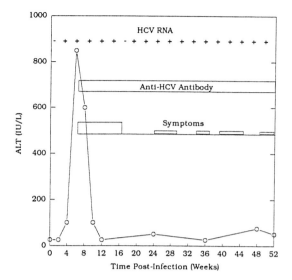

Fig. 4. Time couse of events in chronic hepatitis C infection. (Adapted from Hoofnagle JH. Hepatitis C: the clinical spectrum. Hepatology 1997;26:15S–20S.)

3. A positive test does not correlate with the viral activity in acute, chronic, or resolved HCV infection.
4. The test is neither useful in making treatment decisions nor in assessing recovery after antiviral treatment *(10)*.
5. The assay is not useful in assessing a HCV infection in immunocompromised patients, hemodialysis patients, and HIV-positive patients.
6. Relative cost: $.

2.3.2. RECOMBINANT IMMUNOBLOT ASSAY (RIBA)

2.3.2.1. Principles. In the recombinant immunoblot assay (RIBA), a membrane is coated with stripes of antigens (C100-3, 5-1-1, C-22, C33c, SOD). The battery is larger than EIA. These stripes of antigens are bathed in the serum to be tested, and afterwards a second antibody is added. The antigen–antibody bands are compared with that of positive controls. For the test to be positive, there should be at least two antigen–antibody reaction bands. SOD is added along with other antigens to eliminate false positivity seen in the EIA *(11)*.

2.3.2.2. Clinical Significance.

1. The RIBA II is used to resolve possible false positivity or indeterminate results associated with the EIA.
2. The RIBA II is also performed to confirm the results of EIA in low prevalence groups.
3. The RIBA II is also useful in making a diagnosis of HCV infection in patients with a history of autoimmune hepatitis where false positivity is possible due to hypergammaglobulinemia.
4. The antibody detected is not protective against re-exposure to HCV.

2.3.2.3. Advantages.

1. This test is the most sensitive and specific of the serological tests for HCV infection.
2. RIBA II has an advantage over EIA, because of early seroconversion to some added antigens used in the assay.

2.3.2.4. Limitations.

1. Although superior to EIA, compared to the molecular diagnostic techniques for HCV, this assay is less sensitive and specific *(3)*.

2. This assay has little proven diagnostic value in high prevalence populations, if they are already tested positive by ELISA *(3)*.
3. This test also cannot be used to differentiate between acute, chronic, or resolved HCV infection.
4. The assay can be falsely negative in immunocompromised patients and HIV-positive patients.
5. Relative cost: $$.

2.4. Hepatitis D Virus (HDV, DELTA)

2.4.1. HEPATITIS D VIRUS ANTIBODY

2.4.1.1. Principles. HDV infection always occurs in the presence of HBV infection. Therefore, HDV assays should only be performed in patients who have some evidence of HBV infection. Coinfection is the simultaneous infection by HBV and HDV, whereas superinfection is infection by HDV in patients with pre-existing HBV *(3)*. HDV antigen assays are limited to the research laboratory. The HDV antibody assay is commonly used in clinical practice to diagnose HDV infection *(3,12)*.

2.4.1.2. The HDV Antibody Assays. Two classes of host antibodies, IgM and IgG, can be detected in HDV infection. The presence of the IgM HDV antibody suggests acute HDV infection, whereas the IgG HDV antibody suggests chronic infection. RIA and ELISA are used to detect anti-HDV antibody. In these assays, anti-HDV in sample sera competes for binding to labeled anti-HDV for HDV-antigen *(5)*.

2.4.1.3. Clinical Significance.

1. HBV and HDV coinfection is present if anti-HDV IgM, HBsAg, and HBcAb IgM are present *(2)*.
2. In some patients who are HBsAg negative, but IgM HBcAb positive, markers of acute HDV coinfection may be found. It has been postulated that acute HDV infection decreases the synthesis of HBsAg or masks the detection of HBsAg *(2,3)*.
3. The HDV antibody assay can be used to diagnose acute superinfection if IgM anti-HDV, HBsAg and IgG HBcAb are found positive *(2,3)*.

2.4.1.4. Advantages.

1. The assay is commercially available.
2. Anti-HDV antibody assays are good for screening for HDV infection. The assay is more sensitive and specific, compared to the early indirect immunofluorescent techniques *(2,3)*.

2.4.1.5. Limitations.

1. Seroconversion of anti-HDV IgM may occur weeks after the onset of acute HDV infection. Thus, the test may be falsely negative early in the infection.
2. Seroconversion of anti-HDV IgG usually occurs during convalescence and disappears within 6 mo to 2 yr after the infection *(3)*.
3. Anti-HDV IgM can be absent despite active HDV multiplication. Such cases are diagnosed by HDV molecular diagnostic techniques *(3)*.

2.5. Hepatitis E Virus (HEV)

2.5.1. PRINCIPLES

Enzyme immunoassays (EIA) and Western blot assays have been developed by using synthetic peptides and recombinant viral proteins to determine the presence of antibodies against HEV (IgG, IgM, IgA) in human sera. Current EIA and Western blot assays are more sensitive and specific compared to previous immune electron microscopy and fluorescent antibody assays. Current ELISA techniques are more efficient and can be used for large scale testing of sera from patients in endemic and nonendemic regions of the world *(13)*.

2.5.2. The Assays

For ELISA, HEV recombinant antigens are coated on polystyrene beads. Serum samples are added in serial dilutions to the beads. Captured antibodies are detected by using goat anti-human antibodies *(14)*.

In Western blot assays, antigens are fixed to membranes. Serum samples are incubated with membrane-bound HEV antigens. Bound anti-HEV in serum samples are detected by adding labeled anti-human antibodies *(14)* that produce a color reaction.

2.5.3. Clinical Significance

1. The appearance of anti-HEV antibodies generally coincides with elevated ALT.
2. During the acute phase of HEV infection, anti-HEV IgM predominates, whereas anti-HEV IgG appears during the convalescent phase of the disease.
3. These antibodies are neutralizing antibodies that correlate with the disappearance of the hepatitis E antigen from serum.

2.5.4. Advantages

1. The tests are simple to perform.
2. Relative cost: $.

2.5.5. Limitations

Unfortunately, they are not widely available.

2.6. Cytomegalovirus (CMV)

2.6.1. Principles

In patients with normal immunity, the presence of cytomegalovirus (CMV) in serum is strong evidence of disseminated infection, and can be used to diagnose CMV hepatitis. Noninvasive tests used to diagnose CMV infection include rapid culture methods, CMV antigenemia assay, and PCR techniques.

2.6.2. Rapid Culture Method

2.6.2.1. The Assay. Shell vial centrifugation is used with monoclonal antibodies directed against nuclear protein of CMV. The assay permits early detection (within 48 h) of cytopathic effects of CMV in cell cultures before they become visible to the naked eye *(15)*.

2.6.2.2. Clinical Significance.
This test is used extensively for rapid diagnosis of CMV infection and for making decisions for early treatment *(16)*.

2.6.2.3. Advantages.

1. The test is reasonably specific, and the results frequently can be obtained within 24–48 h.
2. The test has a high positive predictive value (68%) for subsequent disease in immunocompromised patients.
3. Relative cost: $.

2.6.2.4. Limitations.

1. There is a high false-negative rate in 30–40% of patients with CMV infection whose viremia can not be detected by this test.
2. This test is of limited value in monitoring antiviral treatment, because it becomes negative within 2–3 wk after initiation of treatment, regardless of clinical outcome (16).

3. In immunocompromised patients, CMV viremia is found frequently. Therefore, the presence of viremia under these circumstances cannot be used alone to diagnose CMV hepatitis *(2)*.
4. Liver biopsies should be obtained as part of the routine protocol for investigating patients with allografts and other patients with suspected CMV hepatitis. CMV can be detected by immunocytochemical studies in liver biopsy specimens.

2.6.3. CMV ANTIGENEMIA ASSAY

2.6.3.1. The Assay. In this assay, CMV antigens are detected in peripheral leukocytes. This assay consists of direct staining of granulocytes with monoclonal antibodies.

2.6.3.2. Clinical Significance.

Antigenemia assays detect viral antigen and, therefore, indicate the presence of active infection *(16)*.

2.6.3.3. Advantages.

1. The test is widely available.
2. The antigenemia assay is more sensitive and specific compared to culture techniques.
3. The test allows detection of CMV infection earlier than by rapid immunofluorescence culture techniques.
4. The most important feature of this assay is that it can be quantified to correlate with viremia.

2.6.3.4. Limitations.

1. False negatives occur when viral titers are low *(16)*.
2. Although this assay is increasingly used to monitor antiviral therapy, it is considered less sensitive compared to molecular diagnostic techniques *(16)*.
3. Relative cost: $.

2.7. Hepatitis G Virus (HGV)

Hepatitis G is a recently described virus that is related to Hepatitis C. Currently, there are no commercially available serological tests for HGV infection. However, assays are still under development, but can be obtained for investigational use only (Abbott/Boehringer-Ingelheim, Ridgefield, CT).

2.8. Epstein-Barr Virus (EBV)

2.8.1. PRINCIPLES

Several distinct EBV-associated antigens and their corresponding antibodies have been identified. The EBV antigens are classified by the phase of the viral replicative cycle during which they are expressed. The latent phase is characterized by production of Epstein-Barr nuclear antigens (EBNA). Early antigens (EA) are produced during initial stages of viral replication, but prior to viral DNA synthesis. Late antigens are produced after viral DNA synthesis and consist of the structural proteins of viral capsid (viral capsid antigen, VCA) *(17)*.

Heterophile agglutinin is frequently measured in confirming a clinical diagnosis of infectious mononucleosis in otherwise healthy patients. However, this test is not very useful in diagnosing complex cases with immune deficiency and hepatitis as this test is not very sensitive or specific (18).

2.8.2. THE ASSAY

Specific EBV antibodies, anti-EBNP, anti-EA, and anti-VCA *(17)* are detected using immunofluorescence techniques. Fixed cell smears of Raji cells or P3-HR1 cells provide antigens for this assay. The smears are incubated with serum samples, and the presence of bound antibody detected with fluorescein conjugated anti-human antibodies can be observed by fluorescence microscopy *(17)*.

2.8.3. CLINICAL SIGNIFICANCE

1. Acute EBV hepatitis can be diagnosed by the presence of VCA IgM antibodies, which appear within days to weeks after the onset of infection.
2. Patients become positive for anti-EBNA (Epstein-Barr virus nuclear antigen) 2–3 mo after exposure. Appearance of anti-EBNA confirms the diagnosis of primary infection by EBV.
3. VCA IgG antibodies start appearing along with VCA IgM and remain detectable for years after the resolution of infection. VCA-IgG is not useful in making the diagnosis of acute EBV infection.
4. Reactivation or recurrent EBV infection can be diagnosed by viral cultures or by detection of antibodies against early antigens of EBV *(19)*.

2.8.4. ADVANTAGES

1. The assays are widely available.
2. EBV specific antigen/antibody testing is useful in determining susceptibility or immunity to primary EBV infection *(17)*.

2.8.5. LIMITATIONS

1. Antibody response may be low or absent in immunocompromised or immunosuppressed patients. In these cases, a liver biopsy is required to diagnose EBV hepatitis. EBV hepatitis is diagnosed by demonstrating specific nuclear antigens in the liver tissues by immunocytochemical studies.
2. Relative cost: $.

3. MOLECULAR DIAGNOSTIC TECHNIQUES FOR DETECTION OF VIRAL HEPATITIS

Molecular diagnostic techniques are among the most specific and sensitive tests to detect viral infections.

Various molecular diagnostic techniques are available for HBV, HCV, HDV, and CMV. Molecular diagnostic techniques for hepatitis A are not required, because viral titers tend to be low or declining when the diagnosis is likely to be considered *(3)*.

3.1. Hepatitis B Virus

Techniques currently used for the diagnosis of hepatitis include polymerase chain reaction, branched DNA amplification, and ligase chain reaction.

3.1.1. POLYMERASE CHAIN REACTION

3.1.1.1. Principles. Viral DNA is specifically amplified through the use of primers that hybridize to viral DNA. A thermostable enzyme, which is a special DNA polymerase, builds many copies of a specified region of the viral nucleic acid. Through the use of standards, also carried through the same amplification process, quantitation can be achieved *(10,12)*.

3.1.1.2. Clinical Significance. PCR for the diagnosis of HBV is not routinely used in clinical practice. Its use is limited to special clinical circumstances:

1. This test can be useful for the detection of HBV in HBsAg-negative patients with evidence of hepatitis. Previous studies have shown that a small proportion of such patients have HBV DNA sequences in blood, liver, and mononuclear cells *(20)*.
2. PCR is useful for the detection of HBV in patients with chronic hepatitis who have HBsAg, but no HBeAg (precore mutations) *(20)*.
3. The test can be used to follow low level HBV infection in liver transplants.
4. Quantitative PCR can be used to follow the response to antiviral treatment *(20)*.

3.1.1.3. Advantages.
1. PCR is the most sensitive technique for detection of the HBV DNA. PCR can detect trace amounts of viral DNA to a limit of 10–50 HBV particles/mL *(20)*.
2. Because PCR is extremely sensitive, it is useful in detecting early transmission of the virus, e.g., from mother to child *(20)*.

3.1.1.4. Limitations.
1. Samples can be easily contaminated, and care is required for quantitation to be accurate.
2. This technique is not available as a routine procedure in clinical laboratories.
3. Relative cost: $$.
4. It is not widely available.

3.1.2. BRANCHED DNA AMPLIFICATION

3.1.2.1. Principles. This technique to detect HBV DNA is also based on hybridization to viral nucleic acid sequences. However, the sensitivity of the assay is based on amplification of the assay rather than of viral nucleic acid.

3.1.2.2. The Assay. Synthetic oligonucleotides are fixed onto wells in the plates used. The serum containing suspected HBV DNA is then allowed to hybridize with the synthetic oligonucleotides to form an immobilized complex. Then, copies of a DNA molecule already labeled with multiple branches containing alkaline phosphatase are added to the well and allowed to hybridize with additional exposed DNA sequences of the immobilized complex present in the well. Finally, the amplified reaction complex is detected with enzyme-mediated chemiluminescence *(12)*, and the light produced is proportional to the amount of DNA present.

3.1.2.3. Clinical Significance.
1. The test is useful for accurate quantitation of the viral DNA. It can be helpful in detecting extremely low levels of virus in patients on antiviral treatment *(12)*.
2. Very low levels of HBV DNA in patients with HBsAb may not be clinically significant.

3.1.2.4. Advantages.
1. This technique is more likely to be quantitatively accurate than PCR.
2. Like PCR, bDNA technique is more sensitive and specific compared to serological assays used to diagnose HBV infection. This technique can detect up to 1.6 pg/mL of DNA (1 pg = 286,000 genome equivalents) *(12)*.
3. It is particularly useful in detecting HBV DNA in patients without the HBe antigen.
4. Relative cost: $$.

3.2. Hepatitis C Virus

Molecular diagnostic techniques that are available for HCV include bDNA and reverse transcriptase PCR (RT-PCR).

3.2.1. BRANCHED DNA AMPLIFICATION

3.2.1.1. Principles. A signal amplification method or branched DNA chain amplification assay was developed for direct detection of serum HCV RNA. The technique used for this assay is similar to the technique used for HBV bDNA assay (*see* Section 3.1.). It is a solution-phase sandwich hybridization assay coupled with signal amplification employing bDNA based upon specific hybridization of synthetic oligonucleotides (capture extenders and labeling extenders) to the highly conserved 5' untranslated region of HCV RNA, after which the RNA is captured onto the surface of a microwell plate. Synthetic bDNA amplifier molecules and multiple copies of an alkaline phosphatase-linked probe are hybridized to the immobilized complex. Detection is achieved by incubating the complex with a chemiluminescent substrate and measuring the light emission. Since the target is not amplified, the signal is proportional to the level of target nucleic acid. The quantity of HCV RNA in the sample is then determined from a standard curve. This approach should be very reliable for the quantitation of HCV RNA. As a new approach, this assay has not yet reached the sensitivity of RT-PCR.

3.2.1.2. Clinical Significance.

1. This technique is used for quantitative detection, especially for low levels of nucleic acid *(4)*.
2. The technique is useful in pregnant women, who are anti-HCV positive, to assess the risk of transmission to the newborn *(8)*.
3. It is also useful in liver transplantation patients to monitor HCV recurrence.

3.2.1.3. Advantages.

1. The technique is quantitative, simple, and more widely available.
2. It is more sensitive and specific than the serological tests.

3.2.1.4. Limitations.

1. The detection limit of the first generation assay is 350,000 viral genome equivalents/mL of serum and, for the second generation assay, the detection limit is 200,000 genome equivalents/mL.
2. Relative cost: $$$$.

3.2.2. Reverse Transcription Polymerase Chain Reaction

3.2.2.1. Principles. Reverse transcription polymerase chain reaction (RT-PCR) involves reverse transcription of viral RNA followed by amplification of the complementary DNA by the polymerase chain reaction.

3.2.2.2. Clinical Significance.

1. The detection of HCV RNA confirms the diagnosis of active HCV infection *(8–10)*.
2. RT-PCR can also be useful in diagnosing seronegative acute hepatitis in the very early phase, as early as 3–4 d after exposure. HCV infections with low levels of viremia, such as infection from mother to newborn, can also be detected.
3. The technique is useful in detecting HCV infection in immunocompromised patients who cannot mount a detectable antibody response, such as patients with HIV, on hemodialysis, or organ transplant recipients.

3.2.2.3. Advantages.

1. The technique is useful for detection of trace amounts of viral nucleic acids, especially when results of serological assays are negative or indeterminate (RIBA II) *(8,12)*. RT-PCR is the most sensitive technique for HCV detection. It can detect down to about 2000 genomes *(8,12)*.
2. The results of this assay correlate with the active infection and ongoing viral multiplication.

3.2.2.4. Limitations.

1. The test is not widely available.
2. Because of its sensitivity, false positivity is more common due to contamination *(12)*.
3. It is not reliable for detecting < 500–2000 genomes *(8)*.
4. Relative cost: $$$.

3.3. Cytomegalovirus

3.3.1. Principles

After primary CMV infection, the virus is not eradicated from the host. Its DNA persists in a latent form. Serological tests in immunocompromised assay patients are not useful in making the diagnosis of CMV reactivation. On the other hand, detection of CMV viremia in a patient with normal immunity is strong evidence of disseminated infection and can be used to diagnose CMV hepatitis when there is clinical evidence of hepatitis.

3.3.2. THE ASSAYS

The polymerase chain reaction is performed with the basic principle similar to that described earlier for the HBV assay.

3.3.3. CLINICAL SIGNIFICANCE

1. Because of its sensitivity, PCR has been used for early diagnosis of CMV.
2. It is also useful for monitoring antiviral treatment, and detection of gene mutations associated with ganciclovir resistance.
3. PCR of CMV DNA in the plasma may be more predictive of CMV disease than the PCR of CMV DNA on peripheral blood leukocytes *(16)*.

3.3.4. ADVANTAGES

1. The test is widely available.
2. The technique has a higher sensitivity than the CMV culture and antigenemia assay *(16)*.
3. The assay helps in early detection of CMV DNA in patients with subsequent disease *(16)*.

3.3.5. LIMITATIONS

1. The technique has a low specificity as compared to CMV culture, and, therefore, has a low positive and a high negative predictive value for CMV disease *(16)*. CMV viremia, in immunocompromised patients, can not be used to diagnose CMV hepatitis. In such patients, a liver biopsy should be done to diagnose CMV related hepatitis *(19)*.
2. Relative cost: $$$.

SUMMARY

Anti-HAV elevations in patients with clinical evidence of acute hepatitis and elevation in aminotransferases confirm the diagnosis of acute hepatitis A infection.

HBsAg assay is a very sensitive screening test for HBV infection. However, it alone cannot be used to differentiate between various stages of the disease.

HBeAg in the serum correlates with infectivity and the presence of HBV particles in serum.

HBcAb in the serum indicates HBV exposure. However, it alone can not be used to differentiate between acute, resolved, or chronic HBV infection.

HBeAb in the serum indicates declining viremia in most patients with HBV infection.

HBsAb in the serum indicates the presence of immunity in most cases, either due to infection or immunization against HBV infection.

Enzyme Immunoassays-II is a useful screening test for HCV infection in a low prevalence group. However, it cannot be used to distinguish between the various stages of HCV infection and false positive tests.

Recombinant Immunoblot Assay for HCV is superior to EIA, and it is used to resolve false positive or indeterminate results associated with EIA.

Hepatitis D virus antibody assay should only be performed in patients who have some evidence of HBV infection.

Anti-HEV antibodies are neutralizing antibodies. Their rise in serum coincides with elevation in ALT and disappearance of the Hepatitis E antigen from serum.

Cytomegalovirus hepatitis can be diagnosed by PCR, antigenemia assay or rapid culture methods. The latter two tests are more inexpensive and widely available, but less sensitive than the PCR.

PCR for HBV diagnosis is not routinely used in clinical practice. However, it can provide useful information in patients suspected of having HBV infection with negative serum markers.

Branched DNA amplification for HBV is used for quantitative purposes.

RT-PCR for the diagnosis of HCV infection is not routinely used. The test is reserved for research laboratories, but it can be used to diagnose HCV infection in limited circumstances, such as patients with immunocompromised status, equivocal serological test results, and very early infection prior to developing HCV antibodies.

Branched DNA amplification assay for HCV infection is used to quantitate viral load prior to and during treatment.

REFERENCES

1. McMahon BJ, Shapiro CN, Robertson BH. Hepatitis A. In: Haubrich WS, Schaffner F, Berk JE, eds. Bockus gastroenterology, vol. 3, 5th ed. Saunders, New York, 1995, p. 2051.
2. Gerlich WH, Thomssen R. Terminology, structure and laboratory diagnosis of hepatitis viruses. In: McIntyre N, Benhamou JP, Bircher J, Rizzetto M, Rodes J, eds. Oxford textbook of clinical hepatology, vol. 1, Oxford University Press, Oxford, 1991; pp. 537–565.
3. Koff RS. Viral Hepatitis. In: Schiff L, Schiff ER, eds. Diseases of the liver, vol. 1, Lippincott, Philadelphia, 1993; pp. 492–577.
4. Hoofnagle JH. Hepatitis B. In: Haubrich WS, Schaffner F, Berk JE, eds. Bockus gastroenterology, vol. 3, 5th ed. Saunders, New York, 1995; pp. 2062–2081.
5. Hollinger FB, Dreesman GR. Hepatitis viruses. In: Rose NR, Macario EC, Fahey JL, Friedman H, Penn GM, eds. Manual of clinical laboratory immunology. American Society for Microbiology, Washington, 1992; pp. 634–650.
6. Dienstag JL, Wands JR, Isselbacher KJ. Acute hepatitis. In: Wilson, Braunwald, Isselbacher, Martin, Fauci, Root, eds. Harrison's principles of internal medicine, 12th ed. McGraw-Hill, New York, 1991; p. 1324.
7. Neuschwander-Tetri, BA. Common blood tests for liver disease. Postgraduate Medicine. 1995;98:49–63.
8. Davis GL, Lau JY. Hepatitis C. In: Haubrich WS, Schaffner F, Berk JE, eds. Bockus gastroenterology, vol. 3, 5th ed. Saunders, New York, 1995; pp. 2082–3014.
9. Gretch DR, Rosa C, Carithers RL, Willson RA, Williams B, Corey L. Assessment of hepatitis C viremia using molecular amplification technologies: correlations and clinical implications. Ann Int Med 1995;123:327–329.
10. Tedeschi V, Seeff LB. Diagnostic tests for hepatitis C: where are we now? Ann Int Med 1995;123:383–385.
11. Rubin RA, Falestiny M, Malet PF. Chronic hepatitis C: advances in diagnostic testing and therapy. Arch Int Med 1994;154:387–392.
12. Hu KQ, Vierling JM. Molecular diagnostic techniques for viral hepatitis. Gastroenterol Clin North Am 1994;23:479–498.
13. Bradley DW. Hepatitis E virus: a brief review of the biology, molecular virology, and immunology of a novel virus. J Hepatol 1995;22:140–145.
14. Paul DA, Kingge MF, Ritter A. Determination of hepatitis E-virus seroprevalence by using recombinant fusion protein and synthetic peptides. J Infect Dis 1994;169:801–806.
15. Ho M. Cytomegalovirus: principle and practice of infectious diseases. In: Mandell, Douglas, Bennett, eds. Principles and practice of infectious disease. Churchill Livingstone, New York, 1995, pp. 1351–1363.
16. Boeckh M, Myerson D, Bowden RA. Early detection and treatment of cytomegalovirus infections in marrow transplant patients: methodological aspects and implications for therapeutic interventions. Bone Marrow Transplant 1994;14:S66–S70.
17. Sumaya CV, Jenson HB. Epstein-Barr Virus. In: Manual of clinical laboratory immunology. American Society for Microbiology, Washington, 1992; pp. 568–575.
18. Zuckerman AJ, Griffiths P. Infections of the liver caused by viruses other than hepatitis. In: Haubrich WS, Schaffner F, Berk JE, eds. Bockus gastroenterology, Vol. 3, 5th ed. Saunders, New York, 1995; pp. 2141–2150.
19. Griffiths PD. Systemic virosis capable of producing hepatitis as the main clinical picture. In: McIntyre N, Benhamou JP, Bircher J, Rizzetto M, Rodes J, eds. Oxford textbook of clinical hepatology, vol. 1, Oxford University Press, Oxford, 1991; 626–630.
20. Brechot C. Polymerase chain reaction for the diagnosis of viral hepatitis B and C. Gut 1993;Supplement:S39–S44.

4   True Liver Function Tests

Shabbir Chaiwala and George Y. Wu

Contents

1. INTRODUCTION

In Chapter 2, markers of hepatobiliary disease were discussed. Although frequently called liver function tests, they are more properly considered markers of liver damage than function. True liver function tests correlate with hepatic functional capacity and include the galactose elimination, caffeine clearance, prothrombin time (PT), albumin, and cholesterol levels.

2. LIVER FUNCTION TESTS

2.1. Routine Tests That May Reflect Liver Function

2.1.1. Serum Albumin

2.1.1.1. Principles. Albumin is one of the most important plasma proteins synthesized by the liver. Quantitative assessment of plasma albumin is helpful in assessing the synthetic function of the liver *(1)*. In healthy individuals, plasma albumin concentration is normally 35–50 gm/L *(2)*. The average size of the albumin pool in adults is approx 500 g. Normal persons synthesize 12–15 g of albumin a day. Albumin synthesis can double in the face of excessive catabolism or loss of albumin from the body. The normal half-life for albumin is about 20 d *(1)*, but can be decreased to 7 d in nonhepatic febrile illness or trauma *(2)*.

2.1.1.2. The Assay. Serum albumin is determined in most laboratories by automated assays. The assay is based on binding of albumin to a dye (bromocresol green, methyl orange, bromocresol purple) that results in a change in color of the dye. The change in color is read by spectrophotometer and the intensity is proportional to the quantity of albumin in test sample *(3)*.

2.1.1.3. Clinical Significance. Because albumin is the major protein synthesized by the liver, its plasma level is helpful is assessing the severity and chronicity of liver diseases.

2.1.1.4. Advantages.

1. Serum albumin levels can be correlated with the severity of cirrhosis *(1)*.
2. In the absence of inadequate protein intake, loss, or increased degradation, or increased volume of distribution, plasma albumin level is very well correlated with the synthetic function of the liver.

From: *Diseases of the Liver and Bile Ducts: Diagnosis and Treatment*
Edited by: G. Y. Wu and J. Israel © Humana Press Inc., Totowa, NJ

3. The test is widely available in automated analyses.
4. Relative cost: $.

2.1.1.5. Limitations.

1. Factors other than hepatic synthesis, which affect the serum albumin level, include malnutrition, intestinal or renal loss, increased catabolism, increased vascular permeability, and overhydration *(2)*.
2. In acute liver disease, even when the synthetic function is markedly depressed, plasma albumin levels may be normal because of albumin's long half-life *(2)*.
3. In patients with ascites, low plasma albumin levels may be a reflection of abnormal distribution rather than of impaired synthesis *(1)*.
4. The synthesis of albumin may be decreased in certain nonhepatic conditions such as malnutrition, malabsorption, and malignant diseases *(2)*.

2.1.2. Prothrombin Time

2.1.2.1. Principles. Prothrombin Time (PT) is a test used to assess blood clotting. Blood clotting is dependent upon the clotting factors, which are proteins synthesized by the liver. Liver synthesizes factors I (fibrinogen), II (prothrombin), V, VII, IX, and X. Factor VII has the shortest half-life, and it is affected first in liver disease. Abnormalities in the hepatocellular protein synthesis are reflected by elevations in the PT.

2.1.2.2. The Assay. The combined activity of factors I, II, V, VII, and X, which participate in the extrinsic pathway of coagulation are measured. In the assay, the time required for citrated plasma to form a clot in the presence of tissue extract (thromboplastin) and calcium is measured. If any of the factors I, II, V, VII, and X are deficient, singly or in combination, the PT will be prolonged and suggest decreased hepatic synthetic capacity *(1)*.

2.1.2.3. Clinical Significance.

1. Prothrombin time is routinely performed in patients with evidence of any acute or chronic hepatocellular injury to assess the degree of hepatic dysfunction. Conditions in which this test is most useful are acetaminophen toxicity, acute hepatitis, or shock liver *(1)*.
2. This test is useful in assessing the course and outcome of hepatocellular diseases. Prolonged PT indicates poor long-term prognosis in patients with chronic liver disease *(1)*.
3. Prolonged PT in patients with cirrhosis and portal hypertension reflects an increased surgical risk and mortality with a poor outcome from portocaval shunting.
4. Extreme prolongation of PT, particularly in patients with fulminant hepatic failure, is one of the major factors in the decision to proceed with liver transplantation (*see* Chapter 30).

2.1.2.4. Advantages.

1. The test is simple to perform and widely available in clinical chemistry labs *(1)*.
2. This test correlates well with the synthetic function of the liver, and it is useful in assessing the severity of liver disease *(1)*.
3. Relative cost: $.

2.1.2.5. Limitations.

1. Prolongation of PT is not specific for liver disease, as it can be found elevated in patients with hereditary deficiency of clotting factors, and in acquired conditions such as vitamin K deficiency, and consumption coagulopathies. It can also be elevated by vitamin K antagonists such as coumadin. The measurement of factor V can be helpful in differentiating between prolonged PT from vitamin K deficiency vs liver diseases. Factor V will be normal in patients with vitamin K deficiency. Administration of vitamin K can normalize PT by 30% within 24 h in patients with vitamin K deficiency *(1)*.

2. This test can be normal in mild and early hepatocellular injury process. Only significant hepatocellular injury affects its synthetic function and leads to prolongation of PT *(1)*.

3. In patients with significant hepatocellular injury, prolongation of PT can also result from incomplete clearing of activated clotting factors, primary fibrinolysis, impaired plasminogen synthesis, and disseminated intravascular coagulation *(1)*.

2.1.3. SERUM CHOLESTEROL AND LIPOPROTEINS

2.1.3.1. Principles. The liver plays an important role in the synthesis and metabolism of lipids. Abnormal cholesterol and lipoprotein levels can be found in patients with liver disease. However, lipid abnormalities are not specific for liver disease, but provide supportive evidence *(1)*.

2.1.3.2. The Assays. Most patients with acute hepatitis develop elevations of serum triglycerides and free cholesterol. However, there is a decline in cholesterol ester levels. An increase in free cholesterol along with phospholipids is recognized on electrophoresis as an abnormally wide beta band, which represents the presence of an abnormal lipoprotein called lipoprotein X (LPX). The elevation of free cholesterol in the form of LPX is considered to be secondary to a deficiency of lecithin-cholesterol acyltransferase (LCAT), poor handling of LPX by LCAT, and reflux of cholesterol along with bile in patients with cholestasis *(4)*. Free cholesterol in the form of LPX is elevated in 99% of patients with evidence of cholestasis. However, it cannot be used to differentiate between intrahepatic and extrahepatic cholestasis *(4)*. The mechanism for elevation of triglycerides in parenchymal liver disease is poorly understood, but appears to be related to a decrease in hepatic lipase.

2.1.3.3. Clinical Significance.

1. An elevation of free cholesterol is related to a deficiency of LCAT.

2. Lipoprotein electrophoresis is normal in patients with normal LCAT, but as the level of LCAT declines with parenchymal disease, it leads to a loss of the pre-beta band initially and later loss of the alpha band. Alpha and beta bands disappear in acute hepatitis and reappear with the resolution of hepatitis. These parameters can be useful in assessing the prognosis. However, they are not as sensitive or specific as the prothrombin time and bilirubin. The changes in lipoprotein in patients with chronic parenchymal liver disease are similar to those seen in acute liver disease, though less severe *(4)*.

3. Cholesterol levels tend to fall in patients with severe parenchymal liver disease, either acute or chronic. Rebound hypercholesterolemia is seen during the recovery process *(2)*.

2.1.3.4. Advantages.

1. This test is widely available on automated clinical analyzers.

2. Relative cost: $.

2.1.3.5. Limitations. The test is not specific for liver disease.

2.2. Special Liver Function Tests

2.2.1. GALACTOSE ELIMINATION TESTS

2.2.1.1. Principles. The liver plays an important role in the metabolism of galactose. Galactokinase is the major hepatic enzyme responsible for phosphorylation of galactose. Therefore, disappearance of galactose from the blood can be measured as an indication of the functional capacity of the hepatocytes. Galactose elimination is measured by various techniques such as constant infusion, iv bolus injection, and oral loading with simultaneous measurement of plasma galactose or excretion of radioactive CO_2 as a breath test *(1)*. Hepatic clearance of galactose depends on hepatic perfusion and extraction, both of which may be altered by liver disease. Major determinants of hepatic extraction are functional mass of hepatocytes and blood flow to hepatocytes, both of which may be decreased in patients with cirrhosis *(5)*.

2.2.1.2. The Assays.

1. Galactose elimination capacity (GEC): The basis of galactose elimination tests is to saturate the hepatic enzyme galactokinase by various modes of galactose administration and allow elimination of galactose by zero-order kinetics. Galactose elimination capacity (GEC) is proportional to the functional mass of the hepatocytes. Below the enzyme saturation limit, galactose elimination follows first-order kinetics, which are dependent upon hepatic blood flow and can be used to measure hepatic perfusion *(5)*. In a standard galactose elimination test, 0.5 gm/kg of galactose is injected iv and removal of galactose is calculated from four or five blood samples taken at different time intervals during the first hour after injection. Elimination of galactose is plotted on a curve, which can be helpful to calculate the galactose half-life and hepatic functional capacity *(1)*.
2. Galactose single point (GSP): Recently, a galactose single point (GSP) measurement in the assessment of liver function has been described. In this test, the galactose level in plasma is measured 1 h after quick iv infusion and the results correlate very well with GEC. The GSP method is simple, clinically useful, and quantitative for the assessment of liver function *(6)*.

2.2.1.3. Clinical Significance.

1. The GEC is considered to be helpful in differentiating healthy subjects and cirrhotic patients *(1)*. EC is usually not affected by biliary obstruction.
2. The galactose single-point method is useful for quantitative measurement of residual liver function in terms of planning for liver transplantation. The test is also useful for assessing the prognosis of liver disease patients, and for following the patients after liver transplantation *(6)*.

2.2.1.4. Advantages.

1. The GEC and GSP methods are very sensitive in determining functional hepatic mass.
2. These tests are also useful in following the course of the disease along with treatment responsiveness and prognosis.
3. The GSP is simpler to perform than the GEC.

2.2.1.5. Limitations.

1. These tests are not as sensitive as dye tests in detecting subclinical cirrhosis.
2. The galactose extraction by the liver is not 100% (usually approx 94%) *(1)*. The elimination of galactose is not cleared by the liver, but also to some extent by the kidneys *(5)*.
3. Galactose elimination decreases with advancing age in the absence of liver dysfunction *(1)*.

2.2.2. Caffeine Clearance Test

2.2.2.1. Principles. The caffeine clearance test is a quantitative liver function test. Caffeine, *(1,6)* trimethylaxanthine, is metabolized by microsomal enzymes in the liver and excreted in the urine as methylxanthine *(7)*. Since plasma caffeine is extracted (97%) primarily by the liver, it seems to be an ideal compound for the assessment of hepatic metabolic function *(8)*.

2.2.2.2. The Assay. After approx 17 h of caffeine exclusion, about 300 mg of caffeine citrate is given to patients orally. Blood samples are drawn at various time intervals, and plasma caffeine concentrations are measured *(9)*. Because caffeine levels in plasma and saliva are similar, caffeine can be measured in saliva with similar results.

2.2.2.3. Clinical Significance.

1. This test is useful in assessing the functional and metabolic capacity of the liver, and is a particularly sensitive indicator to assess liver function *(8)*.

2. It can also be used to differentiate between hepatocellular disease and simple biliary obstruction as patients with biliary obstruction generally will have a normal caffeine clearance test *(8)*.

2.2.2.4. Advantages.

1. The test is not only quantitative, but also innocuous.
2. Relative cost: $.
3. It can be performed easily, as caffeine is taken orally and its level can be measured either in saliva or blood *(8)*.
4. The sensitivity of this test is approx 89% for all liver diseases and up to 100% for alcoholic liver disease *(8)*.
5. Bcause caffeine is absorbed completely and metabolized primarily by the liver, the test is very useful in assessing hepatic metabolic capacity *(8)*.
6. There is no need for radioisotopes or breath collection (9).

2.2.2.5. Limitations.

1. The specificity of this test is poor, only 62%.
2. Caffeine elimination declines with advancing age and is increased by smoking because of the induction of caffeine metabolizing enzymes. These factors affect the validity of results *(8)*.
3. Validity of caffeine elimination is also affected by drugs such as cimetidine *(8)*.
4. Caffeine clearance is variable between individuals, making the establishment of a clear threshold value for persons without liver disease difficult *(8)*.
5. It is not widely available.

SUMMARY

Serum albumin levels are very well correlated with the synthetic function of the liver, in the absence of processes that cause increased loss of albumin.

Prothrombin time is a routine test for screening the synthetic function of the liver.

Serum cholesterol and lipoprotein levels are commonly found to be abnormal in patients with liver disease; they are not as sensitive or specific as prothrombin time and bilirubin.

The galactose elimination test provides a quantitative measurement of the residual liver function.

The caffeine clearance test is useful for measuring residual functional mass of the liver, and can be helpful in differentiating hepatocellular process from biliary obstruction.

REFERENCES

1. Stolz A, Kaplowitz N. Biochemical tests for liver disease. In: Zakim D, Boyer TD, eds. Hepatology: a textbook of liver disease, 2nd ed. Saunders, New York, 1990; pp. 637–667.
2. McIntyre N, Rosalki S. Biochemical investigations in the management of liver disease. In: McIntyre N, Benhamou JP, Bircher J, Rizzetto M, Rodes J, eds. Oxford textbook of clinical hepatology. vol. 1, Oxford University Press, Oxford, UK, 1991; pp. 293–309.
3. Gendler SM. Albumin. In: Pesce AJ, Kaplan LA, eds. Methods in clinical chemistry. Mosby, New York, 1987, pp 1066–1073.
4. Cooper AD. Hepatic lipoprotein and cholesterol metabolism. In: Zakim D, Boyer TD, eds. Hepatology: a textbook of liver disease, 2nd ed. Saunders, New York, 1990; pp. 96–123.
5. Lauterburg BH, Preisig R. Quantitation of liver function. In: McIntyre N, Benhamou JP, Bircher J, Rizzetto M, Rodes J, eds. Oxford textbook of clinical hepatology, vol. 1, Oxford University Press, Oxford, UK, 1991, pp. 309–314.
6. Tang HS, Hu OY. Assessment of liver function using a novel galactose single point method. Digestion 1992;52:222–231.
7. Boeckh M, Myerson D, Bowden RA. Early detection and treatment of cytomegalovirus infections in marrow transplant patients: methodological aspects and implications for therapeutic interventions. Bone Marrow Transplant. 1994;14:S66–S70.

8. McDonagh JE, Nathan VV, Bonavia JC, Moyle GR, Tanner AR. Caffeine clearance by enzyme multiplied immunoassay technique: a simple, inexpensive, and useful indicator of liver function. Gut 1991;32:681–684.
9. Kaplan MM. Laboratory tests. In: Schiff L, Schiff ER, eds. Diseases of the liver. vol. 1, 7th ed. Lippincott, Philadelphia, 1993, pp. 108–144.

III   Imaging

5

Noninvasive Techniques for the Evaluation of Liver Diseases

Jeff Fidler and David Stark

1. INTRODUCTION

Several techniques are available for noninvasive imaging of the liver. The modality of choice is dictated by the clinical scenario with the objectives of detection, characterization, and staging or quantification of the disease process. The main techniques used in evaluation of the liver include computed tomography (CT), magnetic resonance imaging (MRI), ultrasound, and scintigraphy (nuclear medicine). This chapter will describe these techniques, discuss their indications, limitations, and accuracy in the evaluation of liver disease.

2. MODALITIES

2.1. Computed Tomography

2.1.1. TECHNIQUE

Computed tomography acquires images of the body using a rotating source of ionizing radiation and, by computer assistance, recreates the images based on attenuation differences. Images are acquired by moving the table sequentially through the linear rotating source of radiation at predetermined intervals. This technique is referred to as incremental scanning. Improvements in the mechanical arrays of the detectors, gantry, or ring that orbits the patient, and computer reconstruction techniques have significantly reduced scan times and increased resolution. Slip-ring technology or helical scanning allows scanning of the entire abdomen in a single, screw-like acquisition (spiral CT) with the patient table and radiation source moving continuously.

Because the properties of X-ray attenuation as demonstrated by CT it is often unable to differentiate abnormal from normal tissue, except when there is morphologic distortion. Pharmaceutical-based imaging approaches have been extensively researched to improve lesion

From: *Diseases of the Liver and Bile Ducts: Diagnosis and Treatment*
Edited by: G. Y. Wu and J. Israel © Humana Press Inc., Totowa, NJ

conspicuity. CT scanning of the liver can be performed without any contrast agent. However, in nearly all cases, enteral or parenteral contrast agents, or both, are used.

Parenchymal tissue contrast is improved by the vascular administration of iodinated agents. These agents administered intravenously are designed for rapid excretion, and do not significantly affect body physiology. Binding to blood proteins or cells is negligible, and excretion is by passive glomerular filtration. Thus, these agents will penetrate capillaries and have an extracellular distribution.

Various imaging protocols have been performed to utilize the dual (portal and hepatic arterial) vascular supply of normal liver and improve lesion conspicuity (1,2). Because of the less than optimal results with this dynamic iv bolus technique, other techniques to administer contrast at angiography with selective cannulation of the hepatic artery (CT arteriography, CTA) or by the superior mesenteric artery and splenic artery (CT arterial portography, CTAP) are commonly performed (3,4). These techniques, which examine the arterial and portal venous flow, respectively, generally have greater contrast and improved sensitivity for detecting liver lesions. However, due to variations in the portal venous perfusion of the liver, nonneoplastic perfusion inhomogeneities create numerous false positives, limiting the value of this technique (5–7).

2.1.2. INDICATIONS

CT is indicated for the detection of masses, including metastases and primary liver tumors, characterization of lesions such as hemangioma, and staging of tumors. CT is also indicated in the evaluation of the liver for diffuse disease such as cirrhosis, fatty infiltration and other infiltrative processes in the liver. CT can evaluate the hepatic vascular anatomy and patency. However, Doppler ultrasound is more accurate and cost-effective.

2.1.3. ADVANTAGES

Advantages of computed tomography include the rapidity and visualization of the entire abdomen unimpaired by bowel, gas, or bone. Computed tomography is not operator-dependent and, therefore, the risk of an inexperienced practitioner failing to recognize pathology is minimized. CT can obtain high resolution images as thin as 1 mm, and because of the rapidity, can be acquired during a breath hold with significant improvement in respiratory artifacts. Because spiral CT acquires data in a volume set, three-dimensional reconstructed images can be generated.

2.1.4. LIMITATIONS

The principal limitation of CT is its restriction to acquisition in the transverse plane in the abdomen. When organs or structures have complex shapes oblique to the transverse plane on the CT image, the adjacent structures overlap and their attenuation values are averaged into a single pixel on the image. This can lead to "volume averaging," which can obscure tissue boundaries and mimic pathology. However, the development of spiral CT has largely overcome this limitation. The ability to reconstruct data at narrower intervals, and reconstruct images in various planes helps reduce these volume averaging pitfalls. Solid lesions slightly less than 1.0 cm in size can be detected by using good dynamic technique. Other limitations include those associated with the iv injection of contrast, which can be contraindicated in certain individuals, lead to the development of contrast reactions and, with underlying hemodynamic alterations, may lead to suboptimal enhancement patterns of the visceral organs, including the liver.

2.1.5. RISK

There is no significant risk from computed tomography. The patient will receive a small amount of radiation exposure during the examination, which is approx 15X the effective dose equivalent of a chest X-ray. However, if iv contrast is used, then the associated risks related to iodinated contrast administration, such as anaphylaxis, renal failure, and acute tubular necrosis, are potential complications. Some of these allergic reactions can be reduced or minimized by premedication with steroids. However, patients with a history of contrast allergy or reaction to iodinated agents should avoid them. When required, nonionic contrast media should be used.

2.2. Magnetic Resonance Imaging

2.2.1. TECHNIQUE

Magnetic resonance imaging is performed by placing the patient in a uniform magnetic field, and then applying and sampling repetitive radio frequency waves. When the patient is placed inside the magnetic field, the hydrogen nuclei inside the body align themselves with the magnetic field. To create an image, a radio frequency (RF) pulse must be applied. This RF pulse is generated from a coil and causes the nuclei to be rotated out of alignment. When the RF pulse is terminated, the nuclei attempt to realign with the magnetic field. During this process of "relaxation," a signal is produced in the coil. This signal is then processed and created into an image. Different tissues and pathology have unique times of relaxation. By varying the duration of pulse application and time to listen to the signal (T1 and T2 weighting) these tissues and disorders can be differentiated.

MR technology has rapidly improved over the past several years. Improvements in RF coil technology have led to the development of surface and endoluminal coils, that allow high resolution images with smaller fields of view. Improvements in pulse sequence design have led to faster imaging acquisitions, improved resolution, and increased signal to noise. Improvements in hardware have led to stronger and faster magnets allowing a marked decrease in scan time.

As with CT, various pharmaceutical agents have been evaluated to help improve lesion identification and characterization. The most widely used are the gadolinium chelates, which are extracellular agents. Other agents, such as iron oxide, that are taken up by the reticuloendothelial system and hepatoselective agents, such as mangafodipir trisodium (Mn-DPDP) and certain gadolinium-based agents, are undergoing extensive research.

2.2.2. INDICATIONS

The indications for MRI include lesion identification, characterization and staging; evaluation of the liver in the setting of, or for confirmation of fatty infiltration; evaluation for diffuse infiltrative processes including hemochromatosis; and evaluation of vascular anatomy and patency. Recently, MRI has been shown to be useful in the evaluation of the biliary tract (MR cholangiography) for the detection of choledocholithiasis and bile duct strictures. Images of the biliary system can be obtained using heavily T2-weighted parameters without the injection of contrast. Workstation software allows 3D images of the bile ducts to be reconstructed. Thus, MRI may be a reasonable alternative to direct cholangiography in certain clinical settings. However, the exact clinical role is yet to be defined.

2.2.3. ADVANTAGES

MRI is similar to CT in providing a full view of the entire abdomen and similar anatomic detail (spatial resolution). MR has the further advantage of allowing selection of sagittal, coronal, or oblique planes of acquisition. Three-dimensional volume acquisitions can be performed allowing high resolution images, that can be reconstructed in various planes of view. MRI also has the inherent advantage of improved tissue contrast without the use of iv contrast, which is based on differences in T1 and T2 relaxation processes of the different tissues and pathologic processes within the body. Gadolinium-enhanced MRI has the advantage of being able to be performed in individuals with an iodine allergy or in individuals with impaired renal function. MRI appears more robust than CT, and its technical evolution has outlasted that of CT. Noninvasive angiography by MRI (MRA) has become widely used in the evaluation of abdominal disease. The ability to identify normal blood or CSF flow and measure flow velocities is already affecting the evaluation of neurological, cardiothoracic, and abdominal vascular conditions. There is no exposure to ionizing radiation.

2.2.4. LIMITATIONS

Limitations of MRI include motion artifacts, which are most notable in the upper abdomen and can degrade image quality. This has reduced the utility of MR for many applications. However, with technologic advances to reduce motion artifact and faster imaging (e.g., echo planar technique), which may be obtained in a single breath-hold, this limitation is becoming less significant. By utilizing these improved techniques, resolution can be improved with detection of lesions slightly less than 1 cm in size.

Other MRI limitations include the bore size of the magnet, which decreases the size of patients who can be imaged. Many vendors are currently developing magnets with a wide or open bore that allows scanning of larger patients, reduces claustrophobia, and allows improved access to the patient, allowing the performance of surgical procedures. The magnetic field also limits a select patient population who have contraindications to being placed in a magnetic field.

2.2.5. RISK

There are no known inherent risks to an MRI examination provided the patient does not have one of the contraindications to being placed in a magnetic field, such as an aneurysm clip, recent placement of a vascular clip, certain implants and metallic devices that can be moved by the field, as well as cardiac pacemakers in which a current can be induced. The gadolinium-based contrast agents in clinical use have no measurable toxicity, and have such a low incidence of allergic reactions that they may be administered under some circumstances with no physician present.

2.3. Ultrasound

2.3.1. TECHNIQUE

Sonographic images are obtained by applying and sampling reflected sound waves from the body. These sound waves are generated from a transducer that is placed on the skin surface and transmitted into the body. Sound waves travel at different velocities through different tissues, and are reflected differently by different types of tissue (acoustic impedance). This property allows specific localization and characterization of these different tissues. Because of the speed of transmission, sampling, and reconstruction of the images, imaging can be performed in a real-time setting. Doppler techniques allow determination of flow direction and velocity. This information may be displayed, either as numerical values with statistical analysis or as color representing flow, superimposed on the black and white anatomic background. Various transducers are available, operating at a range of frequencies, including 3.5, 5.0, and 7.0 MHz. Higher frequency transducers offer improved spatial resolution. These, however, suffer from decreased penetration, reducing anatomic coverage. Transducers are available for endoscopic and intraoperative use, allowing proximity to the region of interest and extremely high resolution images. For example, intraoperative ultrasound allows detection of lesions not visible or palpable even during laparotomy.

2.3.2. INDICATIONS

Because of the cost, availability, and versatility of ultrasound, this technique is indicated as an initial screening for most hepatobiliary disorders. Specifically, ultrasound is indicated in the evaluation of liver size, evaluation of the parenchyma for infiltrative processes that can change the echogenicity of the liver, cirrhosis, and lesion detection. Ultrasound is less sensitive than CT or MRI for specific lesion detection. However, it may be useful as some lesions may be more conspicuous on ultrasound when there is underlying parenchymal disease or when ascites or altered portal venous hemodynamics limit CT and MRI examination. Ultrasound is also indicated for vascular evaluation of the liver, including patency, velocity, and directional information of the hepatic artery, portal veins, and hepatic veins. Evaluation for biliary abnormalities should generally begin with ultrasound, which is indicated for the detection of gallstones, evaluation of ductal caliber, and in the evaluation of the gallbladder.

2.3.3. ADVANTAGES

As previously mentioned, ultrasound is more cost effective and more widely available than the other noninvasive techniques. Real-time imaging and the multiplanar capabilities give unique advantages to ultrasound over these other techniques. There is no exposure to ionizing radiation.

2.3.4. LIMITATIONS

Imaging characteristics of sound waves are quite complex. Bowel gas and bone restrict sound wave penetration, obscuring visualization of structures beneath them. Many artifacts can be produced that can mimic pathology. Therefore, expertise of a dedicated sonographer is a necessity to perform high quality sonography. Lesions slightly less than 1 cm in size can be detected, provided there is good contrast in echogenicity between the lesion and normal liver.

2.3.5. RISKS

There are no known risks associated with sonography.

2.4. Scintigraphy

2.4.1. TECHNIQUE

Scintigraphic images of the liver can be obtained by injecting specific radioactive pharmaceuticals that are taken up in the liver. These radiopharmaceuticals are unstable and emit electromagnetic radiation (radioactive decay) that is detected by special scintillation cameras. The scintillation camera contains NaI (Tl), which produces light when exposed to the high-energy radiation. This light is then magnified and created into an image by computer reconstruction. Images are usually acquired in a frontal projection. However, special cameras allow individual slices to be constructed in either coronal, axial, or sagittal planes (single photon emission tomography or SPECT). Various radiopharmaceuticals are available, and the choice depends on the abnormality that is being evaluated. For example, pharmaceuticals that are taken up by the reticuloendothelial system (technetium sulfur colloid) produces a liver/spleen scan that can be used to evaluate focal mass lesions or size and configuration of the liver. Agents, that are taken up by the hepatocytes and excreted into the biliary system, can evaluate the function and excretion of the liver. Blood pool agents (tagged red blood cells) can be used to evaluate for perfusion to specific lesions within the liver.

2.4.2. INDICATIONS

With the advances in CT, MRI, and ultrasound, scintigraphy has a decreasing role in the evaluation of the liver. There are a few indications for lesion characterization, which include the confirmation of hemangioma by using tagged red blood cell scans, and to help confirm the diagnosis of focal nodular hyperplasia (FNH) as an adjunctive imaging technique to CT or MRI. Indications also include the evaluation of hepatic parenchymal perfusion, function and excretion. For example, liver spleen scan is useful for detecting portal hypertension from cirrhosis by demonstrating a shift of colloid to spleen and bone marrow. A bright caudate lobe on liver spleen scan suggests the presence of Budd-Chiari syndrome.

2.4.3. ADVANTAGES

The fundamental advantage of scintigraphy is the selectivity of physiologically targeted radiopharmaceuticals. This method has inherently high sensitivity and can detect nanomolar (10–9) local concentrations of pharmaceuticals, allowing selective targeting of receptors and metabolic processes.

2.4.4. LIMITATIONS

The primary limitation of scintigraphy is the lack of spatial resolution. The use of radiopharmaceuticals as the energy source for imaging, combined with diffuse vascular distribution of the agent, leads to a diffuse signal source, reducing image quality. The sparse and disperse gamma emissions, combined with scatter of the emitted energy by intervening tissues and the use of low-resolution imaging devices, result in grossly inferior spatial resolution. There have been efforts to improve spatial resolution by using SPECT and positron emission tomography (PET). However, these techniques have not significantly changed the approach to imaging of the liver. Lesions that demonstrate increased uptake, such as hemangiomas, can usually be detected at a smaller size than photopenic lesions. Using SPECT techniques, lesions 1.0–1.5 cm in size can be detected.

2.4.5. RISK

The risks associated with scintigraphic examinations include a small radiation exposure to the patient, with a total effective dose slightly less than CT.

3. SELECTED EXAMPLES OF IMAGING OF LIVER DISEASES

3.1. Diffuse Disease

3.1.1. FATTY INFILTRATION (HEPATIC STEATOSIS)

Hepatic steatosis has multiple etiologies. Diagnosis can be confirmed by liver biopsy. However, noninvasive imaging is fairly reliable at diagnosing fatty infiltration of the liver. Comparison of liver-to-spleen attenuation ratios on nonintravenous CT-enhanced images show low attenuation of the liver relative to the spleen with fatty infiltration (Fig. 1). Ultrasound shows diffusely increased echogenicity within the liver in fatty infiltration. However, this finding is nonspecific and can also be seen in hepatic fibrosis.

Occasionally, fatty infiltration of the liver may be focal, and can mimic a liver mass. In these instances, MRI is useful in the confirmation of the etiology of fat. By utilizing chemical-shift imaging, focal fat can be differentiated from certain liver masses.

3.1.2. CIRRHOSIS

Early changes of cirrhosis may consist only of fatty infiltration of the liver. However, in the more advanced cases in which the liver is small and nodular (Fig. 2), both CT and ultrasound are comparable in the diagnosis. Several morphologic parameters have been described in evaluating lobe size by using the principle that in cirrhosis the right lobe and medial segment of the left lobe atrophy with enlargement of the caudate and left lobe. By using these ratios, ultrasound shows a sensitivity and specificity in the 95% range, and CT shows a sensitivity of 84% and specificity of 100% (8). However, in certain types of cirrhosis, the morphologic appearance of the liver may not significantly change, reducing the sensitivity of these examinations.

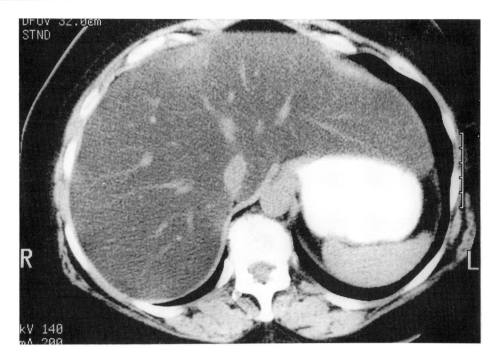

Fig. 1. Fatty infiltration: Unenhanced CT demonstrates diffuse low attenuation of the liver in comparison to the spleen.

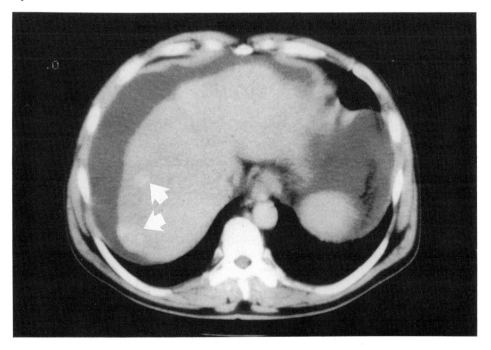

Fig. 2. Cirrhosis: Characteristic findings in cirrhosis include a small liver with a nodular contour. Notice the two hyperenhancing regenerating nodules (arrowhead).

3.1.3. Iron Deposition Disease

Hemochromatosis and hemosiderosis lead to increased iron deposition within the liver. CT and MRI are both capable of diagnosing increased concentrations of hepatic iron. On nonintravenous-enhanced CT images, the liver will have increased attenuation, relative to the density of the spleen. MRI is more sensitive and shows low signal on spin echo and gradient echo images because of a reduction in the T2 and T2* relaxation times secondary to the iron deposition *(9–11)*. MR has been shown to have a sensitivity and specificity of 94% and 90%, respectively. Other organs with increased iron will show similar low signal, which helps evaluate the overall distribution and can help distinguish hemochromatosis from other causes of iron deposition, such as multiple blood transfusions. In hemosiderosis, iron accumulates within the reticuloendothelial system, leading to involvement of the spleen which is usually spared in hemochromatosis.

3.2. Masses

3.2.1. METASTASES

3.2.1.1. Lesion Detection. The accuracy of computed tomography in the detection of metastatic disease is widely debated in the literature. The major problem is the lack of a gold standard in comparing these modalities. It is now generally accepted that CTAP is the most sensitive test, followed closely by MRI. Because most patients with metastatic disease have multiple lesions, the accuracy of CT for distinguishing patients with metastases is greater than 80%. However, for individual lesion detection, the sensitivity is much less. This is because of the enormous biologic variation between tumors and their enhancement patterns. Currently, much research is ongoing evaluating varying scan delays and injection rates on CT to improve lesion conspicuity (Fig. 3).

Because of the availability, cost, and accepted sensitivity in identifying patients with metastases, CT should be the initial study performed. MR should be utilized when there are confusing findings on CT, when there is a contraindication to undergoing a contrasted CT scan, or in the background of fatty infiltration which can limit lesion detection.

In patients who are considered to be surgical candidates, either CTAP, or MR, or a combination of the two studies should be performed because of their improved lesion detection. MR is adjunctive to CTAP allowing possible differentiation of perfusion anomalies from possible neoplastic lesions.

3.2.1.2. Lesion Characterization. Imaging findings may show certain abnormalities suggesting metastases *(12,13)*. These include the demonstration of calcifications seen most often with mucinous carcinomas, such as metastatic colon cancer (Fig. 4). Low density areas may correlate with areas of necrosis. The morphologic pattern of contrast enhancement demonstrating heterogeneity or rings is a useful finding that distinguishes solid neoplasms from cysts from hemangiomas.

3.2.2. PRIMARY LIVER TUMORS

3.2.2.1. Hepatocellular Carcinoma (HCC). Hepatocellular carcinoma is more difficult to detect than metastases or other primary tumors of the liver. The principal reason for this difficulty is that hepatomas most often occur against a background of chronic hepatitis, fatty liver, and cirrhosis (Fig. 5). A wide range of accuracy has been reported in the literature. Biphasic injection techniques (described earlier) may allow improved detection with increased lesion conspicuity on the hepatic arterial phase representative of increased tumor vascularity *(14–16)*.

3.2.2.2. Cavernous Hemangioma. Cavernous hemangioma is a vascular malformation characterized by a cavernous collection of blood spaces. Blood flow is very slow and virtually undetected, except for occasional peripheral site of venous entry. Hemangiomas are exceedingly common, being present in approx 15–20% of the adult population. These lesions are commonly found on imaging techniques. Unfortunately, when these lesions are found in an individual with a malignancy, they can mimic metastases. Although most hemangiomas are confirmed by MRI or tagged red blood cell

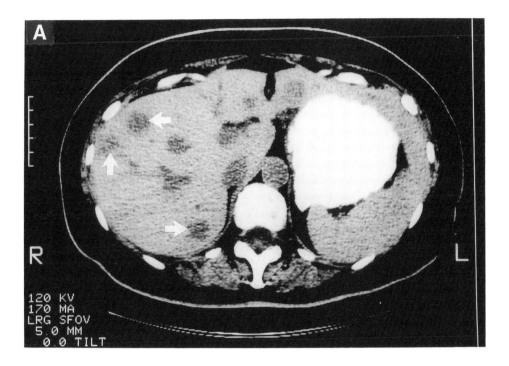

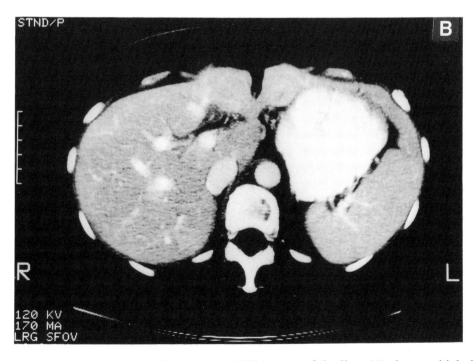

Fig. 3. Hyperenhancing metastases: Noncontrasted CT images of the liver **(A)** show multiple low attenuation lesions consistent with metastases (arrow). On the postcontrast images, the lesions have enhanced to the same degree as the normal liver parenchyma, obscuring their identification **(B)**.

studies, CT can also be used. The classic enhancement pattern of a hemangioma shows peripheral nodular enhancement, centripetal filling, and uniform enhancement with retention of the blood

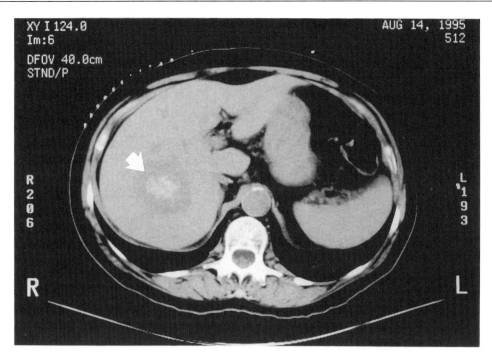

Fig. 4. CT scan of the liver shows a large lesion with central calcification in the right lobe of the liver (arrowhead), a metastasis from mucinous adenocarcinoma of the colon.

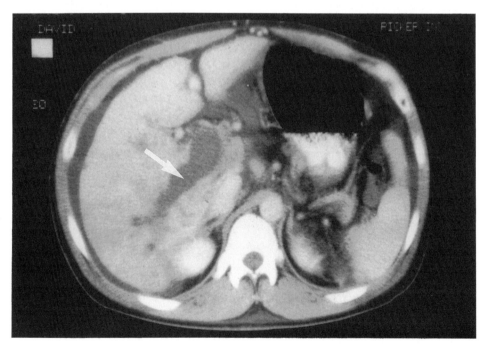

Fig. 5. Hepatocellular carcinoma: Unenhanced CT demonstrates an infiltrative hepatoma in the right lobe of the liver with associated thrombus of the right portal vein (arrow). Vascular invasion is fairly specific for hepatomas.

pool product *(17)* (Fig. 6). By using these criteria, CT has a sensitivity and specificity in the detection of cavernous hemangiomas of approx 80% and nearly 100%, respectively.

The appearance on MR is that of a well-defined lesion with very high signal (equivalent to fluid) on heavily T2-weighted images (Fig. 7). Enhancement with gadolinium is similar to that seen on CT scan *(18–20)*. Using these criteria, the specificity is similar to tagged RBC scans, greater than 95%.

MRI, while more expensive than tagged RBC scans in the confirmation of hemangioma, offers improved evaluation of smaller lesions, lesions near larger vessels, and allows identification of unsuspected lesions.

3.2.2.3. Miscellaneous Tumors. Whereas the sensitivity of CT at detecting other primary tumors of the liver is quite high, many of the imaging features are nonspecific and do not allow definitive characterization. Certain features may be present that can suggest a diagnosis. For example, hepatic adenomas may contain areas of fat, necrosis, and hemorrhage. The presence of a central scar suggests the diagnosis of focal nodular hyperplasia. However, this can also be seen in fibrolamellar carcinoma and adenomas *(21)*.

3.3. Vascular Abnormalities

Ultrasound is the best initial imaging study in the evaluation of the vascular supply to the liver, because of cost, sensitivity, and specificity in the evaluation of the vessels. Several vascular abnormalities can be diagnosed with ultrasound. Ultrasound has a sensitivity of approx 87% in the diagnosis of Budd-Chiari syndrome *(22)*. Certain characteristic abnormal Doppler wave forms combined with hepatic vein distention suggest the diagnosis of passive congestion of the liver. Ultrasound is 100% sensitive, and 93% specific in diagnosing main portal vein thrombus *(23)*. Ultrasound has been shown to be 97% sensitive in diagnosing significant arterial vascular disease (hepatic artery thrombus or stenosis) in post-liver transplant patients *(24)*.

MRI, because of its ability to image flowing blood and determine the direction and velocity of flow, is generally complementary to ultrasound in the evaluation of the hepatic vessels. However, it should be used in selected cases in which ultrasound is nondiagnostic or confusing. Because of its expanded field-of-view, MR shows associated collateral vessels.

With the rapid high resolution images obtained with helical CT, iv-enhanced helical CT scans can exquisitely demonstrate vascular anatomy and patency, especially of the arterial system. Delayed images during the portal venous phase can evaluate the venous structures. However, occasionally flow defects within these vessels can mimic thrombus.

3.4. Biliary Abnormalities

3.4.1. GALLSTONES

The primary modality that should be used to confirm the presence of cholelithiasis is ultrasound. Sonography has a sensitivity of greater than 95% in the diagnosis of cholelithiasis, and can detect approx 70–80% of cases of choledocholithiasis. Gallstones within the distal part of the common bile duct are somewhat more problematic, and difficult to detect secondary to overlying bowel gas. On ultrasound, gallstones appear as echogenic structures with posterior acoustic shadowing. Because of the many possible pitfalls, meticulous technique and knowledge of these pitfalls are a necessity. To allow distention of the gallbladder and improve gallstone detection, patients should be kept fasting for at least 4–6 h prior to the examination.

When using high-resolution technique, CT can detect a significant number of calcified or dense gallstones, because of the contrast between the calcium and bile. However, many stones demonstrate similar attenuation as bile, decreasing their detection rate. Intravenous contrast agents that are excreted in the bile have been evaluated to increase contrast between the stone and surrounding bile and improve detection. However, because of numerous side effects, these agents are not widely used in clinical practice.

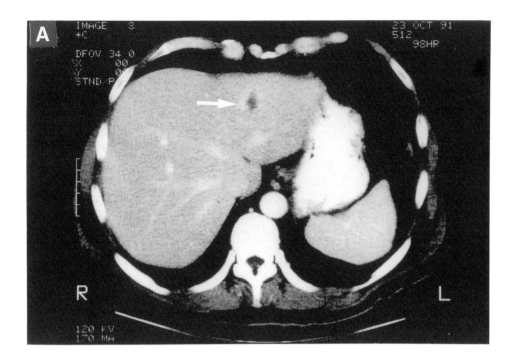

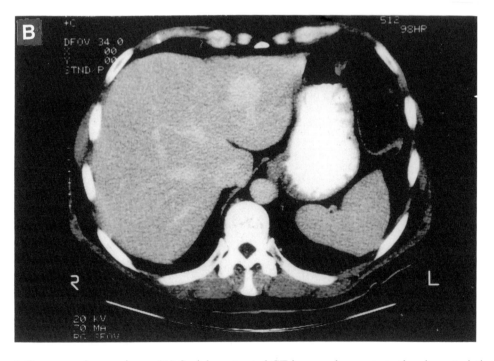

Fig. 6. Cavernous hemangioma: **(A)** Serial-contrasted CT images demonstrate the characteristic enhancement pattern of a cavernous hemangioma. **(B)** Early peripheral nodular enhancement (arrow) with progressive centripetal enhancement and equilibration **(C)** on delayed images.

Recently, MRI (MR cholangiography) has been shown to be useful in the diagnosis of gallstones with a sensitivity for detecting choledocholithiasis of 70–100%.

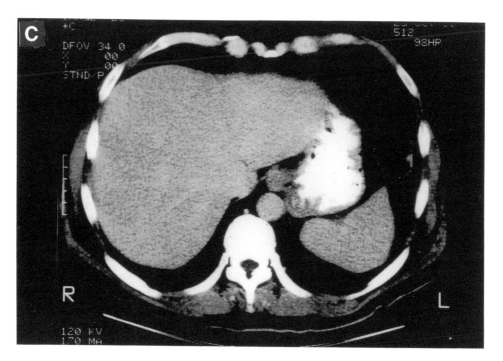

Fig. 6. *(continued)*

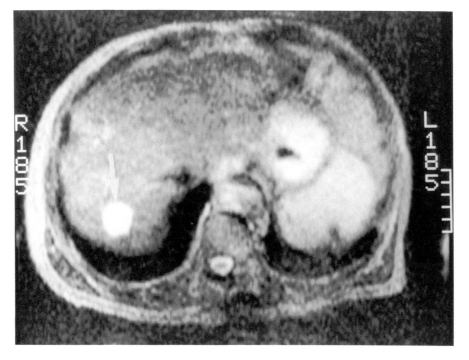

Fig. 7. Cavernous hemangioma: Characteristic MR appearance of a cavernous hemangioma (arrow). The lesion is well defined, with very high signal on T2-weighted images.

3.4.2. ACUTE CHOLECYSTITIS

In patients with suspected acute cholecystitis, sonography or hepatobiliary scintigraphy should be the initial imaging study. An advantage of ultrasound over scintigraphy is that ultrasound allows a generalized screen of the right upper quadrant that may detect other abnormalities mimicking acute cholecystitis. Findings of acute cholecystitis on ultrasound include the presence of gallstones with focal tenderness over the gallbladder ("sonographic Murphy's sign"), gallbladder distention, gallbladder wall thickening, or air within the wall or lumen of the gallbladder, internal membranes, and pericholecystic fluid. The most reliable signs are the presence of gallstones, and a positive sonographic Murphy's sign with a positive predictive value of 92% and a negative predictive value of 95%, respectively *(25)*.

On hepatobiliary scintigraphy (technetium-labeled iminodiacetic acid scans), lack of visualization of the gallbladder is diagnostic of acute cholecystitis. Hepatobiliary scintigraphy also has a high sensitivity and specificity with averages of greater than 95%.

Occasionally, patients may have nonspecific clinical findings and are referred for CT examination. CT findings are similar to ultrasound, including gallbladder wall thickening, pericholecystic stranding, gallbladder distention, pericholecystic fluid, subserosal edema, high attenuation bile, and sloughed membranes. In one study, CT allowed detection of approx 50% of cases of acute cholecystitis. However, the absence of findings does not exclude the diagnosis, and further imaging with ultrasound or scintigraphy should be performed *(26)*.

3.4.3. BILIARY OBSTRUCTION

Biliary obstruction can be due to extrinsic or intrinsic masses, inflammation, and strictures. The evaluation of individuals with suspected biliary obstruction should begin with right upper quadrant sonography. Ultrasound allows detection of bile duct dilatation and can usually determine the site in greater than 90% of the cases, and the cause in greater than 70% of the cases. CT may provide useful information when the ultrasound is inconclusive or incompletely evaluates or stages the abnormality detected. As with choledocholithiasis, MR cholangiography can provide a noninvasive technique to obtain cholangiographic images and the detection of bile duct strictures.

SUMMARY

Because of the cost and wide spread availability, ultrasound generally should be the initial imaging study performed for individuals with suspected hepatobiliary disorders. The average costs of ultrasound, computed tomography (CT), and magnetic resonance imaging (MRI) are $300, $700, and $900, respectively.

Ultrasound should be performed initially to evaluate diffuse diseases such as cirrhosis and in the evaluation of the hepatic vasculature.

CT generally should be the study of choice when evaluating the liver for the detection and staging of masses, with the exception of hepatocellular carcinoma which may be more conspicuous on ultrasound than CT.

MRI is the most sensitive, noninvasive modality to detect focal liver lesions and is complementary to CT arterial portography (CTAP) in the preoperative evaluation.

MR cholangiography is a new, noninvasive technique that may obviate direct cholangiography in certain instances.

REFERENCES

1. Heiken JP, Brink JA, McClennan BL, Sagel SS, Forman HP, DiCroce J. Dynamic contrast-enhanced CT of the liver: comparison of contrast medium injection rates and uniphasic and biphasic injection protocols. *Radiology* 1993;187:327–331.

2. Chambers, TP, Baron RL, Lush RM. Hepatic CT enhancement. *Radiology* 1994;193:513–517.

3. Soyer P, Levesque M, Elias D, Zeitoun G, Roche A. Preoperative assessment of resectability of hepatic metastases from colonic carcinoma: CT portography versus sonography and dynamic CT. *Am J Radiol* 1992;159:741–744.

4. Small WC, Mehard WB, Langmo LS, Dagher AP, Fishman EK, Heiken JP, Bernardino ME. Preoperative determination of the resectability of hepatic tumors: Efficacy of CT during arterial portography. Am J Radiol 1993;161:319-22.

5. Paulson EK, Baker ME, Hilleren DJ, JOnes WP, Knelson MH, Nadel SN, Leder RA, Meyers WC. CT arterial portography: causes of technical failure and variable liver enhancement. *Am J Radiol* 1992;159:745–749.

6. Bluemke DA, Soyer P, Fishman EK. Nontumorous low-attenuation defects in the liver on helical CT during arterial portography: frequency, location and appearance. *Am J Radiol* 1995;164:1141–1145.

7. Soyer P, Lacheheb D, Levesque M. False-positive CT portography: correlation with pathologic findings. *Am J Radiol* 1993;160:285–289.

8. Gore RM. Diffuse liver disease. In: Gore RM, Levine MS, Loufer I, eds. *Textbook of Gastrointestinal Radiology.* Saunders, Philadelphia, 1994; pp. 1968–2017.

9. Siegelman ES, Mitchell DG, Outwater E, Munoz SJ, Rubin R. Idiopathic hemochromatosis: MR imaging findings in cirrhotic and precirrhotic patients. *Radiology* 1993;188:637–641.

10. Siegelman ES, Mitchell DG, Rubin R, Hann HWL, Kaplan KR, Steiner RM, Rao VM, Schuster SJ, Burk DL, Rifkin MD. Parenchymal versus reticuloendothelial iron overload in the liver: distinction with MR imaging. *Radiology* 1991;179:361–366.

11. Gandon Y, Guyader D, Heautot JF, Mohamed-Ihab R, Yaouang J, Buhé T, Brissot P, Carsin M, Deugnier Y. Hemochromatosis: diagnosis and quantification of liver iron with gradient-echo MR imaging. *Radiology* 1994;193:533–538.

12. Hahn PF, Stark DD, Saini S, Rummeny E, Elizondo G, Weissleder R, Wittenberg J, Ferrucci JT. The differential diagnosis of ringed hepatic lesions in MR imaging. *Am J Radiol* 1990;154:287–290.

13. Lee JL, Saini S, Compton CC, Malt RA. MR demonstration of edema adjacent to a liver metastasis: pathologic correlation. *Am J Radiol* 1991;157:499–501.

14. Yamashita Y, Takahashi M, Baba Y, Kanazawa S, Charnsangavej C, Yang D, Wallace S. Hepatocellular carcinoma with or without cirrhosis: a comparison of CT and angiographic presentations in the United States and Japan. *Abdom Imaging* 1993;18:168–175.

15. Kadoya M, Matsui O, Takashima T, Nonomura A. Hepatocellular carcinoma: correlation of MR imaging and histopathologic findings. *Radiology* 1992;183:819–825.

16. Lencioni R, Mascalchi M, Caramella D, Bartolozzi C. Small hepatocellular carcinoma: differentiation from adenomatous hyperplasia with color doppler US and dynamic Gd-DTPA-enhanced MR imaging. *Abdom Imaging* 1996;21:41–48.

17. Quinn SF, Benjamin GG. Hepatic cavernous hemangiomas: simple diagnostic sign with dynamic bolus CT. *Radiology* 1992;182:545–548.

18. McFarland EG, Mayo-Smith WW, Saini S, Hahn PF, Goldberg MA, Lee MJ. Hepatic hemangiomas and malignant tumors: improved differentiation with heavily T2-weighted conventional spin-echo MR imaging. *Radiology* 1994;193:43–47.

19. Semelka RC, Brown ED, Ascher SM, Patt RH, Bagley AS, Li W, Edelman RR, Shoenut JP, Brown JJ. Hepatic hemangiomas: a multi-institutional study of appearance on T2-weighted and serial gadolinium-enhanced gradient-echo MR images. *Radiology* 1994;192:401–406.

20. Whitney WS, Herfkens RJ, Jeffrey RB, McDonnell CH, King CPL, Van Dalsem WJ, Low RN, Francis IR, Dabatin JF, Glazer GM. Dynamic breath-hold multiplanar spoiled gradient-recalled MR imaging with gadolinium enhancement for differentiating hepatic hemangiomas from malignancies at 1.5 T. *Radiology* 1993;189:863–870.

21. Mathieu D, Rahmouni A, Anglade MC, Falise B, Beges C, Cheung P, Mollet JJ, Vasile N. Focal nodular hyperplasia of the liver: assessment with contrast-enhanced TurboFLASH MR imaging. *Radiology* 1991;180:25–30.

22. Boland L, Gainani S, Bassi SL, Zironi G, Bonino F, Brunetto M, Barbara L. Diagnosis of Budd-Chiari syndrome by pulsed Doppler ultrasound. *Gastroenterology* 1991;100:1324–1331.

23. Steiner E, Stark DD, Hahn PF, Saini S, Simeone JF, Mueller PR, Wittenberg J, Ferrucci JT. Imaging of pancreatic neoplasms: comparison of MR and CT. *Am J Radiol* 1989;152:487–491.

24. Dodd GD, Memel DS, Zajko AB, Baron RL, Santaguida LA, Baron RL, Santaguida LA. Hepatic artery stenosis and thrombosis in transplant recipients: doppler diagnosis with resistive index and systolic acceleration time. *Radiology* 1994;192:657–661.

25. Ralls PW, Colletti PM, Lapin SA. Real-time sonography in suspected acute cholecystitis: prospective evaluation of primary and secondary signs. *Radiology* 1985;1455:767–771.

26. Fidler JF, Paulson EK, Layfield L. CT evaluation of acute cholecystitis: findings and usefulness in diagnosis. *Am J Radiol* 1996;166:1085–1088.

SELECTED READINGS

1. Gore RM, Levine MS, Loufer I. Textbook of Gastrointestinal Radiology. Saunders, Philadelphia, 1994.
2. Larson RE, Semelka RC. Magnetic resonance imaging of the liver. Top Mag Reson Imaging 1995;2:71–81.
3. Rofsky NM, Fleishaker H. The liver: diffuse disease and vascular disorders. In: Raymond HW, Zwiebel WJ, Swartz JD, ed. Seminars in Ultrasound, CT and MRI. 1995;1, pp. 16–33.
4. Bluemke DA, Fishman EK. Spiral CT of the liver. *Am J Radiol* 1993;160:787–792.
5. Soyer P, Bluemke DA, Fishman EK. CT during arterial portography for the preoperative evaluation of hepatic tumors: how, when and why? *Am J Radiol* 1994;163:1325–1331.
6. Mitchell DG. Focal manifestations of diffuse liver disease at MR imaging. *Radiology* 1992;185:1–11.

6

Radiologic Interventions
for Liver Disease

Harry H. Chen

1. INTRODUCTION

Interventional radiology in patients with liver diseases involves the use of invasive procedures. These patients often have overt and urgent clinical presentations. For example, jaundice due to biliary obstruction is readily visible in the patient who has been referred for transhepatic cholangiography (THC). The clinical and laboratory evaluation are completed prior to the intervention. For the jaundiced patient, an ultrasound or a computed tomography (CT) scan is used to diagnose biliary ductal dilatation. The precise cause of the obstruction, if not explained by the noninvasive modalities, leads to an invasive procedure. The endoscopic retrograde cholangiopancreatogram (ERCP) is the initial invasive procedure of choice, but failure to catheterize the biliary duct would require a THC.

As always, the objective in the application of an invasive procedure is to provide the patient with a greater benefit than the potential risks of the procedure. Therefore, invasive procedures should be undertaken only after deciding on possible treatment plans once a diagnosis is determined. Invasive procedures should not be employed if the results will not alter patient management.

In contrast to the increased risk of an invasive diagnostic procedure, an invasive *therapeutic* radiological procedure often represents a less invasive alternative to surgery. For example, transjugular intrahepatic portal systemic shunts (TIPS) is less invasive and results in less morbidity than an operative portal caval shunt.

All radiologically guided interventional procedures of the liver have certain common aspects. Visual guidance is often dependent on the experience of the interventionist. Whereas ultrasound (US) will permit real-time visualization of a percutaneously placed needle in a liver lesion, limitations include isoechoic lesions, patient breathing obscuring needle visualization, and rib shadowing. CT guidance permits visualization of the liver, surrounding structures, and a needle with good resolution; again, patient breathing can become a significant limitation.

From: *Diseases of the Liver and Bile Ducts: Diagnosis and Treatment*
Edited by: G. Y. Wu and J. Israel © Humana Press Inc., Totowa, NJ

With ultrafast scans using helical CT, patient breathing motion artifact is less of a problem. Magnetic resonance image (MRI) guidance is rarely used because of the small bore of most diagnostic MRI units. However, there is a subset of liver lesions that are not visualized otherwise. Commonly, fluoroscopy is used with a computerized imaging modality. Initial access is obtained with a computerized image guided technique and additional manipulation is often guided fluoroscopically with the use of iodinated contrast agents.

2. DIAGNOSTIC PROCEDURES

2.1. Hepatic Parenchymal Interventions

2.1.1. PERCUTANEOUS BIOPSY

2.1.1.1. Patient Preparation. For procedures in which sedation is used, the standard patient preparation includes fasting for 4–8 h. Patients should maintain hydration during the period of fasting. Coagulation parameters must be normalized (PT < 15 s, PTT < 1.2 x control) and platelet count >100,000/mL. A cytopathologist must be available for preliminary reading of the cytology.

2.1.1.2. Technique. Penetrating a liver lesion target with a needle requires excellent guidance. Most often, spring-loaded core biopsy needles of at least 18-G size are used. To minimize the risk of bleeding, a 22-G needle can be used for an aspirate rather than to obtain a core biopsy.

2.1.1.3. Indications. The indication for guided liver biopsy is usually to differentiate whether a lesion is benign, malignant, or infectious. Sometimes guided liver biopsies are required even when a lesion has not been visualized, as in cases of diffuse liver disease. In these situations, blind biopsies would be difficult or contraindicated because of anatomical reasons, such as intervening bowel or obesity.

2.1.1.4. Contraindications. The presence of ascites, uncorrected bleeding diathesis, intervening bone or bowel, an uncooperative patient, and previous anaphylactoid reaction to iodinated contrast media are relative contraindications. Ascites usually can be drained immediately prior to biopsy to assure hemostasis postbiopsy. In patients with uncorrectable bleeding diatheses, transjugular biopsy is used to assess diffuse liver processes. Increased sedation will generally control the uncooperative patient.

2.1.1.5. Complications. Complications are uncommon, but the most important are bleeding <2%, infection <2%, and pneumothorax <1% (1). The overall risk of complication is <2%. Needle tract seeding of tumor has been reported (2).

2.1.1.6. Clinical Results. Positive identification of tissue type is made in 80–95% of cases. Reasons for failure are inadequate tissue secondary to size, site, and type of lesion (3,4).

2.1.1.7. Alternative Procedures. When percutaneous hepatic biopsy is unsuccessful, transjugular, laparoscopic, or finally intraoperative biopsies are alternatives.

2.1.2. TRANSVENOUS (TRANSJUGULAR/TRANSFEMORAL) BIOPSY

2.1.2.1. Patient Preparation. Fasting for 4–8 h as required for sedation.

2.1.2.2. Technique. For transjugular biopsy, the right internal jugular vein is accessed. The catheter is advanced through the superior vena cava, and the right atrium to a hepatic vein. The catheter is exchanged over a guidewire for a long needle. In a wedged position, the needle is advanced 3 cm into the liver parenchyma during aspiration to obtain a core of tissue (5). Newer devices have spring-loaded flexible needles that fit coaxially through the guiding cannula for the biopsy. For transfemoral biopsy, a curved sheath is placed into the hepatic vein from a femoral access. Through the sheath, a small biopsy forcep is advanced to the wall of the hepatic vein and several samples along the vein can be obtained.

2.1.2.3. Indications. This procedure is indicated in patients with diffuse liver pathology who have contraindications for percutaneous biopsy: at high risk for bleeding, advanced cirrhosis and portal hypertension, ascites, or marked hepatic insufficiency *(6)*.

2.1.2.4. Contraindications. Transvenous biopsy is contraindicated in cases in which venous access is occluded. The procedure is technically more difficult in the presence of ascites because of the displacement of the liver, but the ascites may be drained prior to biopsy.

2.1.2.5. Complications. Complications are infrequent, but the most important are: hepatic capsular perforation with peritoneal hemorrhage (3%), aneurysm of the hepatic hepatic artery (1–2%), and infection (1–2%) *(6)*.

2.1.2.6. Clinical Results. The technical success rate is 84%. Failures occur due to problems with jugular access, hepatic venous access or needle placement through the catheter *(6)*.

2.1.2.7. Alternative Procedures. Alternative procedures include percutaneous, laparoscopic, or surgical biopsy.

2.2. Biliary Ductal Interventions

2.2.1. Transhepatic Cholangiography (THC)

2.2.1.1. Patient Preparation. Fasting for 4–8 h is required for sedation. Coagulation profile is obtained and any abnormalities are corrected. Broad spectrum antibiotics are given 6–12 h before the procedure to cover gram-negative (*Escherichia coli* and *Enterobacter aerogenes*) and gram-positive species *(Streptococcus fecalis)*. A combination of ampicillin and gentamicin or a third generation cephalosporin, that can penetrate effectively into the bile, is administered.

2.2.1.2. Technique. A thin needle is advanced into the liver from a right 11th intercostal midaxillary approach with fluoroscopic guidance. Once there is bile return, the bile is collected for gram stain and culture. Iodinated contrast is injected to visualize the bile ducts (Fig. 1). Alternatively, access into the left lobe of the liver may be via a left anterior approach using ultrasound guidance.

2.2.1.3. Indications. The major indications for THC are to diagnose the etiology of jaundice, to detect intrahepatic calculi, choledocholithiasis, biliary atresia, choledochal cyst, and to study the biliary system prior to biliary drainage *(7,8)*.

2.2.1.4. Contraindications. Relative contraindications include uncorrectable bleeding diathesis, known hepatic vascular tumor or malformation, previous anaphylactoid reaction to iodinated contrast, or ascites (relative). Anaphylactoid reactions to iodinated contrast can be minimized by pretreatment with Prednisone 50 mg p.o. 13, 7, and 1 h before the procedure, Benadryl 50 mg p.o. 1 h before the procedure, and the use of low osmolar contrast agents.

2.2.1.5. Complications. Complications include bile leak, hemorrhage (0.29%), sepsis, pneumothorax, contrast reaction, hepatic arteriovenous fistulae, and vasovagal reaction. The mortality rate is 0.14%, and overall complication rate is 4.8% *(9)*.

2.2.1.6. Clinical Results. The technical success rate in demonstrating the bile ducts is 90–99% with better results in dilated ducts *(9)*.

2.2.1.7. Alternative Procedures. Alternative procedures include ERCP, cholecystocholangiography, and magnetic resonance cholangiography.

2.3. Hepatic Arterial Interventions

2.3.1. Hepatic Angiography

2.3.1.1. Patient Preparation. Fasting for 4–8 h is required for sedation, and iv hydration during fasting with normal saline is recommended to minimize contrast nephrotoxicity. Coagulation profile is obtained and abnormalities are corrected. Creatinine level is obtained to assess the risk for nephropathy.

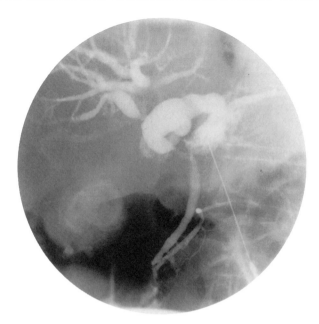

Fig. 1. Transhepatic cholangiogram in a 94-yr-old male who had jaundice for 2 wk. The ERCP failed to cannulate the common bile duct (CBD) and an urgent THC was requested. A 22-G needle was placed into the left lobe hepatic duct by ultrasound guidance. The cholangiogram revealed dilated intrahepatic ducts that were separately occluded at the confluence of the hepatic ducts, a typical picture for a Klatskin tumor. Note the normal-sized common bile duct. There was reflux into the pancreatic duct that was felt to be secondary to post-ERCP sphincter of Oddi edema. Note also the faint density of the large lamellated and rounded gallstone in the gallbladder on the bottom of the image.

2.3.1.2. Technique. Using percutaneous access of the femoral artery, the hepatic artery is catheterized and iodinated contrast is injected during radiographic filming (Fig. 2).

2.3.1.3. Indications. The major indications are to determine the cause of hematobilia, to determine the nature of a liver lesion by its vascular pattern, and to preoperatively map the hepatic arterial tree.

2.3.1.4. Contraindications. The main contraindications are previous anaphylactoid reaction to iodinated contrast, renal insufficiency *(10)*, and coagulopathy (relative) *(11)*.

2.3.1.5. Complications. Complications include hepatic arterial dissection and occlusion, contrast reaction, and contrast nephrotoxicity. The risk of the latter is reduced with adequate patient hydration *(10)*.

2.3.1.6. Clinical Results. The technical success rate is >90% for celiac angiography. In previously embolized hepatic arteries, a more exhaustive search for other feeders is required.

2.3.1.7. Alternative Procedures. Alternative procedures are magnetic resonance angiography, and helical computed tomographic angiography.

2.4. Hepatic Venous Interventions

2.4.1. HEPATIC VENOGRAPHY AND MANOMETRY

2.4.1.1. Patient Preparation. In addition to the standard preparation as described previously, a serum creatinine level is obtained to assess the risk for nephropathy.

2.4.1.2. Technique. The hepatic vein is catheterized via a femoral or a jugular venous approach.

2.4.1.3. Indications. The main indications for this procedure are to measure hepatic venous pressure with and without a wedged catheterization, to visualize the hepatic venogram, and to visualize portal vein by the use of a wedged hepatic venogram.

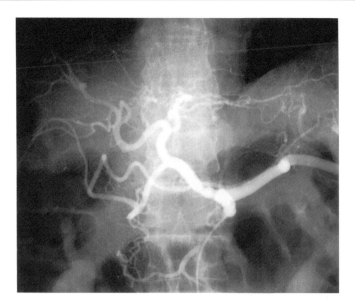

Fig. 2. This is a normal hepatic arteriogram in a patient who was evaluated for vasculitis. There was some spasm of the common hepatic artery from the catheterization and injection. The two branches of the common hepatic artery were the gastroduodenal and proper hepatic arteries. The gastroduodenal artery filled the right gastroepiploic with smaller branches filling the pancreatoduodenal arcade which further fills the inferior pancreaticoduodenal artery. Note that the inferior pancreaticoduodenal artery is the first branch of the superior mesenteric artery (SMA); thus, the major collateral between the SMA and the celiac axis is shown. The branches of the proper hepatic artery are the right and left hepatic artery. The cystic artery is a branch of the gastroduodenal artery (seen in 3%). Refluxed contrast fills the splenic artery.

2.4.1.4. Contraindications. Relative contraindications include renal insufficiency, and previous anaphylactoid reaction to iodinated contrast.

2.4.1.5. Complications. Major complications of this procedure are cardiac arrhythmia due to catheter stimulation of the endocardium, anaphylactoid contrast reaction, and contrast nephrotoxicity.

2.4.1.6. Clinical Results. The technical success rate is 84–100% *(12)*.

2.4.1.7. Alternative Procedures. Magnetic resonance venography, and duplex ultrasound are alternative modalities used to visualize the hepatic and portal veins. CO_2-wedged hepatic venoportogram may be used to visualize the portal veins in a patient with renal insufficiency *(13)* or with a history of previous anaphylactoid reaction to iodinated contrast.

2.5. Portal Venous Interventions

2.5.1. PORTAL VENOGRAPHY

2.5.1.1. Patient Preparation. The standard patient preparation is used as in hepatic angiography.

2.5.1.2. Technique. After superior mesenteric artery (SMA) catheterization, portal venography is obtained as the venous phase of the angiogram.

2.5.1.3. Indications. The major indications for this procedure are to determine portal venous patency prior to hepatic chemoembolization, prior to portal systemic shunt, or prior to hepatic lobectomy, to evaluate for mesenteric varices in a patient with GI bleed and to perform CT portography *(14,15)*.

2.5.1.4. Contraindications. Contraindications are renal insufficiency, and previous anaphylactoid reaction to contrast.

2.5.1.5. Complications. The complication rate is low, but major complications include SMA injury (<1%) *(16)* and nephrotoxicity.

2.5.1.6. Clinical Results. Technical limitations of the procedure are due to portal hypertension with hepatofugal flow. This results in spotty opacification of the portal venous tree. Other anatomical variants, such as a replaced hepatic artery to the SMA, can make superselective SMA catheterization for portal venography more difficult.

2.5.1.7. Alternative Procedures. Doppler ultrasound may be useful in assessing main portal vein patency. Magnetic resonance venography, venous phase of the splenic arteriogram, and transjugular portal venogram are other alternative procedures.

3. THERAPEUTIC PROCEDURES

3.1. Hepatic Parenchymal Interventions

3.1.1. PERCUTANEOUS ALCOHOL ABLATION OF TUMOR NODULES

3.1.1.1. Patient Preparation. Fasting and iv hydration for 4–8 h is required for sedation. Evaluation of coagulation parameters and correction of any abnormalities.

3.1.1.2. Technique. The access with a fine needle (22-G) is the same as that used for ultrasound or CT-guided biopsy. With ultrasound, there is real-time guidance, and the lesion becomes hyperechoic as it is filled with absolute alcohol *(17)*. Under CT guidance, the volume injected is estimated by the lesion size *(18)*. The patient will experience pain during injection, which may last for a few days. To minimize reflux along the track, the needle is left in place for a few minutes. Alcohol enters the hepatocytes by diffusion, producing coagulative necrosis, followed by formation of granulation tissue, fibrosis and partial or complete small vessel thrombosis *(17,19)*.

3.1.1.3. Indications. The indication for this procedure is the presence of hepatocellular carcinomas less than 4–5 cm diameter that are easily detected by ultrasound. Combined therapy with transcatheter embolization *(20,21)* and the presence of liver metastases without localization in other organs or systems are other indications.

3.1.1.4. Contraindications. Lesions that are poorly detected by the guidance system or very close to the dome of liver are poor candidates. The presence of a highly necrotic tumor is also a contraindication because necrotic tumor can provide preferential paths for drainage of the alcohol.

3.1.1.5. Complications. Localized pain and fever are the most common complications. They are self-limited and proportional to the volume injected. A case of tumor seeding along the needle tract has been reported *(22)*.

3.1.1.6. Clinical Results. The procedure has a reasonable success rate for palliation of the carcinoma *(17–19)*. In one report, 18 of 23 hepatocellular carcinomas decreased in size after treatment *(17)*. Some success has been reported for metastases as well *(23)*. For example, 9 out of 11 cases with small metastases (1–2 cm in diameter) had a complete response, in one report, and 4 out of 4 endocrine metastases had a complete response *(23)*.

3.1.1.7. Alternative Procedures. Hepatic chemoembolization, intraoperative cryoablation, and surgical hepatic resection are all alternative procedures.

3.1.2. ABSCESS DRAINAGE

3.1.2.1. Patient Preparation. In addition to the standard preparation antibiotics are added.

3.1.2.2. Technique. After a needle is introduced, a wire is placed, followed by dilatation of the track for abscess catheter placement. The cavity is irrigated with sterile saline and the catheter is connected to a gravity drainage collection bag for daily irrigation until the cavity is collapsed over days to weeks *(24,25)*.

3.1.2.3. Indications. The main indication is the presence of a fluid collection in a patient with fever, leukocytosis, and often localized pain (Fig. 3) *(24)*. Postoperative abscesses with enteric communications *(26)*, and perforated amebic abscess *(27)* are additional indications.

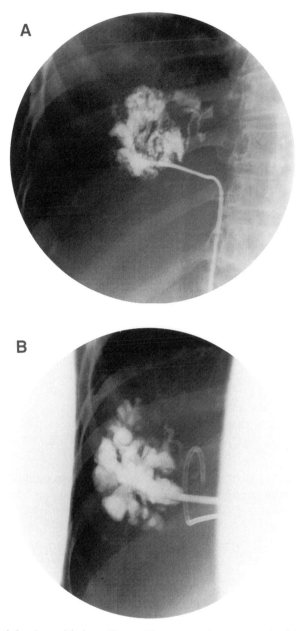

Fig. 3. Bacterial necrotizing hepatitis in a 40-yr-old woman who presented with fever and right upper quadrant pain. After the first drainage catheter was placed, contrast injection showed a complex sinu-soidal filling pattern **(A)**, which was unlike a simple rounded abscess. CT scan showed the catheter in one of two collections, **(B)** a second catheter was placed on the second day after CT scan showed an undrained collection.

3.1.2.4. Contraindications. Contraindications include absence of a safe access route (that avoids pleural space, bowel, major blood vessels, and solid organs), uncorrectable coagulopathy.

3.1.2.5. Complications. Complications include septicemia (4.2%) *(28)*, infection of initially sterile collection, malposition of the tube, hematobilia, bile leakage, hemoperitoneum, and pneumothorax.

3.1.2.6. Clinical Results. Success rates range from 64–77% *(28,29)*. Failure occurs due to multiloculation, phlegmon, improper catheter position, premature catheter removal, or inadequate antibiotic therapy. Drainage of nine echinococcal cysts followed by sclerosis was associated with mild pruritis in two cases; there was no recurrence of cysts at 6 and 12 mo of follow-up *(30)*.

3.1.2.7. Alternative Procedures. Surgical drainage, resection, or debridement are alternative procedures.

3.2. Biliary Ductal Interventions

3.2.1. Biliary Drainage

3.2.1.1. Patient Preparation. Preparation with fasting and antibiotics is the same as for transhepatic cholangiography (THC).

3.2.1.2. Technique. After THC, the type of biliary obstruction (i.e., malignant, benign vs calculus) is determined. The type of lesion will determine whether temporary or permanent biliary drainage is appropriate (i.e., malignant occlusions not amenable to cure will require permanent drainage). A thin guidewire is advanced through the needle into the duct. Once the wire has been securely positioned, the tract is dilated *(31,32)*, and a catheter is introduced (Fig. 4). A biliary drainage catheter is advanced beyond the stenosis *(33)* or a metal stent is placed across the stenosis, depending on the type of lesion.

3.2.1.3. Indications. The main indications for this procedure are palliation for malignant ductal obstruction (permanent metallic stents); benign strictures or anastomotic strictures (cholangioplasty and temporary plastic stents), ascending cholangitis, bile duct stone *(34)*, and access for brachytherapy *(35)*.

3.2.1.4. Contraindications. Relative contraindications include uncorrectable bleeding diathesis and ascites.

3.2.1.5. Complications *(36–38)*. Major complications are biliary sepsis, hematobilia, bile peritonitis, dislodgment of drainage catheter by accidental traction, pancreatitis, duodenal perforation *(39)*, malignant pleural effusion *(40)*, reobstruction, metal stent migration, tumor overgrowth, and ingrowth through the metal stent.

3.2.1.6. Clinical Results. Patency of metallic stents ranged from 20–78% at 25 wk *(38)*. The 25- and 50-wk patient survival for the Wallstent are 42% and 16%, respectively *(38)*. Patency for cholangioplasty of benign strictures such as anastamotic strictures, iatrogenic strictures, and strictures associated with sclerosing cholangioplasty ranged from 42–76% *(32)*.

3.2.1.7. Alternative Procedures. Alternative procedures include ERCP placement of an internal stent, surgical choledochojejunostomy, and cholecystostomy.

3.3. Hepatic Arterial Interventions

3.3.1. Angioplasty

3.3.1.1. Patient Preparation. In addition to standard preparation, adequate renal function should be demonstrated.

3.3.1.2. Technique. After determining the size of the artery by diagnostic angiography, the stenosis is traversed by a size-matched balloon. The balloon is then inflated eliminating the stenosis.

3.3.1.3. Indications. The most common condition in which hepatic angioplasty is necessary is posttransplant hepatic arterial anastomotic stenosis *(41)*.

3.3.1.4. Contraindications. In cases of posttransplant arterial stenosis, marked allograft dysfunction at presentation is a poor prognostic sign *(41)*.

3.3.1.5. Complications. In one report, pseudoaneurysm, and hemoperitoneum were encountered in 21 hepatic angioplasties *(41)*.

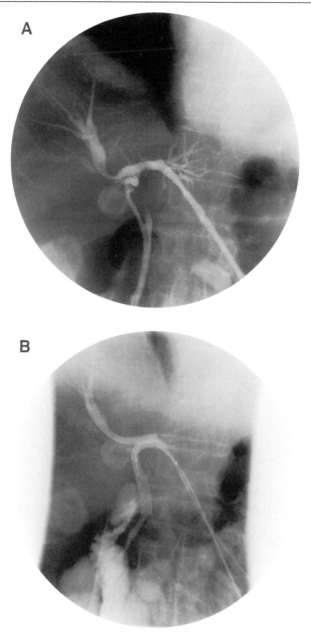

Fig. 4. Biliary drainage (**A**) in the same patient as Fig. 1. One multi-sideholed catheter was placed across the stenosis into the right hepatic duct. A second drainage catheter was placed parallel to the first through the common bile duct ending in the duodenum. Both catheters were connected externally through the same access site into individual drainage bags. Subsequently, metallic internal stents were placed (**B**) which are shown to function well.

3.3.1.6. Clinical Results. A technical success rate of 81% has been reported in allograft hepatic transplants *(41)*.

3.3.1.7. Alternative Procedures. Surgical revision of anastomotic stenoses is an alternative procedure.

3.3.2. EMBOLIZATION

3.3.2.1. Patient Preparation. In addition to standard preparation, adequate renal function should be demonstrated and antibiotics administered.

3.3.2.2. Technique. After selective catheterization of the site of bleeding, polyvinyl alcohol particles (PVA) or Gelfoam pledgets are injected in combination with microcoils or stainless-steel fiber coils *(42)*.

3.3.2.3. Indications. Hematobilia, hematoperitoneum *(43)*, and hepatic hemorrhagic pseudoaneurysm *(44)* are major indications.

3.3.2.4. Contraindications. Anaphylactoid reaction to iodinated contrast, renal insufficiency, and coagulopathy are relative contraindications.

3.3.2.5. Complications. Because of the dual blood supply, hepatic infarction is uncommon with hepatic embolization. However, because the efficacy of embolization is increased with superselective catheterization, arterial injury may occasionally occur, resulting from overly aggressive catheter manipulation.

3.3.2.6. Clinical Results. Technical success is achieved in 88% in cases of bleeding from hepatic vascular injury *(42)*.

3.3.2.7. Alternative Procedures. Surgical ligation is an alternative procedure.

3.3.3. Chemoembolization *(45)*

3.3.3.1. Patient Preparation. Prior to the procedure, a tissue diagnosis, CT/MRI of the liver, and exclusion of extrahepatic disease are required. In addition to standard preparation, adequate renal function should be demonstrated and antibiotics, Decadron, Benadryl, and Zofran are all administered prior to the procedure. Furthermore, tumor markers may be obtained. Finally, a preembolization angiogram of the liver and surrounding organs is required to plan the optimal catheterization for hepatic chemoembolization (HCE), and to confirm patency of the portal vein.

3.3.3.2. Technique. The hepatic artery branch supplying the segment of the lesion is catheterized. A combination of chemotherapeutic agent (mitomycin/adriamycin and cisplatin), lipiodol, iopamidol, and polyvinyl alcohol particles are mixed and injected with fluoroscopic guidance. The volume injected is determined by a slowing of the flow into the lesion (Fig. 5).

3.3.3.3. Indications. The indication for this procedure is the presence of biopsy-proven hepatoma, metastatic neuroendocrine tumor, cholangiocarcinoma, metastatic colon carcinoma, or metastatic ocular melanoma in patients who are not operative candidates. Other than those patients with hepatoma, most have failed iv chemotherapy.

3.3.3.4. Contraindications. Contraindications include severe previous anaphylactoid reaction to iodinated contrast, uncorrectable coagulopathy, severe renal insufficiency, and severe peripheral vascular disease precluding arterial access. In addition, severe thrombocytopenia, leukopenia, cardiac or renal insufficiency are contraindications. Portal venous thrombosis is another contraindication, but in this case, the procedure may be performed if hepatopedal flow is maintained. There is a high risk of hepatic failure following hepatic artery embolization when >50% of liver volume is replaced by tumor, LDH >425 IU/L, AST >100 IU/L, bilirubin ≥ 2 mg/dL. Hepatic encephalopathy or jaundice are absolute contraindications to embolization as is biliary obstruction, even with normal bilirubin.

3.3.3.5. Complications. Major complications (3–4%) include hepatic insufficiency, infarction, hepatic abscess, tumor rupture, surgical cholecystitis, and nontarget embolization to gut, renal insufficiency <1%, anemia requiring transfusion <1% *(45)*.

3.3.3.6. Clinical Results. For hepatoma *(46–48)*, survival at 1 yr post-HCE was reported to be 54–80%, at 2 yr 33–64%, and at 3 yr 18–51%. For colorectal metastases, survival at 1 yr post-HCE was 67%, at 1 yr postdiagnosis is 100% *(45)*. For ocular melanoma, survival for responders is 14 mo. However, for nonresponders, it was only 6 mo. For neuroendocrine tumors *(49)*, survival was 24 mo after embolization, 81 mo postdiagnosis.

3.3.3.7. Alternative Procedures. Alternative procedures include liver transplant, cryoablation, and percutaneous ethanol injection.

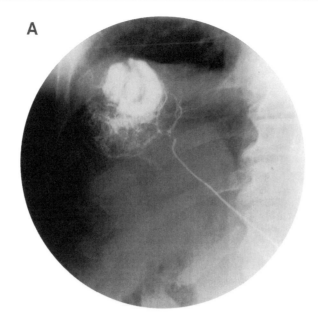

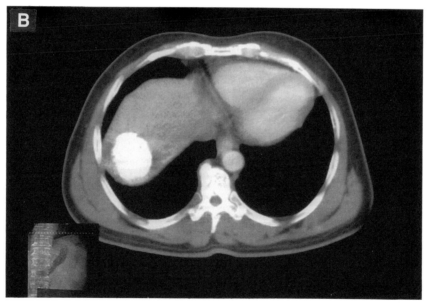

Fig. 5. A 61-yr-old man with cirrhosis. Immediately after selective chemoembolization of a hepatoma in the right hepatic lobe, there was intense opacification of the chemotherapeutic agent casted into the vascular channels and lakes of the tumor (**A**). A CT scan 1 wk later showed a persistent homogeneous chemotherapeutic caste, which may remain for months (**B**).

3.4. Hepatic Venous Interventions

3.4.1. ANGIOPLASTY/STENTING/THROMBOLYSIS

3.4.1.1. Patient Preparation. Preparation is the same as for arterial angioplasty.

3.4.1.2. Technique. The technique is the same as for arterial angioplasty except access is by jugular or femoral vein.

3.4.1.3. Indications. Indications include treatment of hepatic venous webs, stenosis associated with Budd Chiari syndrome *(50–52)*, and combined treatment with thrombolysis,

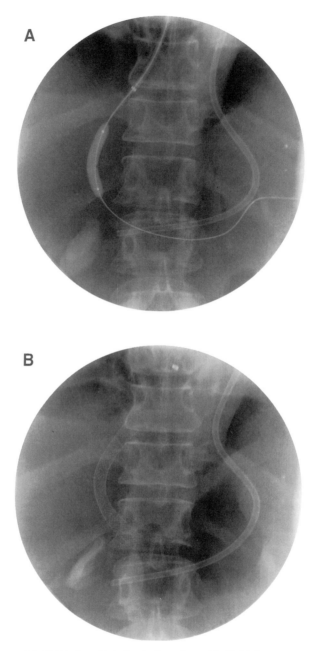

Fig. 6. A 45-yr-old man with Child class C cirrhosis from hepatitis B. He has uncontrollable ascites, and an endstage, shrunken liver. The preshunt portal systemic gradient measured 20 mmHg. After access from the middle hepatic vein to the right vein, the hepatic parenchymal tract was balloon dilated(**A**). A Wallstent was placed to create the permanent portal system shunt (**B**). The angiogram shows a patent shunt with absence of varices (**C**). The postportal systemic shunt gradient measured 11 mmHg.

angioplasty, and intravascular stent *(52)*. Transplant venous anastomotic stenosis *(53)* is another major indication for angioplasty or stenting.

3.4.1.4. Contraindications. Relative contraindications are anaphylactoid reaction to iodinated contrast, renal insufficiency, and coagulopathy.

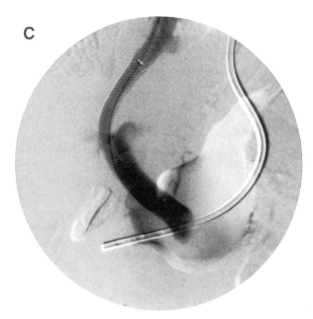

Fig. 6. *(continued).*

3.4.1.5. Complications. No technical complications have been reported in two reported cases. However, transplant anastamotic restenosis has been reported *(53)*.

3.4.1.6. Clinical Results. In hepatic transplants, technical success was reported to be 92%, and the clinical success rate was 75% with 7–33 mo follow up. In Budd-Chiari cases, the duration of clinical efficacy ranged from 2–33 mo *(50,51)* . However, an intravascular stent may be required if there is recurrent restenosis *(8)*.

3.4.1.7. Alternative Procedures. Hepatic transplant, and surgical revision are alternative procedures.

3.5. Portal Venous Interventions

3.5.1. Transjugular Intrahepatic Portosystemic Shunt (TIPS)

3.5.1.1. Patient Preparation. Standard patient preparation including antibiotics is administered prior to procedure.

3.5.1.2. Technique *(54–56)*. Access is achieved via the jugular vein. The right hepatic vein is catheterized, and, with the catheter in a wedged position, iodinated contrast (or carbon dioxide) is injected during digital subtraction angiography to visualize the portal vein. A needle is advanced from the right hepatic vein into the right portal vein. After catheterization of the portal vein, the pressure gradient between the portal vein and the hepatic vein is measured. The portal/hepatic venous track is dilated with a balloon, and a stainless steel stent (i.e., Wallstent) is placed to maintain patency of the track. If the portal vein/hepatic vein pressure gradient is greater than 12 mmHg, the Wallstent is dilated with a larger diameter balloon up to the nominal size of the Wallstent (Fig. 6).

3.5.1.3. Indications. Variceal bleeding is the most common indication for TIPS. Uncontrollable ascites is another condition that can be treated successfully *(57)*. In addition, Budd-Chiari syndrome *(58)* and hepatorenal syndrome are also indications for this procedure.

3.5.1.4. Contraindications. Relative contraindications include significant pressure gradient between the hepatic vein and the right atrium that cannot be resolved with balloon angioplasty. Portal vein thrombosis is another relative contraindication. However, efficacy of TIPS despite portal vein thrombosis has been shown *(59)*.

3.5.1.5. Complications *(60)*. New or worsening encephalopathy occurs in 10–15%, but can be treated successfully with lactulose. Other complications are hepatic capsular perforation in <1% of cases, hepatic vein stenosis with shunt thrombosis in 6–75% (depending on the criteria used), hematobilia 1%, and bacteremia 3%.

3.5.1.6. Clinical Results *(54–57)*. The technical success rate to achieve a gradient <12 mm-Hg was reported to be 96–100%. A second parallel shunt was required in about 10% of cases *(61)*. The 30-d mortality, not necessarily related to procedure, was 13%. Primary shunt patency has been reported to be 75% at 6 mo, 50% at 1 yr, and 32% at 2 yr. Assisted patency has been reported to be 85% at 1 yr *(62)*. Refactory ascetes was controlled in 58% at 8.2 mo (avg) in 50 patients *(62a)*. Elevated creatinine (>1.9 mg/dl) and bilirubin (>3 mg/dl) were associated with treatment failure and early death.

3.5.1.7. Alternative Procedures. Surgical portal systemic shunt, and liver transplant are alternative procedures.

3.6. Percutaneous Cholecystostomy

3.6.1. PATIENT PREPARATION

Preparation is the same as for abscess drainage.

3.6.2. TECHNIQUES

With ultrasound guidance, a needle or sheath needle is advanced into the gallbladder lumen by way of the liver. Once access is achieved, the track is dilated to accommodate a loop-locking drainage catheter.

3.6.3. INDICATION

The presence of an inflamed, obstructed gallbladder in a patient who is a poor surgical risk *(63)* is the primary indication for this procedure. In addition, drainage of the gallbladder in a patient with unexplained infection in whom all other sites of infection except the gallbladder have been eliminated, and obtaining access for gallstone dissolution or percutaneous mechanical lithotripsy *(64,65)* are additional indications.

3.6.4. CONTRAINDICATIONS

The procedure is contraindicated when the gallbladder is inaccessible because of intervening vital structures, and in uncooperative patients.

3.6.5. COMPLICATIONS

Bile leakage resulting in bile peritonitis, and vasovagal effects of the catheter placement are the main complications. Bile leakage has been reported to be associated with early removal (8–10 d) of the catheter before the percutaneous track had adequately matured *(63)*. Complications occurred in 5–10% of patients *(64)*.

3.6.6. CLINICAL RESULTS

Improved clinical condition is seen in 60% of patients drained *(63)*.

3.6.7. ALTERNATIVE PROCEDURES

Operative or laparoscopic cholecystectomy are alternative procedures.

SUMMARY

Radiologic procedures in the liver that have excellent technical and immediate clinical success include: percutaneous abscess drainage, percutaneous biliary drainage, hepatic arterial embolization, hepatic chemoembolization, transjugular intrahepatic portosystemic shunt, and percutaneous cholecystostomy.

The long-term benefits for patients receiving hepatic chemoembolization and transjugular intrahepatic portosystemic shunt are still being evaluated.

All radiologic interventional procedures in the liver begin with the use of a needle, either directly into the liver or into a vessel connected to the liver.

REFERENCES

1. Livraghi T, Damascelli B, Lombardi C, Spagnoli I. Risk in fine-needle abdominal biopsy. J Clin Ultrasound 1983;11:77–81.
2. Smith EH. Complications of percutaneous abdominal fine-needle biopsy. Radiology 1991;178:253–258.
3. Mueller PR, vanSonnenberg E. Interventional radiology in the chest and abdomen. N Engl J Med 1990;322:1364–1374.
4. Welch TJ, Sheedy PF, Johnson CD, Johnson CM, Stephens DH. CT-guided biopsy: prospective analysis of 1,000 procedures. Radiology 1989;171:493–496.
5. Rosch J, Antonovic R, Dotter CT. Transjugular approach to the liver, biliary system and portal circulation. Am J Roentgenol 1975;125:602–608.
6. Goldman ML, Gonzalez AC, Galambos JT, Gordon IJ, Oen K-T. The transjugular technique of hepatic venography and biopsy, cholangiography and obliteration of esophageal varices. Radiology 1978;128:325–331.
7. MacCarty RL, LaRusso NF, Wiesner RH, Ludwig J. Primary sclerosing cholangitis: findings on cholangiography and pancreatography. Radiology 1983;149:39–44.
8. Nichols DA, MacCarty RL, Gaffey TA. Cholangiographic evaluation of bile duct carcinoma. Am J Roentgenol 1983;141:1291–1294.
9. Mueller PR, Harbin WP, Ferrucci JT, Wittenberg J, vanSonnenberg E. Fine-needle transhepatic cholangiography. Am J Roentgenol 1981;136:85–90.
10. Eisenberg RL, Bank WO, Hedgock MW. Renal failure after major angiography can be avoided with hydration. Am J Roentgenol 1981;136:859–861.
11. Wilson NV, Corne JM, Given-Wilson RM. A critical appraisal of coagulation studies prior to transfemoral angiography. Br J Radiol 1990;63:147–148.
12. LaBerge JM, Ring EJ, Lake JR, et al. Transjugular intrahepatic portosystemic shunts: preliminary results in 25 patients. J Vasc Surg 1992;16:258–267.
13. Rees CR, Niblett RL, Lee SP, Diamond NG, Crippin JS. Use of carbon dioxide as a contrast medium for transjugular intrahepatic portosystemic shunt procedures. J Vasc Interv Radiol 1994;5:383–386.
14. Soyer P, Levesque M, Elias D, Zeitoun G, Roche A. Preoperative assessment of resectability of hepatic metastases from colonic carcinoma: CT portography vs. sonography and dynamic CT. Am J Roentgenol 1992;159:741–744.
15. Paulson EK, Baker ME, Hilleren DJ, et al. CT arterial portography: causes of technical failure and variable liver enhancement. Am J Roentgenology 1992; 159:745–749.
16. Sigstedt B, Lunderquist A. Complications of angiographic examinations. Am J Roentgenol 1978;130:455–460.
17. Sironi S, Livraghi T, DelMaschio A. Small hepatocellular carcinoma treated with percutaneous ethanol injection: MR imaging findings. Radiology 1991;180:333–336.
18. Redvanly RD, Chezmar JL, Strauss RM, et al. Malignant hepatic tumors: safety of high-dose percutaneous ethanol ablation therapy. Radiology 1993;188:283–285.
19. Sheu JC, Huang GT, Chen DS, et al. Small hepatocellular carcinoma: intratumor ethanol treatment using new needle and guidance systems. Radiology 1987;163:43–48.
20. Katsuaki T, Nakamura S, Numata K, et al. Hepatocellular carcinoma: treatment with percutaneous ethanol injection and transcatheter arterial embolization. Radiology 1992;185:457–460.
21. Tanaka K, Okazaki H, Nakamura S, et al. Hepatocellular carcinoma: treatment with a combination therapy of transcatheter arterial embolization and percutaneous ethanol injection. Radiology 1991;179:713–717.
22. Cedrone A, Rapaccini GL, Pompili M, et al. Neoplastic seeding complicating percutaneous ethanol injection for treatment of hepatocellular carcinoma. Radiology 1992;183:787–788.
23. Livraghi T, Vettori C, Lazzaroni S. Liver metastases: results of percutaneous ethanol injection in 14 patients. Radiology 1991;179:709–712.
24. Gerzof SG, Robbins AH, Johnson WC, et al. Percutaneous catheter drainage of abdominal abscesses. N Engl J Med 1981;305:653–657.
25. vanSonnenberg E, D'Agostino HB, Casola G, et al. Percutaneous abscess drainage: current concepts. Radiology 1991;181:617–626.
26. Lambiase RE, Cronan JJ, Dorfman GS, et al. Postoperative abscesses with enteric communication: percutaneous treatment. Radiology 1989;171:497–500.
27. Ken JG, vanSonnonberg E, Casola G, et al. Perforated amebic liver abscesses: successful percutaneous treatment. Radiology 1989;170:195–197.
28. Lambiase RE, Deyoe L, Cronan JJ, Dorfman GS. Percutaneous drainage of 335 consecutive abscesses: results of primary drainage with 1-year follow-up. Radiology 1992;184:167–179.
29. Lang EK, Springer RM, Glorioso LW, et al. Abdominal abscess drainage under radiologic guidance: causes of failure. Radiology 1986;159:329–336.

30. Bret PM, Fond A, Bretagnolle M, et al. Percutaneous aspiration and drainage of hydatid cysts in the liver. Radiology 1988;168:617–620.
31. Skolkin MD, Alspaugh JP, Casarella WJ, et al. Sclerosing cholangitis: palliation with percutaneous cholangioplasty. Radiology 1989;170:199–206.
32. Mueller PR, vanSonnenberg E, Ferrucci JT, et al. Biliary stricture dilatation: multicenter review of clinical management in 73 patients. Radiology 1986;60:17–22.
33. Kadir S, Baassiri A, Barth KH, et al. Percutaneous biliary drainage in the management of biliary sepsis. Am J Roentgenology 1982;138:25–29.
34. Clouse ME, Stokes KR, Lee RGL, Falchuk KR. Bile duct stones: percutaneous transhepatic removal. Radiology 1986;160:525–529.
35. Haffty BG, Mate TP, Greenwood LH, et al. Malignant biliary obstruction: intracavitary treatment with a high-dose-rate remote afterloading device. Radiology 1987;164:574–576.
36. Stoker J, Lameris JS. Complications of percutaneously inserted biliary Wallstents. J Vasc Interv Radiol 1993;4:767–772.
37. Lee MJ, Dawson SL, Mueller PR, et al. Palliation of malignant bile duct obstruction with metallic biliary endoprostheses: technique, results and complications. J Vasc Interv Radiol 1992;3:665–671.
38. Rossi P, Bezzi M, Rossi M, et al. Metallic stents in malignant biliary obstruction: results of a multicenter European study of 240 patients. J Vasc Interv Radiol 1994;5:279–285.
39. Gould J, Train JS, Dan SJ, Mitty HA. Duodenal perforation as a delayed complication if placement of a biliary endoprosthesis. Radiology 1988;167:467–469.
40. Anschuetz SL, Vogelzang RL. Malignant pleural effusion: a complication of transhepatic biliary drainage. Am J Roentgenology 1986;146:1165–1166.
41. Orons PD, Zajko AB, Bron KM, et al. Hepatic artery angioplasty after liver transplantation: experience in 21 allografts. J Vasc Interv Radiol 1995;6:523–529.
42. Schwartz RA, Teitelbaum GP, Katz MD, Pentecost MJ. Effectiveness of transcatheter embolization in the control of hepatic vascular injuries. J Vasc Interv Radiol 1993;4:359–365.
43. Rubin BE, Katzen BT. Selective hepatic artery embolization to control massive hepatic hemorrhage after trauma. Am J Roentgenology 1977;129:253–256.
44. Greenstein D, Henderson J, Boyer TD. Liver hemorrhage: recurrent episodes during pregnancy complicated by preeclampsia. Gastroenterology 1994;106:1668–1671.
45. Soulen MC, Dawson SL, Hanks S, Pentecost MJ, Perry LJ. Cancer therapy workshop at the annual meeting of the Society of Cardiovascular and Interventional Radiology 1996.
46. Soulen MC. Chemoembolization of hepatic malignancies. Oncology 1994;8:77–93.
47. Clouse ME, Stokes KR, Kruskal JB, et al. Chemoembolization for hepatocellular carcinoma: epinephrine followed by a doxorubicin-ethiodized oil emulsion and gelatin sponge powder. J Vasc Interv Radiol 1993;4:717–725.
48. Trinchet JC, et al. A comparison of lipiodol chemoembolization and conservative treatment for unresectable hepatocellular carcinoma. N Engl J Med 1995;332;1256–1261.
49. Clouse ME, Perry L, Stuart K, Stokes KR. Hepatic arterial chemoembolization for metastatic neuroendocrine tumors. Digestion 1994;55:92–97.
50. Walker HS, Rholl KS, Rehister TE, van Breda A. Percutaneous placement of a hepatic vein stent in the treatment of Budd-Chiari syndrome. J Vasc Interv Radiol 1990;1:23–27.
51. Savader SJ, Venbrux AC, Klein AS, Osterman FA. Percutaneous intervention in portosystemic shunts in Budd-Chiari syndrome. J Vasc Interv Radiol 1991;2:489–495.
52. Ishiguchi T, Fukatsu H, Itoh S, et al. Budd-Chiari syndrome with long segmental inferior vena cava obstruction: treatment with thrombolysis, angioplasty, and intravascular stents. J Vasc Interv Radiol 1992;3:421–425.
53. Zajko AB, Sheng R, Bron K, et al. Percutaneous transluminal angioplasty of venous anstomotic stenoses complicating liver transplantation: intermediate-term results. J Vasc Interv Radiol 1994;5:121–126.
54. Zemel G, Katzen BT, Becker GJ, et al. Percutaneous transjugular portosystemic shunt. JAMA 1991;266:390–393.
55. Ring EJ, Lake JR, Roberts JP, et al. Using transjugular intrahepatic portosystemic shunts to control variceal bleeding before liver transplantation. Ann of Int Med 1992;116:304–309.
56. Ring E, Lake JR, Sterneck M, Ascher N. Intrahepatic portocaval shunt for variceal hemorrhage prior to liver transplantation. Transplantation 1991;52:160–162.
57. Olafsson S and Blei AT. Diagnosis and management of ascites in the age of TIPS. Am J Roentgenology 1995;165:9–15.
58. Peltzer MY, Ring EJ, LaBerge JM, et al. Treatment of Budd-Chiari syndrome with a transjugular intrahepatic portosystemic shunt. J Vasc Interv Radiol 1993;4:263–267.
59. Radosevich PM, Ring EJ, LaBerge JM, et al. Transjugular intrahepatic portosystemic shunts in patients with portal vein occlusion. Radiology 1993;186:523–527.
60. Freedman AM, Sanyal AJ, Tisnado J, et al. Complications of transjugular intrahepatic portosystemic shunt: a comprehensive review. Radiographics 1993;13:1185–1210.

61. Haskal ZJ, Ring EJ, LaBerge JM, et al. Role of parallel transjugular intrahepatic portosystemic shunts in patients with persistent portal hypertension. Radiology 1992;185:813–17.
62. Haskal ZJ, Pentecost MJ, Soulen MC, et al. Transjugular intrahepatic portosystemic shunt stenosis and revision. Am J Roentgenol 1994;163:439–444.
62a. Nazarian GK, Bjarnason H, Dietz CA, Ferral H, Bernadas CA, Hunter DW. Journal of Vascular and Interventional Radiology (supplement) 1997;8:227.
63. Boland GW, Lee MJ, Leung J, Mueller PR. Percutaneous cholecystostomy in critically ill patients. Am J Roentgenology 1994;163:339–342.
64. VanSonnenberg E, DíAgostino HB, Casola G, et al. Interventional radiology in the gallbladder: diagnosis, drainage, dissolution, and management of stones. Radiology 1990;174:1–6.
65. VanSonnenberg E, Casola G, Zakko SF, et al. Gallbladder and bile duct stones: percutaneous therapy with primary MTBE dissolution and mechanical methods. Radiology 1988;169:505–509.

IV Hepatocellular Diseases

7

Hepatic Steatosis and Alcoholic Hepatitis

Mark R. Versland

CONTENTS

1. INTRODUCTION

The liver normally contains lipid equal to approx 5% of its weight. These lipids are composed of triglycerides, phospholipids, cholesterol, and cholesterol esters. Hepatic steatosis, or fatty liver, results from excess accumulation of lipid, primarily triglycerides, but also phospholipids. It may be clinically insignificant or lead to development of cirrhosis.

2. NORMAL LIPID METABOLISM

2.1. Fatty Acids

Fatty acids may be obtained from exogenous sources (i.e., dietary intake and adipose tissue), or to a lesser extent, synthesized *de novo* from glucose. Following a meal, triglyceride-rich lipoproteins (chylomicrons) are formed at the intestinal epithelial surface and gain access directly to the systemic circulation via lymphatic channels. Chylomicrons are then metabolized to fatty acids throughout the body on vascular endothelial surfaces containing lipoprotein lipase (LPL) *(1)*. Fatty acids can then undergo three possible fates: They may be used directly as a source of fuel by tissue such as muscle, esterified to triglycerides in adipose cells and stored, or transported to the liver where they enter various biochemical pathways. Uptake of free fatty acids by the liver is proportional to the concentration of fatty acids in the portal vein. This is directly influenced by the amount of triglyceride in the diet *(2)*.

Storage and lipolysis of triglyceride in adipose tissue are under both neural and hormonal controls. Glucose and insulin are critical to the process of triglyceride synthesis in adipose tissue. Triglyceride cannot be formed without intracellular glucose. Insulin regulates glucose entry into adipose cells, and also inhibits lipolysis by blocking formation of cyclic AMP (cAMP) that controls a hormone-sensitive lipase. Insulin response to blood glucose levels is an important determinant of whether fatty acid storage or triglyceride lipolysis predominates. For example, insulin deficiency in diabetes results in significant lipolysis of stored triglyceride

From: *Diseases of the Liver and Bile Ducts: Diagnosis and Treatment*
Edited by: G. Y. Wu and J. Israel © Humana Press Inc., Totowa, NJ

and delivery of large amounts of free fatty acid to the liver. Excess triglyceride synthesized from these fatty acids is stored, resulting in increased lipid accumulation in the liver.

In the fasting state, fatty acids are mobilized from adipose tissue. Epinephrine, norepinephrine, ACTH, thyroxin, corticosteroids, and glucagon regulate this process by increasing cAMP activity and, as a result, lipolysis. Low glucose levels also contribute primarily to lipolysis, as they are also associated with low insulin levels in the fasting state.

Fatty acids taken up by the liver are esterified in hepatocytes to triglycerides. As in adipose tissue, glucose and insulin also regulate triglyceride synthesis in the liver. Insulin affects both glucose removal by the liver and inhibition of glucose release by the liver. Fatty acids entering the liver may also be oxidized for use as fuel. Oxidation is an important means of controlling excess fat accumulation in the liver. Finally, fatty acids may be incorporated into phospholipids that are used in cell membrane formation.

Triglyceride can be stored or released into the circulation as very low density lipoproteins (VLDL). This provides another source of fatty acids for use as fuel by tissues, storage in adipose cells, or they may recirculate back to the liver. The influx of fatty acid into the liver, storage and transport of triglycerides, and fatty acid oxidation are all in dynamic equilibrium. Factors that upset this balance may result in hepatic steatosis *(3)*.

2.2. Lipoproteins (1)

Lipoproteins function to transport lipids in the plasma. Except for chylomicrons, the liver is the main source of lipoproteins. Lipoproteins themselves are composed of apoproteins that surround a core of lipid. Apoproteins are important constituents of lipoproteins, in that they help regulate the metabolism of the lipid core and also control transport. There are three major classes of hepatic lipoproteins: very low density lipoproteins (VLDL), low density lipoproteins (LDL), and high density lipoproteins (HDL).

Chylomicrons are synthesized in enterocytes and consist of a core of triglyceride and a small amount of cholesterol encased in an apoprotein coat. The apoprotein coat is important for trafficking and also hydrolysis of chylomicrons by activating endothelial LPL. Following hydrolysis, chylomicron remnants are removed by the liver via a receptor-mediated mechanism. Cholesterol in the remnants regulates the intracellular synthesis of cholesterol by its action on HMG-CoA reductase. Other portions of the degraded chylomicron are then used in the formation of other lipoproteins, particularly HDL.

VLDLs are triglyceride-rich lipoproteins secreted by the liver. They are important in maintaining lipid equilibrium in the liver. When VLDLs enter the plasma compartment, they are hydrolyzed much like chylomicrons by the action of LPL. VLDL remnants, depleted of triglyceride, and high in cholesterol concentration, enter two possible pathways. Most are taken up by the liver via a receptor-mediated pathway, and the components used in HDL synthesis. The remainder are further degraded to LDL particles.

LDL are formed from the degradation of VLDL. They function to transport cholesterol to peripheral tissues. About a quarter of the LDL released into the plasma are taken up by a receptor-mediated process in the peripheral tissues. Most of the LDL, however, returns to the liver again via the LDL receptor on hepatocytes. The cholesterol contained in the LDL is then hydrolyzed, and can either be re-esterified and stored, utilized in membranes, or secreted again. The intracellular stores of cholesterol are critical for regulation of new cholesterol synthesis and for synthesis of new LDL receptors.

HDL functions primarily to transport cholesterol from peripheral sites back to the liver where it is metabolized. They are synthesized in the liver *de novo* or formed from the catabolic products of VLDL and chylomicron particles. HDL is critical for the process of reverse transport of cholesterol back to the liver from peripheral tissues, because the liver is the only organ capable of excreting cholesterol.

2.3. Mechanisms of Fatty Liver

Theories regarding development of hepatic steatosis center around increases in fatty acid supply to the liver or alterations in the synthesis and secretion of lipoproteins. It is likely that different mechanisms, or a combination of the above, play a role in the development of hepatic steatosis, depending on the cause.

2.3.1. Increased Fatty Acid Supply

Increases in fatty acid supply can originate from exogenous sources such as dietary intake or adipose tissue or, alternatively, from decreased oxidation of fatty acids by hepatic mitochondria. Experimental data on fatty livers indicate that much of the lipid that accumulates in the liver originates from adipose tissue (4). Manipulations that interfere with mobilization of fatty acids prevent development of fatty liver. Hepatic steatosis that develops as a consequence of increased supply of fatty acids probably reflects the inability of the normal compensatory mechanisms, such as oxidation of fatty acids and secretion of triglycerides, to keep up with the increased synthesis of triglyceride by the liver.

2.3.2. Abnormal Synthesis or Secretion of Lipoproteins

Secretion of triglyceride from the liver occurs via VLDL particles. Factors or agents interfering with protein synthesis may result in production of fatty liver secondary to deficiency in apoproteins needed for packaging and secretion of triglycerides in VLDL. An example of this is orotic acid (5). This agent blocks secretion of VLDL, resulting in massive fatty liver. The actual mechanism, however, is unclear and other agents that interfere with secretion produce only minimal accumulations in hepatic triglyceride. Nutritional deficiencies have also been implicated in animal models of hepatic steatosis. This is, again, presumably related to alterations in VLDL packaging and secretion of triglyceride. The best studied model is choline deficiency that results in fatty liver and cirrhosis, as well as affecting other organ systems. The importance of some of these mechanisms in humans is not clear, however (6).

2.4. Pathology

Except for acute fatty liver of pregnancy, hepatic steatosis often results in an enlarged liver, and triglyceride may comprise 25% of the weight (3,7). Histologically, a variety of abnormalities may be found in addition to lipid. Mallory bodies may be seen both in alcoholic and nonalcoholic steatohepatitis. Inflammatory infiltrates, both polynuclear and lymphocytic, may be present. The entire spectrum of liver injury up to and including cirrhosis may be seen. Triglyceride may be present in either large droplets (macrovesicular steatosis) or small droplets (microvesicular steatosis) (3). Macrovesicular steatosis is easy to identify by the presence of large ballooned cells. Microvesicular steatosis may be more difficult to recognize, and may require the use of special stains, such as oil red O, to confirm the diagnosis. Both patterns of triglyceride deposition can be seen together. However, one form generally predominates, and can suggest a diagnosis. Some conditions associated with the two different patterns are listed in Table 1.

3. CONDITIONS AND AGENTS CAUSING HEPATIC STEATOSIS

3.1. Alcohol

Alcohol and its metabolites are common causes of hepatic steatosis. This may occur over a period of days to weeks. Alcohol does not appear to affect intestinal absorption of lipids or lipoprotein synthesis. It does increase lipolysis in peripheral adipose tissue, resulting in increased delivery to the liver. This primarily occurs at high blood concentrations of alcohol.

Table 1

Some Causes of Microvesicular and Macrovesicular Steatosis

Macrovesicular	Microvesicular
Starvation	Reye's syndrome
Obesity	Acute fatty liver of pregnancy
Diabetes mellitus	Hepatitis C
Jejunoileal bypass	Wilson's disease
Parenteral alimentation	
Alcohol	
AIDS	

Alcohol also increases fatty acid synthesis by decreasing the nicotinamide adenine dinucleotide (NAD) to NADH ratio and damaging mitochondria. Ethanol inhibits the tricarboxylic acid cycle resulting in increased production of acetate that can be used as substrate for fatty acid synthesis. Mitochondrial injury also decreases oxidation of fatty acids in the liver. Fatty acid oxidation is inhibited by acetaldehyde, the major metabolic product of ethanol. Ethanol also replaces fatty acids as the primary source of reducing hydrogen ion for NAD. As a result, less is hydrolyzed. Finally, alcohol also induces the microsomal enzyme system that is responsible for esterification of fatty acids to triglycerides. Ethanol-induced hepatic steatosis is likely a multifactorial process with no single particular mechanism consistently predominating. Different effects occur with acute high serum levels of alcohol and with long-term chronic use *(6)*.

3.2. Nonalcoholic Hepatic Steatosis

Nonalcoholic hepatic steatosis can be divided into four major etiologic categories: metabolic causes, nutritional causes, drugs, and infections. The differentiation from alcohol-induced hepatic steatosis is primarily based on an absence of a significant alcohol history. In some cases, though, histologic features characteristic of certain drugs or disease processes can also help to define the cause *(8)*.

3.2.1. METABOLIC CAUSES

3.2.1.1. Obesity. Steatosis and, to a lesser degree, steatohepatitis are common in obese patients and tend to be more so in women than men. As the mass of peripheral adipose tissue increases, so does the release of fatty acids. Also, dietary intake of fat may be higher in obese individuals. Fatty acid substrates in the serum tend to diminish the need for glucose and result in higher serum concentrations. This, in turn, results in increased insulin release. In general, insulin decreases free fatty acid levels. However, in the obese patient, the mass of adipose tissue overwhelms the regulatory effect of insulin (insulin resistance). Even with normal serum glucose, many obese patients can be demonstrated to have abnormal glucose tolerance tests *(8)*.

3.2.1.2. Diabetes Mellitus. Hepatic steatosis is relatively common in diabetes, affecting about half of patients with the disease. The relationship of the diabetes itself to fatty liver is not clear, as it is uncommon in Type I diabetes. Most cases of fatty liver occur in obese women with Type II diabetes. Close regulation of blood sugars seems to have little effect. It appears that obesity, rather than the diabetes, may be more important in the development of steatosis or steatohepatitis in this group *(9)*.

3.2.1.3. Acute Fatty Liver of Pregnancy. Acute fatty liver of pregnancy is a condition of unknown cause occurring in the third trimester of pregnancy (*see* Chapter 26). This condition results in acute liver failure, and has a high mortality if the fetus is not delivered. The condition must be distinguished from pre-eclampsia/eclampsia and viral hepatitis. This can generally be accomplished by the time course, laboratory features, and, at times, histology. Generally the patient recovers completely. Unlike most instances of steatosis in which the liver is normal or enlarged, the liver in acute fatty liver pregnancy is small and shrunken due to hepatocyte drop out *(7)*.

3.2.1.4. Wilson's Disease. Wilson's disease is an inherited condition in which there is an overload of copper in the body (*see* Chapter 21). Microvesicular steatosis can be seen in Wilson's disease before the development of cirrhosis or other features. In a young person without other causes for fatty liver, this diagnosis should be considered and serum ceruloplasmin levels and urinary copper determined *(10)*.

3.2.2. NUTRITIONAL CAUSES

3.2.2.1. Protein-Calorie Malnutrition. Protein calorie malnutrition is a broad term applied to two conditions: kwashiorkor and marasmus. Classically, kwashiorkor results from a deficiency of dietary protein, and marasmus from deficiency in both protein and calories. Kwashiorkor is defined by the presence of edema, skin depigmentation, and hepatomegaly. Marasmus is defined as body weight less than 50% of expected without edema or skin changes. Approximately 10% of cases can be described purely as kwashiorkor, and approx 20% of cases purely as marasmus. The majority are an overlap between the two conditions. In classic marasmus, significant hepatic steatosis is not seen. Massive hepatic steatosis in protein-calorie malnutrition can be reversed with the addition of adequate protein to the diet. In these individuals, there are high circulating levels of fatty acids, but low VLDL and triglyceride levels. This suggests that hepatic steatosis may result from both increased influx of fatty acids, and the inability to secrete triglyceride. This is reversed by protein administration. It should be noted that cirrhosis does not develop in this condition, suggesting that factors other than fat alone are responsible for development of steatohepatitis *(11)*.

3.2.2.2. Starvation. Starvation may result in hepatic steatosis, but depends on the magnitude of fasting. Fatty acid mobilization occurs during fasting. However, in severe fasting states, increased utilization of lipids for fuel prevents the development of fat accumulation in the liver. If some carbohydrates are consumed, however, the oxidation of fatty acids is markedly reduced and triglyceride will accumulate due to the increased influx of fatty acids *(3)*.

3.2.2.3. Surgery for Obesity. Jejunoileal bypass is a technique for control of morbid obesity in which most of the small bowel surface is bypassed by anastomosing the proximal 30–40 cm of jejunum to the distal 15–20 cm of ileum. Postoperatively, changes in the liver, ranging from asymptomatic steatosis to steatohepatitis with liver failure, may be seen. These changes generally occur within 6 mo of surgery. In the ensuing years, the degree of fat accumulation in the liver may return to presurgical levels. The only way to reliably follow these individuals postoperatively is with serial liver biopsies. The explanation for the fat accumulation and liver disease is not clear. However, it is not simply a result of increased fatty acid mobilization from adipose tissue. Dieting and other forms of obesity surgery, such as gastric partitioning, do not cause these changes. Also, changes can be improved or prevented with the use of antibiotics, suggesting that factors resulting from bacterial overgrowth in the excluded loop are likely responsible. Reversal of the bypass procedure will reverse the changes in the liver. Because of these complications, jejunoileal bypass has all but been abandoned over the past 15 yr *(12)*.

3.2.2.4. Parenteral Alimentation. Patients receiving parenteral alimentation may develop elevations in their aminotransferases, alkaline phosphatase, and bilirubin. Liver biopsy may reveal macrovesicular steatosis. This appears to be a result of administration of excessive calories. However, it may also result from increased fatty acid synthesis by the liver *(13)*.

3.2.3. Drugs

Numerous drugs and toxins have been implicated in the development of hepatic steatosis. The more common of these are listed along with other causes in Table 1 (*see* Chapter 13).

3.2.3.1. Corticosteroids. Fatty liver is a common finding in patients with Cushing's syndrome. In patients on steroids, fatty liver only appears to occur at high doses. Experimentally, this seems to occur due to increased influx of free fatty acids into the liver serving as substrate for increased triglyceride synthesis *(14)*.

3.2.3.2. Methotrexate. Methotrexate is a folic acid antagonist used in the management of oncologic, dermatologic, and rheumatologic diseases. It has been implicated in the development of hepatic fibrosis in a dose-dependent manner. In those individuals that develop liver toxicity, biopsy will often show the presence of macrovesicular fat in the specimen. Liver biopsy is the only reliable way to confirm liver toxicity *(15)*.

3.2.3.3. Valproic Acid. Valproic acid is an antiseizure medication that may rarely cause acute hepatocellular injury and liver failure. This is most commonly seen in children. Liver biopsy shows central necrosis and the presence of microvesicular steatosis *(16)*.

3.2.3.4. Tetracycline. Historically, large iv doses of tetracycline have resulted in a syndrome of acute fatty liver, hepatocellular necrosis, and death. Histologically, microvesicular steatosis is seen, and is indistinguishable from that in acute fatty liver of pregnancy. The mechanism is likely a combination of increased hepatic synthesis of triglyceride, and impaired secretion due to interference with formation of lipoproteins. This condition is not seen with the usual oral doses of the antibiotic used today *(17)*.

3.2.3.5. Amiodarone. Amiodarone is an iodinated benzofuran derivative used primarily in the treatment of refractory cardiac arrhythmias. The drug may produce hepatotoxicity, as well as affecting other organ systems such as the lungs and thyroid. The most common lesion affecting the liver is a chronic hepatitis that on biopsy resembles alcoholic hepatitis with macrovesicular steatosis and Mallory bodies. This may progress to cirrhosis. Discontinuation of the drug then needs to be balanced against the need for treatment of the cardiac arrhythmia *(18)*.

3.2.4. Infections

3.2.4.1. Hepatitis C. Unlike other forms of viral hepatitis, hepatitis C infection may result in a moderate microvesicular steatosis. This is not the main feature of the disease, however, and other evidence of infection is usually present on examination of liver biopsy specimens *(19)*.

3.2.4.2. Reye's Syndrome. Reye's syndrome is a condition in which a viral prodrome is followed by progressive liver failure. It generally occurs in children, and is rare in adults. The trademark feature of the syndrome is that most affected individuals have taken aspirin during their viral syndrome. Liver failure can develop rapidly following the viral prodrome. Hepatomegaly is common and, histologically, microvesicular steatosis is present *(20)*.

3.2.4.3. HIV. Liver biopsy specimens will commonly demonstrate the presence of a macrovesicular steatosis along with numerous other abnormalities. This hepatic steatosis is likely multifactorial, resulting from factors such as malnutrition, alcohol use, and parenteral hyperalimentation *(21)*.

3.2.5. Natural History of Nonalcoholic Fatty Liver

Excluding patients with steatohepatitis from conditions known to result in hepatocellular failure such as acute fatty liver of pregnancy, Reye's syndrome, hepatitis C, and toxin-induced injury, the most common presentation of hepatic steatosis is in an obese, middle-aged woman with glucose intolerance and/or hyperlipidemia. These individuals almost always have a benign course. Studies involving serial biopsies have demonstrated that, in the absence of pre-existing fibrosis on a biopsy, it is extremely rare to progress to clinically important liver disease. This type of individual fortunately makes up the large predominance of patients seen with nonalcoholic steatohepatitis. There is some data, though, suggesting there may be a subset of patients with nonalcoholic steatohepatitis that have or go on to develop cirrhosis. These individuals are characterized by fibrosis on their initial liver biopsy, and may not fit the typical profile. They are more often male, and may not have hyperlipidemia or hyperglycemia. It is not known whether the steatohepatitis is a cause or is a result of some other unknown condition affecting the liver (8,22).

3.2.6. Diagnosis

Most patients with hepatic steatosis are asymptomatic and come to clinical attention based on an enlarged liver, abnormal "liver function tests" found on a laboratory profile, or findings on an imaging study performed for other reasons. Elevations in the aminotransferases, alkaline phosphatase, gamma glutamyl transferase, and bilirubin may all be seen and are nonspecific. The magnitude of the laboratory abnormalities does not correlate with the severity of the underlying liver disease. There are no specific symptoms.

Fatty infiltration of hepatocytes alters the normal density of the liver and, thus, imaging studies can suggest the presence of excess fat in the liver. Generally, hepatic steatosis is a diffuse process, but it may also produce focal lesions. Ultrasound can reveal increased echogenicity of the liver parenchyma and CT scanning can detect lower attenuation due to the lower density of the lipid. MRI is more expensive than the other two modalities, but can provide an even more accurate assessment of the presence of hepatic steatosis as MRI takes advantage of the difference in water content between fat and water-filled cells (23) (see Chapter 5 for more detail and examples). For most cases, ultrasound is the imaging study of choice, because of its relatively lower cost.

The question of when to do liver biopsy in a patient with suspected hepatic steatosis is a difficult one. In those patients with normal liver chemistries, in whom the diagnosis of fatty liver is suggested, for example, by an ultrasound performed for other reasons, biopsy is not required. For all others, the decision to perform liver biopsy should be made based on the need to confirm the diagnosis or potential findings that would alter the management of a patient; for example, continuing or stopping a drug such as methotrexate. If, in the opinion of the clinician, biopsy findings will not alter the current management of the patient, it is not necessary to obtain the biopsy.

3.2.7. Treatment

Treatment of hepatic steatosis is directed at the underlying cause. For the most common scenario, i.e., the obese individual with hyperglycemia/lipidemia, treatment involves weight loss and control of hyperlipidemia. Individuals with biopsy-proven nonalcoholic steatohepatitis may benefit from treatment with ursodeoxycholic acid (24).

4. ALCOHOLIC HEPATITIS

Alcoholic hepatitis is a form of toxin-induced liver disease that runs a wide clinical spectrum from subclinical disease diagnosed only on liver biopsy, to cirrhosis, and fulminant hepatic failure. The term "alcoholic hepatitis" was first used to describe the clinical presentation of alcoholic patients with jaundice (25). Excessive alcohol intake over a long period of time is necessary for development of alcoholic hepatitis with cirrhosis. Whereas there is considerable variation, at least 40–60 g of ethanol per day for more than 15 yr is required for the development of alcoholic hepatitis with cirrhosis. This is equal to about six, 12-oz beers per day, 4 glasses of wine, or three, 2-oz shots of whiskey. Women may develop disease with smaller amounts due to their smaller body size, hormonal differences, and less prehepatic metabolism of ethanol by gastric alcohol dehydrogenase (ADH) (26–28).

4.1. Metabolism of Alcohol

There are two predominant pathways for alcohol metabolism in the hepatocyte: the ADH pathway in the cytosol of the cell, and the microsomal ethanol oxidizing system (MEOS) located in the endoplasmic reticulum. Both pathways result in production of acetaldehyde that is the toxic intermediate in alcohol metabolism. The ADH system is the predominant mode of metabolism, and occurs mainly in the liver. ADH is also located in the stomach, to varying degrees, and metabolism that occurs here may affect liver toxicity by decreasing the amount of alcohol reaching the liver. Differences in gastric ADH may explain, in part, the observation that some individuals develop toxicity from smaller amounts of alcohol than others. For example, women tend to have lower rates of gastric alcohol metabolism than men, and may develop liver injury from alcohol at lower doses than men *(28)*.

When ethanol is oxidized by ADH, acetaldehyde is produced, and reducing equivalents are transferred to nicotinamide adenine dinucleotide (NAD), converting it to a reduced form, NADH. Acetaldehyde is then metabolized to acetate by the enzyme aldehyde dehydrogenase (ALD), releasing additional reducing equivalents. The release of a large number of reducing equivalents tends to overwhelm the hepatocyte's ability to maintain a normal redox state. This results in several disorders. Metabolic acidosis develops due to increased levels of lactic acid. Hyperuricemia results from the acidosis inhibiting renal excretion, as well as from increased formation of uric acid from purines generated by increased ATP breakdown. This may help explain the observation that excessive alcohol intake may aggravate or precipitate attacks of gout. The decreased NAD/NADH ratio also contributes to triglyceride accumulation in the hepatocytes.

The MEOS is part of an inducible P450 enzyme system that oxidizes ethanol to acetaldehyde. This is a secondary system to the ADH system. However, the effect of alcohol on this inducible system has potentially important clinical ramifications. For example, with acute alcohol intake, there is competition between alcohol and other drugs such a phenobarbital, dilantin, and coumadin for enzyme-binding sites. This results in a decreased rate of metabolism of the medications and, thus, higher blood levels. This explains the increased toxicity of drugs taken together with alcohol during suicide attempts. During the chronic phase of alcohol intake, however, induction of this enzyme system results in increased metabolism of the drugs and, as a result, more drug is needed to maintain normal levels. This can be deleterious, in that drugs such as acetaminophen in alcoholics may be more rapidly metabolized to toxic intermediates, resulting in hepatotoxicity at lower doses *(29)*.

4.2. Pathology

Histologic diagnosis of alcoholic hepatitis requires three features: ballooning degeneration of hepatocytes with areas of necrosis, inflammatory cell infiltration that is predominately composed of neutrophils, and fibrosis. The injury tends to be seen first, and is most severe in the centrilobular region of the liver. Fatty infiltration is extremely common, and the term alcoholic steatohepatitis is a more accurate description of the process. Steatohepatitis is not unique, however, to alcoholic liver injury. Mallory bodies or alcoholic hyalin are also often present and tend to be in greatest number near the areas of most intense inflammation. Mallory bodies are histologically identified as a collection of purple-red material near the nucleus of the hepatocyte when viewed with hematoxylin and eosin stain. Mallory bodies are felt to be formed from collections of intermediate filaments. The original, and most popular, postulate is that alcohol metabolites inhibit the normal microtubular transport mechanism in the hepatocyte, causing accumulation of the filaments and production of Mallory bodies. Another theory proposes that Mallory bodies are the product of a gene that normally is suppressed, but somehow becomes activated during the course of toxic injury to the hepatocyte. Mallory bodies were once considered diagnostic of alcoholic liver injury, but they have since been demonstrated in nonalcoholic steatohepatitis.

Cholestatic changes are also commonly seen with bile stasis, plugging, and, at times, destruction of bile ductules in the portal triads. This is most commonly due to an intrahepatic process and reflects direct toxin injury and also possibly mechanical compression of small ducts from hepatocyte swelling and fatty infiltration (25).

4.3. Pathogenesis of Alcoholic Hepatitis

Most of the toxic effects of alcohol on the liver are felt to be mediated through production of acetaldehyde. Acetaldehyde is produced mainly through the action of ADH. However, with chronic alcohol intake, induction of the MEOS also contributes. Acetaldehyde levels are controlled by ALD located in the mitochondria. Chronic alcohol intake inhibits ALD, resulting in further elevation of acetaldehyde.

The balloon-like hepatocytes seen in alcohol-induced liver injury are believed to result from impairment by the acetaldehyde of the microtubular transport system of the hepatocyte. This results in accumulation of lipoproteins and other proteins made by the cell. The result of this process is swelling of the cells and eventual destruction. Free radicals are also generated by parts of the MEOS. These free radicals react with unsaturated fatty acids present in cellular organelles and membranes. Unstable intermediates are produced in this way that then undergo peroxidative degeneration. This results in changes in membrane fluidity, and loss of enzyme function that ultimately leads to cell death. Acetaldehyde also probably promotes lipid peroxidation through inactivation of free radical scavengers. With chronic alcohol use, lipocytes in the liver transform into myofibroblast-like cells that produce collagen and, ultimately, cirrhosis. Acetaldehyde may further enhance this situation by up-regulating the production of collagen.

Immune mechanisms may also play a role in alcohol-related hepatotoxicity. Mallory bodies can bind to immunoglobulins and, when released from dying hepatocytes, are complexed with these immunoglobulins and with tissue and serum carbohydrates. In this form they possess chemotactic properties and may help explain the neutrophilic inflammatory infiltrate seen in alcoholic hepatitis. Circulating cytotoxic T-cells sensitized to hepatocytes have been found in chronic alcohol abusers, particularly those with cirrhosis. This would help explain the portal inflammatory changes (mainly T-cells) noted histologically, and also the fact that liver injury may progress over time even if the alcohol is stopped (6,30).

Finally, alcohol and its metabolites, particularly acetaldehyde, are responsible for the significant lipid accumulation characteristic of alcoholic hepatitis. This occurs by several mechanisms. Lipolysis is increased in peripheral adipose tissue, resulting in increased delivery to the liver. This primarily occurs at high blood concentrations of alcohol. Acetaldehyde also increases fatty acid synthesis by increasing the NADH/NAD ratio and damaging mitochondria. The tricarboxylic acid cycle is inhibited, resulting in increased production of acetate that can be used as substrate for fatty acid synthesis. Mitochondrial injury also decreases oxidation of fatty acids in the liver. In addition, ethanol replaces fatty acids as the primary source of reducing hydrogen ion for NAD. As a result, less is hydrolyzed. Finally, alcohol also induces the microsomal enzyme system that is responsible for esterification of fatty acids to triglycerides (6).

4.4. Incidence of Alcoholic Hepatitis

Due to the large number of individuals who have only mild symptoms, the true incidence of alcoholic hepatitis can only be estimated, as most of these cases will not be brought to medical attention and liver biopsy would be necessary to establish the diagnosis. There also appears to be a variation in incidence in different nationalities. In Denmark, a study of patients who were admitted for alcohol detoxification and treatment showed changes on liver biopsy consistent with alcoholic hepatitis in about 20% *(25)*. In a United States study involving veterans with liver disease, who underwent liver biopsy, approx 35% had changes consistent with alcoholic hepatitis. These were skewed populations, however, in that these were patients seen in the hospital. Persons with mild asymptomatic disease would not be detected, and, thus, the figure of 35% likely underestimates the true incidence in the population *(31)*.

4.5. Factors Influencing Alcohol-Induced Liver Injury

4.5.1. NUTRITIONAL FACTORS

Alcoholic hepatitis was originally felt to be a nutritional problem based on the observation that most patients presenting with moderate to severe disease were malnourished. It has subsequently been shown that alcoholic hepatitis and cirrhosis could develop despite adequate nutritional support. The mechanism of malnutrition in alcoholic liver disease is multifactorial. The heavy drinker may consume nearly half of his daily caloric intake in the form of ethanol. Whereas the total number of calories may be nearly adequate, the ethanol provides mainly "empty" calories. Patients with this condition are often in a net catabolic state. Protein intake may be inadequate to meet the needs of cellular repair. In addition, alcohol intake produces anorexia, further complicating the situation. Lastly, the effects of alcohol on other organ systems, such as the pancreas, may result in malabsorption. It is not known, though, whether malnutrition plays a role in the liver injury or if it is simply a condition associated with alcoholism *(6)*.

4.5.2. GENETICS

There is evidence for a genetic predisposition for alcohol-induced liver injury. Ethanol is metabolized predominantly in the liver. After ingestion, ethanol is rapidly absorbed from the stomach and small intestine. Serum levels are then determined by the rate of oxidative metabolism of ethanol by the liver. Acetaldehyde and the production of reducing agents, mainly NADH, are felt to be the primary contributors to liver injury. The two enzymes primarily involved in ethanol metabolism are ADH and ALD. Multiple isoenzymes of ADH and ALD have been discovered. These isoenzymes have a different predominance in different populations and function differently. For example, the flushing phenomenon is commonly seen in people with a particular subtype of ALD that results in slow metabolism of acetaldehyde. This is common in Asians. Variation in the metabolism of ethanol as a function of these genetic differences may explain the higher prevalence of alcoholic liver injury in some populations *(32)*.

4.5.3. CYTOKINES

Cytokines are a group of soluble polypeptides that act as modifiers of biologic responses by regulating gene expression, differentiation and proliferation of cells. They are secreted by cells into the microenvironment where they interact with various receptors, and the end result is often a function of a cascade of cytokines. Various cytokines have been examined for their possible role in alcoholic hepatitis. These include the interleukins, tumor necrosis factor, colony-stimulating factors, and transforming growth factor *(32)*. These cytokines have been implicated in induction and continuation of the inflammatory response and stimulation of cells that lead to increased production of extracellular matrix and, ultimately, fibrosis and cirrhosis. It is not known, however, whether these agents are directly regulated by ethanol and its metabolites or whether the increased expression of these agents is a function of the underlying inflammatory response *(32)*.

4.5.4. Hepatitis C Virus

The interaction of alcohol and hepatitis C is not clear. It is known, however, that alcoholics with more severe liver disease are more likely to have concurrent infection with hepatitis C. Histologically, the liver damage contains both alcoholic and viral features, suggesting one superimposed on the other *(30)*.

4.6. Diagnosis of Alcoholic Hepatitis

Clinical signs and symptoms of alcoholic hepatitis vary from asymptomatic to acute liver failure. In asymptomatic individuals, one of the most common findings is an enlarged liver (greater than 12 cm in the mid-clavicular line). Cirrhosis is commonly seen in biopsies from patients with alcoholic hepatitis. However, unlike other processes that produce cirrhosis, the liver in alcoholic hepatitis often remains enlarged, as opposed to becoming small and shrunken. Evidence of liver failure may be present as portal hypertension with ascites and varices, and encephalopathy. It is important to recognize that alcoholic hepatitis by itself, without cirrhosis, may produce these findings, and that this is a potentially reversible condition. Liver biopsy is the only reliable way to establish whether the patient has underlying cirrhosis.

Laboratory findings are varied and reflect underlying liver damage as well as nutritional deficits, and a direct toxic effect of alcohol on the bone marrow. A macrocytic anemia is commonly seen. This may result from both the changes induced in red cell membranes, and also from folate deficiency that is common in alcoholics. Vitamin B12 levels are usually increased, reflecting release from the damaged liver. Liver enzyme tests generally show a pattern in which the aspartate aminotransferase (AST) and alanine aminotransferase (ALT) are both elevated with the AST greater than ALT. The greater elevation in AST probably reflects its greater concentration in the centrilobular region of the liver where alcohol-induced liver injury is more severe. Despite a significant amount of inflammation seen histologically, it is very unusual for the AST to exceed levels greater than 200 IU/L or 5 times the upper limit of normal. Elevations greater than 300 IU/L should raise suspicion of another or concurrent process affecting the liver. Classically, it has been taught that an AST/ALT ratio of greater than 2 is diagnostic of alcoholic hepatitis. However, this ratio is seen in only about half the patients, generally those with the most severe disease. Alcoholic hepatitis is a cholestatic form of liver disease, and the alkaline phosphatase and bilirubin may be elevated out of proportion to the aminotransferases. This feature, along with the leukocytosis and fever that can be present, may present diagnostic problems trying to distinguish this entity from gallbladder and biliary tract disease. This is an important distinction, as operating on a patient with severe alcoholic hepatitis carries a significant risk of morbidity and mortality. The GGT is generally high. This is not very useful as a test, because it reflects microsomal enzyme induction as well as liver injury. Alterations in the prothrombin time and albumin may be seen reflecting both hepatic synthetic dysfunction as well as nutritional deficiency *(33,34)*.

Imaging studies are generally not helpful in diagnosing alcoholic hepatitis. They invariably show an enlarged, fatty-appearing liver. They are more helpful in eliminating other or concurrent problems, such as biliary tract disease and pancreatitis. Even in this capacity, care must be taken in their interpretation or they may suggest an incorrect diagnosis. For example, the HIDA scan used to help confirm a diagnosis of cholecystitis may also show nonvisualization of the gallbladder (a positive scan) in alcoholic hepatitis despite the absence of a blocked cystic duct *(35,36)*.

There are no specific recommendations regarding the use of liver biopsy in alcoholic hepatitis. In severe alcoholic hepatitis, the biopsy may be relatively contraindicated because of a coagulopathy or thrombocytopenia. The diagnosis is often not difficult in these cases, and can generally be established by a history of long-term, heavy alcohol use, serologic tests, and noninvasive imaging studies to help rule out biliary tract obstruction. Biopsy is useful in the patient who has recovered from a bout of severe alcoholic hepatitis or in the patient with mild disease to determine if the patient has cirrhosis. It should be kept in mind that this will not significantly alter management of the patient. From the standpoint of management, liver biopsy is probably most useful in the patient who may have multiple potential causes of liver disease, such as drugs other than alcohol. Approximately 20% of alcoholic patients who have clinical and laboratory features suggesting alcoholic hepatitis will have another cause found on liver biopsy (37). Biopsy may also occasionally be useful in the patient who does not admit to significant drinking. Findings on the biopsy showing alcoholic hepatitis may be helpful in forcing the patient to confront a potential problem before it becomes more serious.

4.7. Prognostic Features in Alcoholic Hepatitis

Typical patients who present with severe alcoholic hepatitis have generally stopped drinking several days to a week prior to presentation. Their illness will commonly worsen over the next 10–14 d despite cessation of drinking. Most of the early mortality from alcoholic hepatitis occurs during this time period. The prognosis regarding acute 30-d mortality depends on the severity of the hepatitis at the time of admission. Various methods have been employed for evaluation. However, currently the most widely used and best predictor of severity is the so-called Maddrey discriminate function. This is an objective measure of severity of alcoholic hepatitis based on two laboratory criteria, the prothrombin time and bilirubin. Prothrombin time and bilirubin were found to be the two best predictors of survival. The discriminate function is equal to 4.6 X (prothrombin time - control) + bilirubin (mg/dL). Values greater than 32 indicate severe disease with a significant 30-d mortality (38).

Beyond the initial acute phase of alcoholic hepatitis, there is little long-term data regarding mortality. One study followed patients with serial liver biopsies. No patients that continued to drink recovered, and about a third of these progressed to cirrhosis. Of those that stopped drinking, after a year, half still had alcoholic hepatitis, a quarter had progressed to cirrhosis, and the remainder had healed (39).

4.8. TREATMENT

Abstinence is the mainstay of treatment of alcoholic liver disease. However, in practice this may be difficult to achieve. In one study only approx 10% of chronic alcohol users were able to maintain complete abstinence over a 2 yr period (40). An approach to treatment is outlined in Fig. 1.

4.8.1. NUTRITION (41)

The role of nutrition in patients with alcoholic hepatitis has been extensively studied, with the rationale being that almost all these patients are malnourished. This is particularly true in patients requiring hospitalization. In most, voluntary food intake is not adequate to meet their nutritional needs. These patients must then catabolize protein stores in order meet their basal energy requirements. This is not a desirable situation, and most of these patients will require additional nutritional support, either enterally or parenterally. Both modes have been studied with each showing the ability to establish a positive nitrogen balance. The enteral route is preferred. However, if this is not possible, parenteral alimentation should be used. The goal of nutritional therapy should be to establish a positive nitrogen balance. The approximate daily needs of the patient can be estimated at about 30 cal, and 1 g/kg body wt of protein. A common mistake is to restrict protein to avoid inducing or worsening hepatic encephalopathy. Adequate protein is necessary to establish a positive balance, and no studies have shown this to worsen encephalopathy to any significant degree. Whereas dietary supplementation will improve

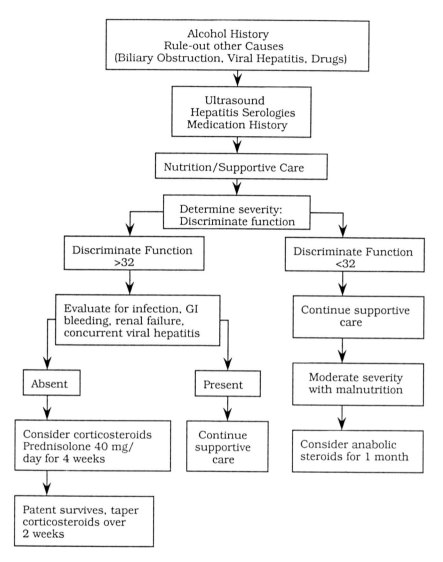

Fig. 1. A scheme for the treatment of alcoholic hepatitis.

various clinical parameters in patients with alcoholic hepatitis, it has, however, been difficult to demonstrate any significant effect on acute mortality. Two specific nutrients that are of interest are polyunsaturated lecithin and diets high in saturated fats. Polyunsaturated lecithin can inhibit the formation of cirrhosis in animal models. This may occur by stimulation of collagenase activity that offsets the acetaldehyde-induced increase in collagen production. Of interest is one study suggesting a diet high in saturated fats may be advantageous in alcoholic hepatitis *(42)*. Application of this to humans still awaits study.

4.8.2. Medications (*see* Table 2)

4.8.2.1. Corticosteroids *(38,43)*. There have been many trials examining the role of corticosteroids in the treatment of alcoholic hepatitis. The rationale for their use is the acute inflammatory reaction observed histologically in the liver. Corticosteroids at a dose equal to 40 mg/d

29. Lieber CS. Biochemical factors in alcoholic liver disease. Seminars in Liver Dis 1993;13:136–153.
30. Pares A. Hepatitis C virus antibodies in chronic alcoholic patients: association with severity of liver injury. Hepatology 1990;12:1295–1299.
31. Mendenhall CL. Veterans Administration Cooperative Study Group on Alcoholic Hepatitis. Alcoholic hepatitis. Clin Gastroenterol 1981;10:417–441.
32. Arron R. Molecular biological aspects of alcohol-induced liver disease. Alcoholism: Clin Exp Res 1995;19:247–256.
33. Goldberg SJ. Veterans Administration Cooperative Study Group on Alcoholic Hepatitis IV: Describing the population with minimal hyperbilirubinemia. Am J Gastro 1986;11:1024–1037.
34. Mendenhall CL. Protein calorie malnutrition associated with alcoholic hepatitis: Veterans Administration Cooperative Study Group on Alcoholic Hepatitis. Am J Med 1984;76:211–222.
35. Garner WL. Cholescintigraphy in the critically ill. Am J Surg 1988;155:727–729.
36. Shuman WP. PIPIDA scintigraphy for cholecystitis: false positives in alcoholism and total parenteral nutrition. Am J Radiol 1982;138:1–6.
37. Mezey E. Treatment of alcoholic liver disease. Sem Liver Dis 1993;13:210–216.
38. Carithers RL. Methylprednisolone therapy in patients with severe alcoholic hepatitis: a randomized multicenter trial. Ann Int Med 1989;110:685–690.
39. Galambos JT. Alcoholic hepatitis: its therapy and prognosis. Prog Liver Dis 1972;4:567–588.
40. Orrego H. Long-term treatment of alcoholic liver disease with propylthiouracil. NEJM 1987;317:1421–1427.
41. Morgan TR. Treatment of alcoholic hepatitis. Sem Liver Dis 1993;13:384–394.
42. Nanji AA. Dietary fatty acids: a novel treatment for alcoholic liver disease. Gastroenterology 1995;109:547–554.
43. Mathurin P. Survival and prognostic factors in patients with severe alcoholic hepatitis treated with prednisolone. Gastroenterology 1996;110:1847–1853.
44. Krom RAF. Liver transplantation and alcohol: who should get transplants. Hepatology 1994;20:28S–32S.

8

Self-Limited Viral Hepatitis: A, E, CMV, EBV

Enrique J. Martinez and Lennox Jeffers

1. INTRODUCTION

The term self-limited viral hepatitis refers to diseases caused by a special group of viruses that have a tendency to attack liver. Although they have the potential to cause significant morbidity and mortality in the acute phase of their illness, they never cause chronic hepatitis. Infections tend to be more severe in immunocompromised individuals.

2. HEPATITIS A

Hepatitis A is an RNA virus that accounts for 26–28% of all acute hepatitis cases reported each year to the Centers for Disease Control *(1–3,4)*. It is the most common cause of viral hepatitis in the United States *(5)* and is endemic to Central and South America, North Africa, and Asia *(6)*.

2.1. Epidemiology

Poor sanitation plays a major role in the spread of hepatitis A infections, as it is primarily spread via a fecal-oral route. Fecal-oral spread can occur via contaminated sources, such as water, and ingestion of raw or undercooked bivalve mollusks from contaminated waters. The virus is inactivated by boiling water, but can survive 12 wk to 10 mo in water at room temperature *(7)*.

Epidemics related to mollusks can be devastating *(8)*. Salads, cold meats, hamburgers, orange juice, pastries, and raw milk have all been reported as sources. Most cases of HAV, in the United States, are diagnosed in patients within 8 wk of travel to an endemic area. In

From: *Diseases of the Liver and Bile Ducts: Diagnosis and Treatment*
Edited by: G. Y. Wu and J. Israel © Humana Press Inc., Totowa, NJ

developed countries with temperate climates, epidemic waves can be seen every 7 yr, as this is the time required to develop a sufficient number of susceptible hosts. Day care center outbreaks among children and adult parents or caretakers of the children account for 15% of the hepatitis A cases in the United States, with the parents or adults being more likely to manifest symptoms of disease *(9,10)*. Among infants and adolescents, 80% are asymptomatic and anicteric, whereas over 80% of adult cases are icteric. Humans who have had close contact with infected primates also have been infected *(11)*. Percutaneous spread is possible, but infrequent. Maternal-neonatal spread is not generally noted, but there has been a case report of a woman with acute hepatitis A who experienced a placental abruption and delivered an asymptomatic infant. However, several other infants and staff in the hospital became secondarily infected *(11)*. Saliva, semen, and urine infectivity is uncertain. The overall attack rate for hepatitis A in the United States is 9 cases per 100,000 *(5,12)*, but the rates vary with ethnicity. In the United States, hepatitis A occurs in decreasing frequency as follows: Native Americans, Hispanics, Blacks, Whites, and Asian Americans. Secondary attack rates in households of clinical disease is 20% *(13)*, but subclincal attack rates may be even higher. The most common identifiable risk factor (24–47%) is household or sexual contact with someone with hepatitis A *(14)*. Other significant factors and their risks are: day care center contact, 15%; foreign travel, 6–15%; association with food or waterborne sources, 5–19%; intravenous drug abuse, 2%. In 40% of cases, no risk factor can be identified.

2.2. Characteristics of Hepatitis A Infections

HAV occurs more commonly in late autumn and early winter, particularly in children. Following entry into the body, the liver serves as the replication source of the virus. Symptoms develop with an incubation time ranging from 15–50 d, with a mean of 30 d. The onset of disease is usually abrupt. Fecal shedding occurs for 2–3 wk prior to development of symptoms and persists until the transaminases peak. Shedding diminishes as HAV IgM appears. No human intestinal carrier state has been identified. Hepatitis A does not appear to be more severe in HIV infected individuals, but this depends on their overall state of health and immune function *(15)*. The majority of hepatitis A cases recover in 4–6 wk, but some prolonged cases of up to 1 yr may be seen.

2.3. Cardinal Symptoms and Signs

2.3.1. SYMPTOMS

A prodrome often precedes the full onset of symptoms. This period is characterized by malaise and weakness, with associated abdominal discomfort, anorexia, fever, nausea, and vomiting. Fever to > 38°C is common. Less commonly, chills (27%), headaches (22%), and myalgias (32%) have also been reported. Within a few days to a week, the majority of the patients will develop dark urine (81%), jaundice (71%), and pruritus (29%). Anorexia may persist as the remainder of the prodromal symptoms diminish. Extrahepatic symptoms are uncommon, but include arthralgias, 11–40%; diarrhea: 24%; transient rash, 1–14%; sore throat, 7%; hyposmia (e.g.m cigarette smoke aversion), uncommon; arthritis, rare *(16,17)*.

2.3.2. ATYPICAL CLINICAL MANIFESTATIONS

Atypical clinical manifestations of hepatitis A have been reported and fall into five major categories *(18–20)*:

2.3.2.1. Cholestatic. Acute cholestatic hepatitis A is present when the serum bilirubin remains >171 umol/L (10 mg/dL) for over 12 wk in the absence of hemolysis or renal failure. Most patients have aminotransferases <500 IU/L.

2.3.2.2. Relapsing. A biphasic or relapsing form of hepatitis A is seen in 6–10% of patients, and typically occurs 4–15 wk after the initial episode. In this condition, normal aminotransferases can be noted during remission. The relapse can be more or less severe than the initial episode, with aminotransferases usually >1000 IU/L. The full duration of illness ranges from 16–40 wk. Hepatitis A IgM persists throughout this course. Patient feces and serum remains infectious during the relapse. Fecal virus levels disappear within 30 d, but HAV RNA levels in stools can be detected for months. The mechanism responsible for relapses is probably immunologically mediated, but the exact mechanisms remain unclear. Nevertheless, HAV never progresses to chronic hepatitis.

2.3.2.3. Extrahepatic. Extrahepatic manifestations caused by immune complex disease are rare with HAV. Typically, they are seen when the illness becomes protracted, either with cholestasis or relapse. Cutaneous vasculitis can manifest as an erythematous maculopapular eruption involving the lower extremities and can be associated with purpuric lesions. On skin biopsy, IgM anti-HAV and complement may be noted in the blood vessel walls. Cryoglobulinemia due to IgM anti-HAV has also been reported. Arthritis when noted, generally also involves the lower extremities.

2.3.2.4. Autoimmune. HAV-induced autoimmune hepatitis type 1 has been reported. Antibodies to asialoglycoprotein and defects in the T-cell suppressor-inducer cells have been implicated *(21,22)*.

2.3.2.5. Renal Failure. Renal failure in the absence of fulminant HAV has been noted in a few cases. The exact mechanism of the renal failure is unclear, but tends to parallel the course of the liver disease.

2.3.3. Physical Examination

On physical exam, findings are typical for a liver-related process (*see* Chapter 1). A mildly enlarged liver with mild to moderate tenderness to palpation is typical. However, the liver span is less than 12 cm in 78–85% of cases *(17)*. Splenomegaly can be seen in 7–15% *(16,17)*, and posterior cervical adenopathy in 4–15%.

2.4. Laboratory

Typically, viremia precedes clinical disease. Serum alanine and aspartate aminotransferase activities tend to increase during the prodromal period to levels frequently well above 500 IU/L *(16)*. Bilirubin levels peak at <170 umol/L (10 mg/dL) shortly after the aminotransferases peak. Mean presenting levels of laboratory parameters include total bilirubin, 85.5 umol/L (5 mg/dL); alkaline phosphatase, 269 U/mL; AST, 1442 mIU/mL; and ALT, 1952 IU/mL *(23)*.

Levels of AST and ALT decrease by 75% per week for the first few weeks. In two thirds of patients, this is followed by a slower descent to normal within 2 mo. Eighty five percent will be normal by 3 mo, and nearly all will be normal by 6 mo *(16)*. Delayed normalization of aminotransferase levels beyond 12 mo is rare. Bilirubin levels decline more slowly than aminotransferase levels. Eighty-five percent of cases remain jaundiced for > 2 wk *(16)*. Two thirds of patients have normal bilirubin levels by 2 mo. Atypical lymphocytes are seen in 7% of cases.

2.5. Diagnosis

Whereas a variety of detection techniques exists for identifying hepatitis A in serum, stool, and liver tissue, the diagnosis is confirmed primarily by serological testing, *see* Fig. 1 (diagnostic algorithm). Levels of IgM against HAV peak during the acute and early convalescent stages, and usually become undetectable in 4 mo. In 25% of cases, the HAV-IgM persists for

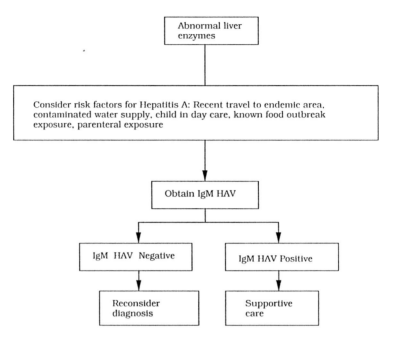

Fig. 1. A schematic plan for the diagnostic evaluation of hepatitis A.

more than 6 mo *(24)*. Persistence beyond 12 mo is rare. Levels of IgG against hepatitis A peak during the convalescent phase and usually remain detectable in declining levels for decades.

Noninvasive imaging studies that are normal make invasive tests unnecessary. A liver biopsy is usually not required to make the diagnosis. Histology often demonstrates marked centrilobular cholestasis and portal inflammation.

2.6. Treatment

For most patients with HAV, treatment is supportive, (*see* Fig. 2; treatment). Patients should be advised to abstain from alcohol, as this may be associated with relapse of jaundice *(25–27)*. Participation in contact sports should be avoided during the symptomatic period. Prolonged cholestasis may require fat-soluble vitamin supplementation. Persistently rising serum bilirubin levels, prolonged prothrombin time, evidence of hepatic encephalopathy, or other evidence of liver decompensation suggest the need for hospitalization. HAV-infected patients who develop fulminant hepatitis can be considered for liver transplantation. Clinical HAV hepatitis in transplanted patients is rare, and when seen, is usually mild.

2.7. Prognosis

For the vast majority of patients, prognosis is good. Disease morbidity and mortality correlate with age *(4)*. Case fatality rates in infants and children up to age 14 yr is 0.1% *(28–30)*. For adolescents and young adults age 15–39 yr, the rate is 0.4%, whereas for adults above age 40 yr it is 1.1–2.7%. Superimposition of hepatitis A on chronic hepatitis B disease leads to higher peak aminotranferase levels, more severe disease, and may also increase the mortality rate *(31,32)*. In the United States there is up to a 58-fold increase in mortality with superimposed disease.

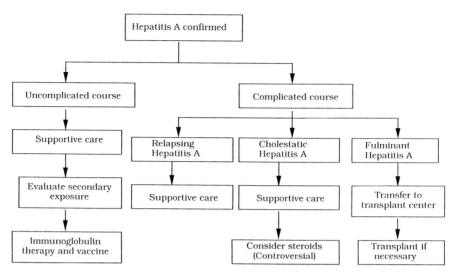

Fig. 2. A schematic plan for the treatment of hepatitis A.

2.8. Prevention

2.8.1. PASSIVE IMMUNIZATION (HUMAN SERUM IMMUNE GLOBULIN)

Human serum immune globulin is of greatest value when used before or within 2 wk of exposure to hepatitis A. It is not indicated for people who already have clinical manifestations of hepatitis A. The recommended dose for adults with travel plans to an endemic area is as follows: for a travel period of less than 3 mo: 0.02 mL/kg given intramuscularly; for a period of 3 mo or more: 0.06 mL/kg given intramuscularly. Doses should be repeated every 4–6 mo of stay, and doses over 10 mL should be divided over several sites. Human immune globulin decreases both the number and severity of infections when given according to this protocol.

2.8.2. ACTIVE IMMUNIZATION (HEPATITIS A VACCINE)

The recent development of an HAV vaccine makes prevention of this infection possible. Two formulations of hepatitus A vaccines are now available: a) Havrix by SmithKline Beecham Biologicals (Philadelphia, PA); b) Vaqta by Merck and Company: pediatric dose 0.5 mL (25 U) followed by a booster of 0.5 mL dose 6–18 mo later. Adults age 18 yr and older should receive a single 0.1 mL (50 U) dose followed by a booster 6 mo later. Immunity against HAV with the current vaccine is estimated to last 15–20 yr.

The vaccine is currently recommended for travelers going to an endemic area, especially military personnel. Other potential susceptible targets include day care center staff, health care workers, homosexual men who are sexually active, iv drug users, and family members of children in day care facilities.

2.9. Indications for Consulting the Subspecialist:

A gastroenterologist/hepatologist should be consulted when a patient with HAV infection develops encephalopathy or other signs of liver failure, has a chronic infection with hepatitis B, develops autoimmune hepatitis, or deteriorates for unclear reasons.

3. HEPATITIS E

3.1. Epidemiology

Hepatitis E is an RNA virus closely related to the calcivirus family. It is endemic to Asia, India, Mexico, Middle East, Pakistan, and the former Soviet Union, but is rare in the United

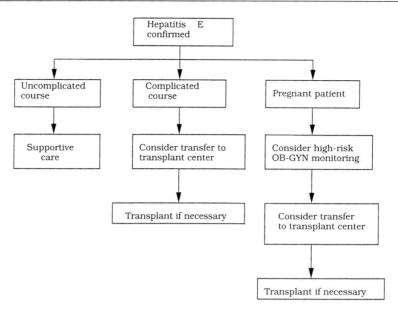

Fig. 4. A schematic plan for the treatment of hepatitis E.

that hepatitis E antibodies in affected individuals are protective against repeat exposure *(46)*. Travelers to endemic areas should be cautioned regarding consumption of water and salads from affected areas. Vaccine development efforts are underway, but not currently available.

3.8. Indications for Consulting the Subspecialist

Because of the high mortality, pregnant women suspected of having hepatitis E should be cared for in an institution capable of handling a high risk pregnancy with potential for liver failure. Any patient who exhibits signs of progressive liver decompensation should be referred to a subspecialist (*see* Chapter 30).

4. CYTOMEGALOVIRUS

4.1. Epidemiology

Cytomegalovirus (CMV) is a DNA virus that belongs to the herpes virus family. It requires close contact for transmission, so that crowded conditions are associated with increased rates of transmission of CMV. CMV can be acquired *in utero*, perinatally, intrafamilial, during transfusion or transplantation, or sexually *(47–49)*. In neonates, 1% of infections are acquired *in utero*, with 3–30% infected at birth *(47,48)*. Perinatal transmission may be acquired by ingestion of genital secretions during birth or by breast feeding from a CMV-excreting mother *(49,50)*. This perpetuates infection, since asymptomatic children can then transmit CMV via secretions to other susceptible hosts. Transmission via saliva on toys is possible *(9)*. In day care centers, shedding of CMV has been noted in up to 57% of children vs 8% in children cared for at home *(9)*. Once infected, the CMV DNA incorporates itself into the host cells and remains latent. Intermittent asymptomatic reactivations with viral shedding in urine and saliva are common. Host defenses control these reactivations in most cases. In pregnant patients, this can lead to fetal infection, but is felt to be less likely than with a primary infection. CMV can cause mild hepatitis in immunocompetent individuals, but tends to be more severe in immunocompromised patients. Prevalence of antibody to CMV is seen in over 80% of adults over age 40 yr. Reinfection of individuals with prior exposure is possible, particularly with a different strain of CMV.

4.2. Cardinal Signs and Symptoms

4.2.1. SYMPTOMS

Most cases are asymptomatic. Neonates with congenital exposure can present with hepatosplenomegaly and elevated aminotransferases. Hemolytic anemia may precipitate jaundice in patients with CMV hepatitis *(46)*. Some adult cases can be similar to infectious mononucleosis (IM). Fatigue, fever, and malaise are common *(51)*. In these cases, other somatic symptoms overshadow the CMV hepatitis. After primary infection, viral DNA persists and can reactivate at different times through out the patient's life, particularly when host immune systems are not able to keep the virus in check. Different CMV strains can cause disease flares in patients who are immune to other strains. Most infected infants will have no symptoms at birth, with only 5–10% exhibiting classic signs of infection. Classic CMV features include hepatosplenomegaly (75–90%), jaundice (60%), and thrombocytopenic purpura. Associated features include *(52)*, chorioretinitis, deafness, hemolytic anemia, low birth weights, microcephaly, periventricular calcifications, psychomotor retardation. CMV neonatal liver disease is seen 1 in 5000 births *(52,53)*.

4.2.2. PHYSICAL EXAMINATION

On physical examination, the liver tends to be smooth in contour. Pharyngitis and lymphadenopathy are less common than with mononucleosis. Portal hypertension without cirrhosis has been reported *(54)*. In neonates, congenital infections may manifest with hepatosplenomegaly (75–90%), jaundice (60%), and thrombocytopenic purpura lesions (*see* Section 4.2.1.).

4.3. Diagnosis

Diagnosis rests on changes in antibody status, virus isolation from tissue culture, or virus detection in blood, urine, saliva, or tissue samples in the presence of elevated liver serum enzymes (Fig. 5, diagnosis). The preferred method of detection in neonates is isolation of CMV from urine. Urine often contains the highest titers of the virus, and offers a simple source. Tissue biopsies and cultures of infected organs are particularly useful for the diagnosis in immunocompromised hosts. CMV cultures are done primarily on fibroblast monolayers. Evidence of CMV is provided by detection of its typical cytopathologic effect, but can take several weeks to be present. Liver serum enzyme tests can be mild to moderately elevated *(55)*. Elevated serum levels of both conjugated and unconjugated bilirubin are seen. Infected children are six times more likely to demonstrate abnormal serum liver tests *(56,57)*. Atypical-appearing lymphocytes can be seen on peripheral smears.

A liver biopsy can be helpful if classic "owl's eye" nuclear inclusions *(46)* are seen. Noncaseating granulomas and multinucleated giant cells have also been noted. Overall, the liver biopsy may demonstrate a nonspecific giant cell neonatal hepatitis-like picture *(47)*. Paucity of bile ducts has been associated with some cases of CMV infection *(56,58)*.

Patients who are infected congenitally are best diagnosed by detection of CMV in urine, thus avoiding the confounding issue of maternal antibodies. CMV IgM antibodies may also be used to detect acute infection or titers of CMV IgG may be followed. With recurrent infections in immunocompetent patients, IgM antibodies are not detected. However, in recurrent infections in renal transplant recipients, up to one third develop IgM antibodies.

4.4. Treatment

Congenital CMV and acquired CMV infections are both best treated with supportive measures (Fig. 6, treatment). Hospitalization may be required if there are persistently rising serum bilirubin levels, prolonged protime levels, evidence of hepatic encephalopathy, or other evi-

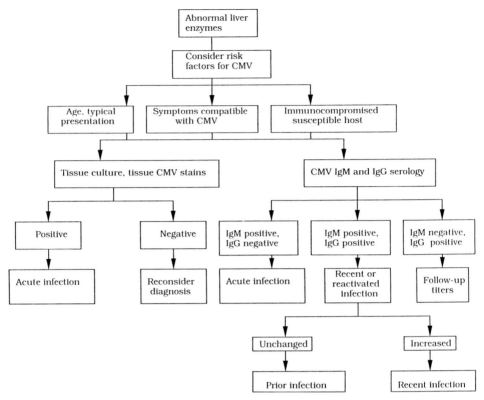

Fig. 5. A schematic plan for the diagnostic evaluation of CMV hepatitis.

dence of liver disease decompensation. Whether immunocompetent individuals with CMV hepatitis should be treated with specific anti-CMV medications is unclear *(59)*. In immunocompromised patients, treatment with such agents may be worthwhile. In transplant recipients, response rates of 70% have been reported *(59,60)*.

4.5. Potential Complications

The majority of neonatal cases recover without untoward effects, although a case of noncirrhotic portal hypertension has been described and a role in bile duct paucity has been suggested. Fatal cases of CMV hepatitis have been reported *(61,62)*. In addition, CMV-related biliary tract disease is not an uncommon presentation in HIV patients *(15)*. CMV hepatitis is uncommon in HIV-infected patients, but if present, is generally mild.

4.6. Prognosis

For the vast majority of immunocompetent patients, prognosis is good. Immunodeficient patients may have a more severe course due to lack of host immune factors. Pregnancy is a special situation because there is a 33% chance of CMV crossing the placenta, and a subsequent 10–15% chance of adversely affecting the fetus. In neonates, the disease usually resolves by the first year of life. CMV does not appear to be associated with progression to chronic liver disease.

4.7. Prevention

Because most infected patients are asymptomatic and may shed intermittently even after recovery, it is difficult to prevent exposures. Caregivers of identified infants should practice precautions if they are pregnant or immunocompromised.

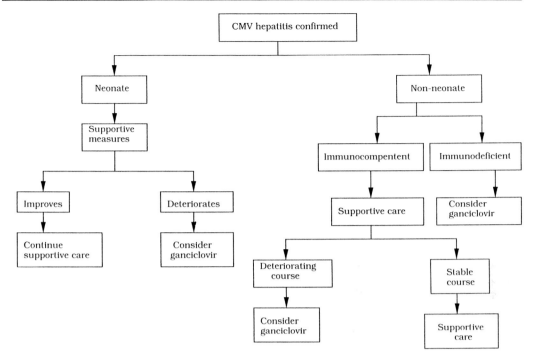

Fig. 6. A schematic plan for the treatment of CMV hepatitis.

4.8. Indications for Consulting the Subspecialist

Because of the extensive differential diagnosis of neonates with jaundice, these patients should be sent to a specialist. In older patients, only those who follow an atypical or fulminant course should be referred to a specialist.

5. EPSTEIN-BARR VIRUS

5.1. Epidemiology

Epstein-Barr virus (EBV), the causative agent of infectious mononucleosis, is a DNA virus and belongs to the herpes virus family. Saliva appears to be the primary vehicle for spread of EBV. Oral secretions contain the virus in 80% of patients with acute infectious mononucleosis *(63–65)*. Up to 20% of healthy adults have the virus detected in their saliva. Viral infection probably involves infection of oropharyngeal epithelial cells with secondary spread to B-lymphocytes. Free viral particles or B-lymphocytes then carry the infection to other organs. Typically, the viremia precedes clinical disease. There have been rare reports of transfusion-related disease acquisition *(66,67)*. EBV has been isolated from genital tract cultures, suggesting a possible sexual route for exposure as well *(68)*. Natural infection with EBV occurs during childhood. Severe disease is unusual but can be noted, especially with older patients. The incubation period is 4–7 wk in older children, but is shorter in infants. In the rare cases of hematological spread, incubation periods of 2–5 wk have been reported.

Infection occurs in younger age groups in underdeveloped countries and later in more developed countries. This explains the higher incidence in the latter areas of infections in patients who are in their late teens. Although the disease is endemic in some areas, no epidemics have been reported. Little data exists concerning the incidence of EBV hepatitis in HIV-infected individuals, but disease may be more severe in immunodeficient individuals.

Jaundice from EBV infection is infrequent and occurs in only 5% of patients, which is similar to the frequency with which it occurs in hepatitis A and hepatitis E *(69)*. In patients with depressed cell-mediated immunity, EBV hepatitis may cause life-threatening illness. EBV DNA persists for life in the host and can be detected during reactivations. Unlike the other self-limited viruses, EBV is linked to Burkitt's B-cell lymphoma and nasopharyngeal carcinoma as a causative agent.

5.2. Cardinal Signs and Symptoms

5.2.1. Symptoms

Most commonly, clinical EBV infection begins with the syndrome of infectious mono-nucleosis. Onset of symptoms typically involves a 3–5 d prodrome of anorexia, headache, malaise, and myalgias, followed by more pronounced signs of disease *(69,70)*. Fevers of 38–40°C are nearly always present. Chills may be reported. Sore throat, with exudative pharyngitis is seen in up to half of the patients. In adults over age 40 yr, atypical presentation of EBV infection with abdominal pain, and biliary tract like disease can be seen *(71–73)*. Liver involve-ment occurs in 90% of adolescents, but is overshadowed by complaints of fever, fatigue, sore throat, and lymphadenopathy *(70)*. Jaundice is not common. A rare case of severe cholestatic hepatitis from IM with a bilirubin of 658 μmol/L (38.5 mg/dL) has been noted due to a combination of hepatitis and hemolytic anemia *(67)*.

5.2.2. Physical Examination

Lymphadenopathy is primarily present in the posterior cervical area. Splenomegaly is detectable in up to 50% of patients by the second week. Other physical findings include periorbital edema in 20%, jaundice in 5–10%, hepatomegaly in 10–15%, and palatal petechiae in up to one third of the patients. Variable, transient generalized morbilliform rash, lasting 1–2 d is seen in 3–10%. Ampicillin use causes rash in 90%. Patients above age 30, may present with more atypical features, particularly, with jaundice, and may prompt work-up for extrahe-patic biliary obstruction *(71)*.

5.3. Diagnosis

The diagnosis rests on the demonstration of active or recent EBV infection and abnormal liver serum enzymes (Fig. 7, diagnosis). Laboratory parameters follow a typical hepatitis course with modest elevations in 80% of patients with AST and ALT of generally less than 500 IU/L. Total bilirubin levels range from 17–137 umol/L (1–8 mg/dL) *(74–76)*, and peak from the second to fourth week of disease. Alkaline phosphatase is generally mildly elevated. IgM-EBV viral capsid antigen (VCA) develops quickly and persists for weeks to months. The IgM-EBV VCA titer may be missed in up to 85%. IgG-EBV VCA may be detectable for life. The detection of IgM and IgG-EBV VCA antibodies in the absence of IgG-EBV nuclear antigen is diagnostic of primary infection.

Heterophile antibody tests rely on the detection of IgM to EBV. Seventy-five percent of patients have detectable levels of this antibody by the end of the first week of illness. By the third week, 85–90% will become positive *(70,77)*. The heterophile antibody test will remain positive for weeks to months after acute EBV infection. Monospot (hetero-phile agglutinin) testing can be negative in up to one sixth of patients in EBV hepatitis. Monospot testing can take up to 2–3 wk after symptoms to be positive and then persist positive up to 9 mo. Sensitivity of testing is only 80%, but specificity is 99%. Unlike CMV, EBV cannot be routinely cultured.

Leukocytosis can be seen in the range of 10,000–20,000/mm³. Atypical lymphocytes, also known as Downey cells, can compose 10–40% of the leukocyte count. Mild thromobocytopenia

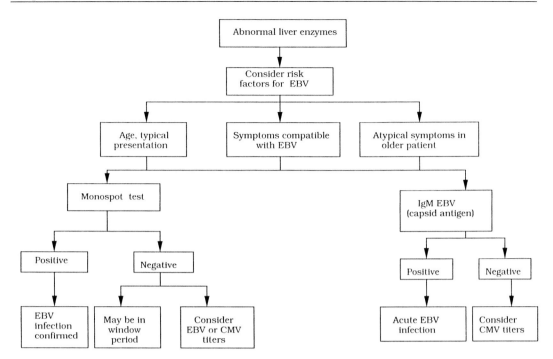

Fig. 7. A schematic plan for the diagnostic evaluation of EBV hepatitis.

of 50,000–200,000/mm^3 is seen in less than one half of the cases (69,70). Serologic diagnostic techniques are widely available and generally detectable within the second week of disease.

A liver biopsy is usually not necessary. However, if liver histology is obtained, the main feature is a pleomorphic cellular infiltrate that can be found to be expanding the portal tract and may extend into the sinusoid. Small areas of focal necrosis may be seen. Occasionally, large atypical lymphocytes may be present. Multinucleated giant cells are not seen. A distinguishing feature vs other hepatitis is the focal distribution of the necrosis. Cirrhosis has not been reported *(78)*.

5.4. Treatment

There is no specific therapy for mononucleosis. Treatment is generally supportive (Fig. 8, treatment). Acetaminophen should be used for symptom relief and aspirin should be avoided due to reports of Reye's syndrome being noted in patients with EBV *(79)*. Acyclovir does not appear to affect the course of illness *(80–84)*. In the rare case of impending airway obstruction, severe hemolytic anemia, or thrombocytopenia, prednisone at 40–60 mg/d for 5–7 d, then tapered over 2 wk may improve symptoms *(79)*. It is not clear if transplantation of a patient in the rare event of fulminant EBV infection would lead to predisposition to posttransplant immunoproliferative disorders.

5.5. Potential Complications

Fifty deaths from infectious mononucleosis have been reported, but hepatitis has been associated with only nine of these cases *(69,70)*. Congenital EBV is a potential result of development of primary EBV infection during a first trimester pregnancy, although only one case has been reported *(85–87)*. Fulminant EBV hepatitis has been reported, but is exceedingly rare. Abdominal complication, especially rupture of enlarged organs has been documented *(88)*.

22. Ramahan SM, Chira P, Koff RS. Idiopathic autoimmune hepatitis triggered by hepatitis A. Am J Gastro 1994;89:106-108.
23. Tong MJ, El-Farra NS, Grew MI. Clinical manifestations of hepatitis A: recent experience in a community teaching hospital. J Inf Dis 1995;171:S15-18.
24. Karayiannis P, Chitranukroh R, Fry M, Petrovic LM, Moore D, Scheuer PJ, Thomas HC. Protracted alanine aminotransferase levels in tamarins infected with hepatitis A virus. J. Med Virol 1990;30:151-158.
25. Brunt PW. Alcohol and chronic liver disease. J. Roy Coll Phys Lond. 1974;8:45-51.
26. Anonymous, How long should patients keep off alcohol after infectious hepatitis? Drug Ther Bull 1975;13:87,88.
27. Krieg D, Weigl E, Bach H. Prognosis of chronic hepatitis. Acta Hepatogastroenterol 1976;23:168-172.
28. McNeil M, Hoy JF, Richards MJ. Aetiology of fatal viral hepatitis in Melbourne: a retrospective study. Med J Aust 1984;141:637-640.
29. Papaevangelou G, Tassopoulos N, Roumeliotou-Karayannis A, Richarson C. Etiology of fulminant hepatitis in Greece. Hepatology 1984;4:369-372.
30. O'Grady J. Management of acute and fulminant hepatitis. Vaccine 1992;10:S21-23.
31. Zuckerman AJ. Viral hepatitis. Transfus Med 1993;3:7-19.
32. Keefe EB. Is hepatitis A more severe in patients with chronic hepatitis B than other chronic liver diseases? Am J Gastroenterol 1995;90:201-205.
33. Agarwal R, Naik SR. Hepatitis E: intrafamilial versus waterborne spread. J Hepatol 1994;21:718-723.
34. Wald A. Hepatitis E. Adv Pediatr Infect Dis 1995;10:157-166.
35. Bradley DW. Enterically transmitted non-A, non-B hepatitis. Br Med Bull 1990;46:442-461.
36. Velasquez O, Stetler HC, Avila C, Ornelas G, Alvarez C, Hadler SC, Bradley DW, Sepulveda J. Epidemic transmission of enterically transmitted non-A, non-B hepatitis in Mexico, 1986-1987. JAMA 1990;263:3281-3285.
37. Kane, MA, Bradley DW, Shrestha SM, Maynard JE, Cook EH, Mishra RP, Joshi DD. Epidemic non-A, non-B hepatitis in Nepal; recovery of a possible etiologic agent and transmission studies in marmosets. JAMA 1984;252;3140-3145.
38. Khuroo MS, Dar MY, Hepatitis E: evidence for person-to-person transmission and inability of a low dose immune serum globulin from an Indian source to stop it. Indian J. Gastroenterol 1992;11:113-116.
39. Mahon JB, Chernesky MA. Vertical transmission of viral hepatitis. Transfus Med Rev 1993;7:112-120.
40. Robson SC, Adams S, Brink N, et al. Hospital outbreak of hepatitis E. Lancet 1992;339:1424,1425.
41. Nanda SK, Ansari IH, Acharya SK. Protracted viremia during acute sporadic hepatitis E virus infection. Gastroenterology 1995;108:225-230.
42. Chauhan A, Jameel S, Dilwari JB, Chawla YK, Kaur U, Ganguly NK. Hepatitis E virus transmission to a volunteer. Lancet 1993;341:149,150.
43. Khuroo MS, Teli MR, Skidmore S, Sofi MA, Khuroo MI. Incidence and severity of viral hepatitis in pregnancy. Am J Med 1981;70:252-255.
44. Khuroo MS, Kamili S, Jameel S. Vertical transmission of hepatitis E Virus. Lancet 1995;345:1025,1026.
45. Arankalle VA, Jha J, Favoroc MO, Chaudhari A, Fields HA, Banerjee K. Contribution of HEV and HCV in causing fulminant non-A, non-B hepatitis in western India. J Viral Hep 1995;2:189-193.
46. Bryan JP, Tsarev SA, Iqbal M, Ticehurst J, Emerson S, Ahmed A, Duncan J, Rafiqui AR, Malik IA, Purcell RH;et al. Epidemic hepatitis   E in Pakistan patterns of serologic response and evidence that antibody to hepatitis E virus protects against disease. J. Infect Dis 1994;170:517-521.
47. Griffiths PD. Cytomegalovirus and the liver. Sem Liver Dis 1984;4:307-313.
48. Alford CA. An epidemiological review of intrauterine and perinatal infections of man. Mead Johnson Symp Perinat Dev Med 198;21:3–11.
49. Reynolds DW, Stagno S, Hosty TS, Tiller M, Alford CA Jr. Maternal cytomegalovirus excretion and perinatal infection. N Eng J Med 1973;289:1-5.
50. Satgnos S, Reynolds DW, Pass RF, Alford CA. Breast milk and the risk of cytomegalovirus infection. N Eng J Med 1980;302:1073-1076.
51. Weller TH. The cytomegaloviruses, ubiquitous agents with protean clinical manifestations. N End J Med 1971;285:203-224.
52. Hanshaw JB. Cytomegalovirus In: Remington JS, Klein JO, eds. Infectious Diseases of the Fetus and Newborn Infant. 2nd ed. Saunders, Philadelphia, 1983.
53. Danks DM, Campbell PE, Jack I. Studies of the aetiology of neonatal hepatitis and biliary atresia. Arch Dis Child 1977;52:360-367.
54. Dresler S, Linder D. Noncirrhotic portal fibrosis following neonatal cytomegalic inclusion disease. J. Pediatr 1978;93:887,888.
55. Hanshaw JB, Betts RF, Simon G, Boynton RC. Acquired cytomegalovirus infection: association with hepatosplenomegaly and abnormal liver-function tests. N Engl J Med 1965;272:602-609.

56. Oppenheimer EH, Esterly JR. Cytomegalovirus infection: a possible cause of biliary atresia. Am J Pathol 1973;71:2a.
57. Felber S, Sinatra F. Systemic disorders associated with neonatal cholestasis. Sem Liver Dis 1987;7: 108-118.
58. Finegold MJ, Carpenter RJ. Obliterative cholangitis due to cytomegalovirus: a possible precursor of paucity of intrahepatic bile ducts. Hum Pathol 1982; 13:662-665.
59. Erice A, Jordan MC, Chace BA, Fletcher C, Chinnock BJ, Balfour HH Jr. Ganciclovir treatment of cytomegalovirus: a possible precursor of paucity of intrahepatic bile ducts. Hum Pathol 1982;13:662-665.
60. Shaefer MS, Stratta RJ, Markin RS, Cushing KA, Woods GL, Reed EC, Wood RP, Langras AN, Ganciclovir therapy for cytomegalovirus disease in liver transplant recipients. Transpl Proc 191;23:1515,1516.
61. Shusterman NH, Frauenhoffer C, Kinsey MD. Fatal Massive hepatic necrosis in cytomegalovirus mononucleosis. Ann Intern Med 1978;88:810-812.
62. Tucciarone L, Felici W, Nigro G. Un caso di malattia citomegalica acquisita a decorso fatale. Riv Ital Pediatr 1989;15:643-646.
63. Henle W, Henle G. Epstein-Barr virus and infectious mononucleosis. N Engl J Med 1973;288:263-264.
64. Golden HD, Chang RS, Prescott W, Simpson E, Cooper TY. Leukocyte transforming agent: prolonged excretion by patients with mononucleosis and excretion b normal individuals. J Infect Dis 1973;127;471-473.
65. Niederman JC, Miller G, Pearson HA, Pagano JS, Dowaliby   JM. Infectious mononucleosis. Epstein-Barr virus shedding in saliva and oropharynx. N Engl J Med 1976;294:1355-1359.
66. Corey L, Stamm WE, Feorino PM, Bryan JA, Weseley S, Gregg MB, Solangi K. HBS Ag negativve hepatitis in a haemodialysis unit: relation to Epstein-Barr virus. N Engl J Med 1975; 293:1273-1278.
67. Madigan NP, Newcomer AD, Campbell DC, Taswell HF. Intense jaundice in infectious mononucleosis. Mayo Clin Proc 1973;48:857-862.
68. Durbin WA, Sullivan JL. Epstein-Barr virus infection. Ped Rev 1994;15:63-68.
69. White NJ, Juel-Jensen BE. Infectious mononucleosis hepatitis. Sem Liver Dis 1984;4:301-306.
70. Brady M. Epstein-Barr virus infection in children: implications for the treatment of infectious mononucleosis. J Pediatr Health Care 1994;8:233-235.
71. Horowitz CA, Henle W, Henle G. Infectious mononucleosis in older patients age 4-72 years. Report of 27 cases including three without heterophile antibody response. Medicine 1983;62:256-262.
72. Ansari A, Grotte M. Acute hepatitis as a primary manifestation of infectious mononucleosis in a 53 year old man. Am J Gastroenterol 1984;79:471-473.
73. Jacobson IM, Gang DL, Shapiro RH. Epstein-Barr viral hepatitis: an unusual case and review of the literature. Am J Gastroenterol 1984;79:628-632.
74. Hoagland RJ. Infectious mononucleosis. Grune and Stratton, New York 1967.
75. Kilpatrick ZM. Structural and functional abnormalities of liver in infectious mononucleosis. Arch Intern Med 1966;117:47-53.
76. Nelson RS, Darragh JH. Infectious mononucleosis hepatitis. Am J Med 1950;21:26-33.
77. Powell MA. Question and Answer. Infectious mononucleosis. J Am Acad Nurse Pract 1993;5:89-91.
78. Wadsworth RC, Keil PG. Biopsy of the liver in infectious mononucleosis. Am Fam Phys 1994;49:879-885.
79. Bailer ER, Diagnosis and treatment of infectious mononucleosis. Am Fam Phys 1994;49:879-885.
80. Andersson J, Ernberg I. Management of Epstein-Barr virus infections. Am J Med 1988;85:107-115.
81. Andersson J, Britton S, Ernberg I, Andersson U, Henle W, Skoldenberg B, Tisell A. Effect of acyclovir on infectious mononucleosis: a double-blind, placebo-controlled study. J Infect Dis 1986;153:283-290.
82. Andersson J, Skoldenberg B, Henle W. Acyclovir treatment in infectious mononucleosis: a clinical and virological study. Infection 1987;15:S14-20.
83. Van der horst C, Joncas J, Ahronheim G, Gustafson N, Stein G, Gurwith M, Fleisher G, Sullivan J, Sixbey J, Roland S, et al. Lack of affect of peroral acyclovir for the treatment of acute infectious mononucleosis. J Infect Dis 1991;164:788-792.
84. Lowe L, Hebert AA, Duvie M. Gianotti-Cristi syndrome associated with Epstein-Barr virus infection. J Am Acad Dermatol 1989;29:336-338.
85. Costa S, Barrasso R, Terzano P, Zerbini M, Carpi C, Musiani M, et al. Detection of active Epstein-Barr virus infection in pregnant women. Eur J Clin Microbiol 1985;4:335, 336.
86. Goldberg GN, Fulginiti VA, Ray CG, Ferry P, Jones JF, Cross H, Minnich L. In utero Epstein-Barr virus (infectious mononucleosis) infection. JAMA 1981;246:1579-1581.
87. Joncas JH, Alfieri C, Leyritz-Wills M, Brochu P, Jasmin G, Boldogh I, Huang ES. Simultaneous congenital infection with Epstein-Barr virus and cytomegalovirus. N Engl J Med 1981;304:1399-1403.
88. Robinson RG. Abdominal complications of infectious mononucleosis. J Am Board Fam Pract 1988;1:207-210.
89. Sakamoto T, Uemure M, Fukui H, Yoshikawa M, Fukui K, Kinoshita K, Kojima H, Matsumori T, Tsujii T, Sumazaki R. Chronic active Epstein-Barr hepatitis in an adult. Intern Med 1992;31:1190-1196.
90. Haines JD Jr. When to resume sports after infectious mononucleosis. How soon is safe? Postgrad Med 1987;81:331-333.

9 Acute and Chronic Hepatitis B and D

Steven A. Rogers and T. Jake Liang

CONTENTS

1. INTRODUCTION

Viral hepatitis represents a diverse spectrum of clinical syndromes caused by a group of distinct viruses. All of the five well-characterized hepatitis viruses (A through E) are associated with acute hepatitis, whereas only hepatitis B virus (HBV), hepatitis C virus (HCV), and hepatitis D virus (HDV, delta agent) can cause chronic hepatitis (Table 1).

2. EPIDEMIOLOGY

HBV and HDV are percutaneously transmitted viruses. Transmission of HBV occurs through exposure to infectious blood, blood products, and contaminated instruments. Sexual contact in both heterosexual and homosexual populations is the most commonly recognized mode of transmission. Specific populations at high risk of exposure to HBV include iv drug users, homosexual men, individuals engaged in promiscuous heterosexual contact, health care workers, and children born to chronically infected mothers. However, the prevalence of infection with HBV among the general population is quite high; it is estimated that in volunteer blood donors the prevalence of exposure to HBV (i.e., prevalence of anti-HBs) ranges from 5–10% in the United States (1). The probability of progression from acute hepatitis B to chronic infection varies widely depending upon the age and the immune status of the infected individual. Whereas an immunocompetent adolescent or middle-aged individual has approx a 5–10% chance of developing chronic infection, a baby born to a mother with chronic hepatitis B (HBeAg+) has about a 90% chance of developing chronic infection (2). Additionally, immunosuppressed patients or individuals with comorbid illnesses are at greater risk of developing chronic hepatitis B infection.

Transmission of HDV is similar to HBV, although is far less prevalent than HBV worldwide. Approximately 5% of HBV carriers worldwide are infected with HDV (3). Although

From: *Diseases of the Liver and Bile Ducts: Diagnosis and Treatment*
Edited by: G. Y. Wu and J. Israel © Humana Press Inc., Totowa, NJ

Table 1

Characteristics of Hepatitis B and D

	Hepatitis B	Hepatitis D
Nucleic acid	DNA (Partially double stranded)	RNA (Circular)
Viral structural proteins	Surface (HBsAg), Core (HBcAg)	HDAg
Transmission	Percutaneous	Percutaneous
Chronic infection	Yes (5–90%)	Yes
Fulminant hepatitis	<1%	Up to 15%

percutaneous transmission is the primary mode of transmission, in Mediterranean countries, HDV infection is endemic among those infected with HBV, and transmission is frequently by nonparenteral routes, particularly close contact. In the United States, outbreaks of coinfection with HBV and HDV in urban areas have been reported in iv drug users and their sexual partners *(4)*. Interestingly, the course of disease in these outbreaks was very severe with a high incidence of fulminant hepatitis *(5)*.

3. CLINICAL SYNDROMES

3.1. Acute HBV Infection

3.1.1. CARDINAL SIGNS AND SYMPTOMS

3.1.1.1. Symptoms. The clinical presentation of uncomplicated acute viral hepatitis is similar, regardless of viral etiology. However, in the vast majority of cases, acute HBV infection is clinically silent, particularly when acquired early in life. When symptoms do occur, they are usually self-limited, lasting less than 4–6 mo in most immunocompetent adults. After an incubation period of approx 2–3 mo, prodromal symptoms occur including general malaise, anorexia, nausea, vomiting, low-grade fever, alteration in taste and smell, and right upper quadrant or epigastric discomfort. After approximately 2 wk, these symptoms abate and jaundice may develop. Typically, jaundice is mild and lasts no longer than 1 mo.

3.1.1.2. Physical Examination. Physical examination is often unrevealing. Lymphadenopathy, hepatomegaly, and splenomegaly are occasionally present, but marked organomegaly is unusual. Patients tend to have right upper quadrant tenderness. Icterus is only seen in patients with moderate to severe hepatitis (total bilirubin >3 mg/dL). Low grade fever is common in acute phase. Nonspecific rash is occasionally present and spider angioma is rarely found in self-limited acute hepatitis. In patients presenting with fulminant hepatitis, abnormal neurological examinations including asterixis, and fetor hepaticus are often present. Skin rashes typical of immune complex diseases can be the only physical findings of acute HBV infection.

3.1.2. CLINICAL VARIANTS

Unusual clinical variants of acute hepatitis B have been described. A prolonged period of jaundice during acute, self-limited hepatitis (cholestatic hepatitis) has been reported. Additionally, immune complex phenomenon has been associated with acute hepatitis B *(6)*. A serum sickness-like syndrome has been recognized occurring before jaundice *(7)*. Polyarteritis nodosa characterized by generalized vasculitis can appear in the course of infection. Glomerulonephritis has been associated with both chronic and acute infection, particularly in children.

3.1.3. COMPLICATIONS

Fulminant hepatitis with acute liver failure occurs in less than 1% of all cases of acute hepatitis B *(8)*. It is characterized by sudden and progressive liver dysfunction and massive necrosis of liver tissue with a mortality of approx 85%. Occurrence of encephalopathy within 8 wk of the onset of symptoms defines fulminant hepatitis.

3.2. Chronic HBV Infection

3.2.1. CARDINAL SIGNS AND SYMPTOMS

3.2.1.1. Symptoms. Chronic infection with HBV has been defined serologically by persistence of HBsAg for 6 mo after the onset of acute infection. In the majority of cases, chronic hepatitis B infection is asymptomatic, often coming to medical attention when serum liver enzymes tests are obtained during a routine examination or during a screening evaluation for insurance eligibility. When symptoms accompany chronic infection, they are often nonspecific with fatigue, general malaise, and anorexia being the most common presenting complaints. Occasionally, the patient might experience persistent or intermittent jaundice after a recognized attack of acute hepatitis.

3.2.1.2. Physical Examination. Physical findings in patients chronically infected with HBV are rather variable, mostly depending on severity of liver diseases and other associated conditions. Chronic stigmata of liver diseases including spider angiomas, palmar erythema, peripheral edema, ascites, splenomegaly (hepatomegaly is often absent in patients with cirrhosis), and gynecomastia are commonly present in patients with decompensated liver disease. Skin rashes consistent with immune complex disease can be seen in patients with associated hematological conditions, such as mixed cryoglobulinemia.

3.2.2. COMPLICATIONS

A serious complication of chronic infection is the development of cirrhosis with decompensated liver disease, which may occur in up to 25% of those chronically infected with HBV. The clinical signs of cirrhosis usually develop 10–30 yr after the onset of hepatitis B infection. When superinfection with HDV occurs, a more rapid progression to cirrhosis generally occurs. A more serious complication of chronic hepatitis B infection is hepatocellular carcinoma (HCC). Risk factors associated with the development of HCC include acquisition of hepatitis B infection early in life, pre-existing immunocompromised condition, and male gender (9). In the United States, HCC occurs almost exclusively in patients who have already progressed to cirrhosis. In endemic areas, HCC can occur in the absence of cirrhosis, whereas it is often associated with other risk factors for HCC, such as aflatoxin and HCV coinfection.

3.3. Hepatitis D Virus Infection

3.3.1. CARDINAL SIGNS AND SYMPTOMS

3.3.1.1. Symptoms. HDV requires the helper function of the hepatitis B virus and, therefore, does not by itself cause infection. The presence of hepatitis D virus can alter the clinical expression of disease in an individual infected with HBV (4). Acute infection from HDV can either occur concurrently with acute hepatitis B infection (coinfection) or superimposed upon chronic HBV infection (superinfection). Coinfection is often clinically and biochemically identical to acute HBV infection, although coinfection has been associated with a higher incidence of severe and fulminant hepatitis (10). Overall, mortality rates of coinfected patients are higher than in acute hepatitis B infection alone. Interestingly, coinfection is not associated with a higher frequency of progression to chronic infection. However, coinfected individuals who progress to chronic hepatitis are more likely to develop cirrhosis than individuals chronically infected with HBV alone (11).

Acquisition of HDV in an individual chronically infected with HBV (superinfection) is often clinically apparent by a sudden, unexplained clinical and biochemical deterioration in a previously stable patient. As with coinfection, the likelihood of severe hepatitis and fulminant hepatitis are increased in superinfection.

3.3.1.2. Physical Examination. Physical findings are similar to those of acute and chronic HBV infection. There are no distinguishing features.

3.3.2. COMPLICATIONS

Superinfection has been associated with more severe hepatitis and a higher frequency of fulminant hepatitis than infection with HBV alone and coinfection. The role of HDV in the development of HCC is unclear. Theoretically, it can act as a promoting factor by potentiating the progression to cirrhosis.

4. DIAGNOSIS

4.1. Laboratory Features

In acute hepatitis B infection, there are both virus-specific and nonspecific laboratory features. The aminotransferases are usually elevated as in other forms of hepatic inflammation and injury, but the degrees can be quite variable. The earliest abnormality tends to be elevation of the serum aminotransferase levels (ALT, AST), which reflect hepatic inflammation in the prodromal phase of infection. During acute viral hepatitis, the ALT levels are usually greater than the AST levels, and peak ALT values can be greater than 1000 IU/L. Following these elevations is a gradual rise in the serum bilirubin level with jaundice becoming apparent when the level exceeds 2.5 mg/dL. In severe hepatitis, hepatic synthetic function may be impaired resulting in reduced serum albumin level and prolongation of the prothrombin time can be observed.

Serologic markers are diagnostic for HBV infection (Table 2). The earliest marker of acute infection, preceding most biochemical abnormalities and clinical signs of infection, is the surface antigen of the virus, HBsAg (*see* Chapter 3). The serologic detection of this antigen usually precedes all other biochemical features by several weeks. In a typical case of acute hepatitis B, resolution of infection is heralded by the disappearance of HBsAg, and the appearance of antibody to HBsAg (anti-HBs). Anti-HBs is a neutralizing antibody to HBV, and is the sole antibody produced during vaccination. Approximately 2 wk after the appearance of HBsAg in the serum, the next viral-specific marker is the antibody to the viral core protein (anti-HBc). During acute hepatitis B, the anti-HBc is of the IgM class; as the infection resolves, the IgG class predominates and remains detectable for years. Detecting anti-HBc can be clinically useful in two clinical situations. First, IgM anti-HBc may help differentiate acute HBV from chronic HBV infection presenting with another cause of acute hepatitis—drugs, other hepatitis viruses, and so on. Detecting IgM anti-HBc will be diagnostic for acute HBV infection, whereas in chronic HBV infection, only IgG anti-HBc will be present. Second, unusual cases of acute hepatitis have been reported in which the HBsAg level is undetectable or there is a prolonged delay between the disappearance of HBsAg and the detection of anti-HBs in the "window period." In these situations, acute hepatitis B infection can be diagnosed by detecting IgM class of anti-HBc.

Another useful serologic marker in acute and chronic HBV is hepatitis e antigen (HBeAg). Its detection in serum implies active viral replication and high infectivity to individuals who do not possess immunity to HBV (i.e., who are anti-HBs negative). During typical acute infection, HBeAg is present early, about the same time as HBsAg, and disappears within several weeks as the illness resolves with seroconversion to anti-HBe. This serologic marker is particularly valuable in patients with chronic infection, because it indicates active viral replication, ongoing liver injury, and a highly infective state. As patients respond to treatment or spontaneous improvement, HBeAg disappears from serum and antibody to it (anti-HBe) becomes detectable suggesting a quiescent state of the infection.

Table 2

Common Serologic Patterns of HBV and HDV Infection

	HBsAg	Anti-HBs	Anti-HBc	HBeAg	Anti-HBe	Anti-HDV
Acute hepatitis B	+	-	+ (IgM)	+	-	-
Resolved Hepatitis B	-	+	+ (IgG)	-	+	-
HBV vaccine response	-	+	-	-	-	-
Chronic HBV infection (high infectivity)	+	-	+ (IgG)	+	-	-
Chronic HBV infection (low infectivity)	+	-	+ (IgG)	-	+	-
Acute coinfection with HBV and HDV	+	-	+ (IgM)	+	-	+
Superinfection with HBV and HDV	+	-	+ (IgG)	-	+/-	+

Complementing the traditional serologic and biochemical tests of HBV infection are commercially available molecular assays used to detect HBV DNA in the serum. Direct determination of the titer of HBV DNA in the serum gives a quantitative measurement of the level of HBV replication and can be used to monitor a patient's response to treatment. The powerful technique of polymerase chain reaction (PCR) which can amplify trace quantities of viral DNA has been adapted to HBV diagnosis. In some cases, low levels of persistent HBV infection can only be diagnosed through the use of this sensitive technique.

Specific viral markers of HDV infection are limited to the detection of antibodies to HDV antigen (anti-HDV) (Table 2). Generally, no distinction is made between classes of antibodies, and total anti-HDV levels are routinely reported by most commercial laboratories. During coinfection with HBV, level of anti-HDV might only be detected transiently, and at low titer making diagnosis difficult. In superinfection, anti-HDV is easily detectable early in infection and remains in the serum for a prolonged period of time.

4.2. Virologic Variants

It had previously been assumed that the clinical course of hepatitis B virus infection is solely dependent upon the host's immune response to the virus and not to specific characteristics of the virus itself. An exception to this has been the demonstration of the impact of a mutant form of hepatitis B virus on disease expression. A HBV mutant, particularly prevalent in the Mediterranean regions, leads to an altered serologic pattern during infection and is possibly associated with a more severe form of chronic infection (12). This mutant results from a single nucleotide alteration in the viral genome that leads to a premature termination signal of the precore region, thus preventing HBeAg synthesis. The rather atypical serologic features of infection with this precore mutation are high levels of HBV DNA, the absence of HBeAg, and the presence of anti-HBe in the serum. For unclear reasons, infection with this HBV mutant has been postulated to be associated with severe chronic hepatitis B, an accelerated course to cirrhosis, and a poor response to antiviral therapy.

5. PREVENTION

Currently there are two forms of immunization against HBV infection: active vaccination with recombinant HBsAg (13) and passive immunization is available with high-titer anti-HBs immune globulin (HBIG) (Table 3). Standard vaccination involves three intramuscular injec-

Table 3

Recommendation for Immunoprophylaxis after Percutaneous Exposure

Status of exposed individual	Status of exposure source	Treatment
Unvaccinated	HBsAg (+)	HBIG and HBV vaccine
	HBsAg (-)	HBV vaccine
	Unknown HBV status	HBV vaccine
Previously vaccinated	HBsAg (+)	Check serum anti-HBs titer. If <10, treated as if unvaccinated
	HBsAg (-)	No treatment
	Unknown HBV status	No treatment

tions (deltoid, not gluteal) of HBV vaccine at 0, 1, and 6 mo. It should be given to high risk individuals, including health care workers, dialysis patients, hemophiliacs, iv drug users, individuals with a history of sexual promiscuity, and close contacts of chronic HBV carriers. Because vaccination strategies targeting high risk individuals have been largely successful, it is now recommended that HBV vaccination be incorporated into the standard immunization program for all infants in the United States.

The HBV vaccine currently available is a recombinant vaccine, and the recommended dose for each injection is 10–20 mg for adults and 40 mg for immunosuppressed individuals *(14)*. Anti-HBs titers should be determined in all immunized individuals approx 1 mo after the third injection to confirm seroconversion. Side-effects from the vaccine are infrequent and include soreness at the injection site, malaise, and rarely low-grade fevers. It is generally recommended that anti-HBs titer should be checked 5–10 yr after adequate immunization and, if the titer falls below 10 IU/L, a booster dose should be given. For those who do not respond to standard HBV vaccine (5%), a new vaccine including additional viral antigens will soon be available.

Active HBV immunoglobulins (HBIG) are recommended for nonimmune individuals who are exposed to HBV contaminated fluids or material. HBIG in a dose for adults of 0.06 mL/kg given intramuscularly is given along with a complete course of HBV vaccine as soon as possible after exposure. Concurrent administration of the first dose of the vaccine and HBIG is advisable as long as different sites of immunization are used. These guidelines are also applicable to individuals exposed by sexual contact to a chronic HBV carrier as well as infants born to HBsAg-positive mothers. If an individual sustains an exposure to a source for which the HBV status is unknown, a complete course of HBV vaccine is recommended. Previously vaccinated individuals should have the serum anti-HBs titer determined after exposure. If their antibody levels are below 10 IU/L, a complete course of HBV vaccine is indicated. For HBsAg-positive patients undergoing liver transplantation, administration of high dose HBIg has been recommended to prevent re-infection of the transplanted liver and to reduce mortality *(15,16)*. The recommended dose is 10,000 IU iv HBIG perioperatively during the anhepatic phase, and 10,000 IU iv during each of the first 6 d postop. 10,000 IU anti-HBs Ig were given iv whenever the circulating anti-HBs antibody concentration fell below 100 IU/L during follow-up.

6. TREATMENT

6.1. Acute Infection

Acute infection with HBV is usually a self-limited illness and can be managed as an outpatient. The cornerstone of treatment of acute hepatitis B infection is supportive, as no specific therapy exists in this setting. Management consists of maintaining adequate nutrition, palliating symptoms, avoiding and limiting spread of infection to contacts. Hospitalization is generally limited to severe cases characterized by marked prolongation of the prothrombin time (>5 s above control), encephalopathy, ascites, edema, inability to maintain adequate hydration, hypoglycemia, or hypoalbuminemia. Additionally, individuals with debilitating comorbid illness, and immunocompromised or elderly patients might be easier to manage as inpatients. No specific diet appears to alter the course of acute infection, although a high-calorie diet is recommended. Exercise can be continued as tolerated, although most patients prefer bed rest. Corticosteroid therapy is not indicated in acute hepatitis B and, in some cases, might exacerbate the course of disease. Any potentially hepatotoxic medication should be avoided, including alcohol and acetaminophen. Oral contraceptives can be continued.

Certain medications can be safely administered in acute hepatitis B infection, particularly to alleviate the symptoms of nausea, vomiting and, occasionally, pruritus. Antiemetics can be used judiciously. Agents such as trimethobenzamide (Tigan) or metoclopramide (Reglan) should be used instead of phenothiazines which have been associated with cholestatic hepatitis in up to 1% of patients. In those patients with cholestasis and pruritus, cholestyramine (Questran) at doses of up to one packet mixed in water four times a day is often effective.

Although every effort should be made to limit the spread of infection to contacts, it is not necessary to isolate patients with acute hepatitis B infection. Caregivers should avoid direct contact with blood or body fluids and sexual activity should be avoided until the illness completely resolves.

For outpatients, regular assessment of severity of symptoms and identification of complications should be performed on each office visit. Laboratory data useful to follow in acute infection include the serum aminotransferase levels that correlate with ongoing inflammation, and the prothrombin time and serum albumin that reflect hepatic synthetic function. HBsAg should be repeated after clinical resolution of acute infection, and followed until seroconversion to anti-HBs. In patients with persisting HBsAg for longer than 6 mo after onset of acute infection and with sustained elevation of liver function tests, a liver biopsy should be considered.

6.2. Chronic Hepatitis

Currently interferon-α is the only approved medication for the treatment of chronic viral hepatitis. Interferons are a family of cytokines that produce a variety of immunomodulatory and antiviral effects. By binding to specific receptors on the cell surface, interferons increase the activity of macrophages and cytotoxic T-cells, which mediate the destruction of virus-infected cells. Additionally, interferons directly inhibit viral replication in infected cells.

Interferon-α given intramuscularly at either 5 million units (MU) five times a week or 10 MU three times a week for 4 mo induces a remission in approx 30% of treated patients with chronic hepatitis B infection (17) (Table 4). Side effects are common in patients on this dosage. For patients with intolerable side effects, dosage can be reduced to five million units three times a week for 6–12 mo with similar efficacy. Remission has traditionally been defined as the loss of HBeAg, and HBV DNA, and is associated with biochemical, histological, and clinical improvement. A true cure of the HBV infection is the elimination of HBsAg from the serum and the appearance of anti-HBs, which eventually occurs in approx 65% of the responders at 5 yr after treatment (9). Typical of a response to interferon is an elevation of the serum aminotransferase levels approx 8–10 wk after treatment (18). This response likely reflects immune clearance of infected hepatocytes and often predicts a long-term remission.

Several factors have been identified that predict a high likelihood of response to interferon. These include a serum alanine aminotransferase level greater than 100 IU/L, a serum HBV DNA level less than 200 pg/mL, female gender, onset of disease in adulthood, liver histology without cirrhosis, and absence of antibody to HIV and anti-HDV.

Table 4

Recommended Dosing of Interferon-Alpha for Chronic Hepatitis B

Dose: 5 million units five times a week or 10 million units three times a week.

Duration: 4–6 mo.

However, intolerable side effects are common with these regimens. Side effects are common in patients on this dosage. For patients with intolerable side effects, dosage can be reduced to 5 million units three times a week for 6–12 mo with similar efficacy.

Monitoring: complete blood counts weekly for 4 wk, then monthly serum aminotransferases; HBeAg, HBV DNA, HBsAg, and anti-HBs at completion of course. Thyroid function tests should be obtained at the pretreatment stage as well as half-way during the treatment.

Side effects from interferon treatment are quite common, but minor, and only in less than 1% of the cases requires discontinuation of therapy. The most common side effects include flu-like symptoms which are dose-dependent and often respond to acetaminophen treatment given before each dose of interferon. Other side effects include diarrhea, alopecia, lethargy, nausea, and a variety of neuropsychiatric effects such as irritability, insomnia, difficulty concentrating, and depression (17). Additionally, interferon treatment can induce autoimmune thyroiditis. Thyroid function tests should be obtained at the pretreatment stage as well as half-way during the treatment. Because granulocytopenia and thrombocytopenia can occur during treatment, blood counts need to be monitored during interferon therapy. The interferon dose should be decreased by 50% if the granulocyte count drops below $750/mm^3$ or the platelet count drops below $50,000/mm^3$. Interferon should be stopped if these counts fall below $500/mm^3$ and $30,000/mm^3$, respectively. Retinal hemorrhage and hearing impairment are major, but uncommon complications.

Attempts to augment the effectiveness of interferon have included adding other agents to the standard interferon regimen. One popular approach has been to add a tapering course of prednisone for 6 wk prior to the institution of interferon treatment (19). Particularly in patients with serum aminotransferase levels less than 100 IU/L, prednisone priming may enhance viral replication and immune responsiveness to interferon therapy. Such an approach must be undertaken only with extreme caution as steroid use in the setting of chronic hepatitis B may precipitate deterioration of liver function, leading to increased fatality. Higher doses of interferon have also been used in patients who fail to respond to standard doses. This approach, however, is associated with greater toxicity and only marginally increases the response rate.

Other agents being investigated include interferon-β, thymosin, and nucleoside analogs. The nucleoside analog, lamivudine, administered as an oral agent, has shown considerable promise in clinical trials (20).

Liver transplantation is recommended for end-stage liver disease. One-year survival in patients transplanted for chronic HBV is worse than in patients transplanted for other liver diseases, mainly because of increased morbidity and mortality associated with reinfection of the graft. However, re-infection appears to be less common in patients with fulminant hepatitis B. Immunoprophylaxis is recommended to prevent of reinfection (see Section 5.).

Treatment for HDV infection is generally targeted at the HBV coinfection. Therefore, treatment options are similar to those outlined for HBV; however, only interferon-alpha has been shown to have some benefits. In general, HDV infection appears to be more resistant to treatment.

SUMMARY

Acute infection with hepatitis B virus is usually self-limited or asymptomatic. However, it can lead to chronic illness with progressive liver injury.

Hepatitis D virus requires HBV coinfection and it can cause chronic hepatitis.

Simultaneous acquisition of HBV and HDV (coinfection) is associated with severe or fulminant hepatitis and a higher fatality rate than infection with HBV alone.

Clinical deterioration in a patient with chronic HBV infection should raise the possibility of HDV superinfection.

Acute and chronic HBV infection can be diagnosed by the use of specific, widely available serologic tests.

A vaccine against HBV is available and is safe and highly effective in preventing HBV and HDV infection.

Treatment for acute HBV infection is supportive; treatment of chronic HBV infection with IFN-α is successful in approx 30% of individuals.

REFERENCES

1. Margolis HS, Alter MJ, Hadler SC. Hepatits B. Evolving epidemiology and implications for control. Sem Liver Dis 1991;11:84–92.
2. de Franchis R, Meucci G, Vecchi M. The natural history of asymptomatic hepatitis B surface antigen carriers. Ann Int Med 1993;118:191–194.
3. Dusheiko G. Rolling review–the pathogenesis, diagnosis and management of viral hepatitis. Alimentary Pharmacol Therapeut 1994;8:229.
4. Lattau L, McCarthy J, Smith M. Outbreak of severe hepatits due to delta and hepatitis B viruses in parental drug abusers and their contacts. N Eng J Med 1987;317:1256.
5. Hadler S, DeMonzon M. Delta virus infection and severe hepatits: an epidemic in Yupca Indians of Venezuela. Ann Int Med 1984;100:339.
6. Gocke D. Immune complex phenomena associated with hepatitis. In: Vyas CS, Schmid R, eds. Viral hepatitis: a contemporary assessment of etiology, epidemiology, pathogenesis and prevention. Franklin Institute Press, Philadelphia; 1978; p. 277.
7. Shusterman N, Landon WT. Hepatitis B and immune complex disease. N Eng J Med 1984;55:19–35.
8. Katelaris P, Jones D. Fulminant hepatic failure. Med Clin North Am 1989;73:1989.
9. Koprenmann J, Baker B, Waggoner J, Everhart J, DiBisceglie A. Long-term remission in chronic hepatitis B after alpha interferon therapy. Ann Int Med 1991;114:629–634.
10. Hoofnagel J. Type D (delta) hepatitis JAMA 1989;261:1321.
11. Smedile A, Verme G, Cargnel A. Influence of delta infection on severity of hepatitis B. Lancet 1982;2:945.
12. Liang TJ, Hasegawa K, Rimon N, Wands JR, Ben-Porath E. A hepatitis B virus mutant associated with an epidemic of fulminant hepatitis B. N Engl J Med 1991;324:1705–1709.
13. Dienstag J, Werner B, Polk B. Hepatitis B vaccine in health care personnel: safety, immunogenicity, and indicators of efficacy. Ann Int Med 1984;101:34–40.
14. Szmuness W, Stevens C, Harley E. Hepatitis B vaccine: demonstration of efficacy in a controlled clinical trial in a high-resk population in the United States. N Engl J Med 1980;303:833.
15. Samuel D, Bismuth A, Mathieu D. Passive immunoprophylaxis after liver transplantation in HBsAg-positive patients. Lancet 1991;337:813–815.
16. Samule D, Muller R, Alexander G. Liver transplantation in European patients with hepatitis B surface antigen. N Engl J Med 1993;329:1842–1847.
17. Renault P, Hoofnagle J, Park T. Psychiatric complications of long-term interferon alpha therapy. Arch Int Med 1987;147:1577–1580.
18. Lai C, Lok A, Lin H. Placebo-controlled trial of recombinant alpha-2 interferon in Chinese HBsAg carrier children. Lancet 1987;2:877–880.
19. Perrillo R, Regenstein F, Peters M. Prednisone withdrawl followed by recobinant alpha interferon in the treatment of chronic type B hepatitis: a randomized, controlled trial. Ann Int Med 1988;109:95–100.
20. Dienstag JL, Perrillo RP, Schiff ER, Bartholomew M, Vicary C, Rubin M. A preliminary trial of lamivudine for chronic hepatitis B infection. N Engl J Med 1995;333:1657–1661.

10   Hepatitis C and G

Gabu Bhardwaj, Gary L. Davis,
and Johnson Y. N. Lau

CONTENTS

1. INTRODUCTION TO THE HEPATITIS C VIRUS

After the discovery of hepatitis B and A viruses in the 1960s and early 1970s, it became obvious there still were many cases of clinical viral hepatitis, particularly posttransfusion hepatitis, that could not be accounted for by either of these viruses. Hence, the term non-A, non-B hepatitis (NANBH) was coined to represent those as yet unidentified hepatitis viruses. In the late 1970s and early 1980s, a series of elegant experiments, done mainly by Bradley et al. at the Centers for Disease Control and Prevention *(1,2)*, established the transmissibility and the physicochemical properties of this infectious parenteral NANB hepatitis agent. In 1986, interferon-alpha was reported to be useful in patients with chronic NANB hepatitis, even before the etiologic agent was identified. In 1989, the major parenteral NANB hepatitis agent, now designated as hepatitis C virus (HCV) was identified *(3)*. The disease non-A, non-B hepatitis is now called hepatitis C.

2. VIROLOGY

HCV is an RNA virus and a member of the flaviviridae family that includes members such as yellow fever, dengue, and Japanese encephalitis viruses (Fig. 1). Because of its diversity, HCV has been classified into six different genotypes and a series of subtypes *(4)*. The nomen-

From: *Diseases of the Liver and Bile Ducts: Diagnosis and Treatment*
Edited by: G. Y. Wu and J. Israel © Humana Press Inc., Totowa, NJ

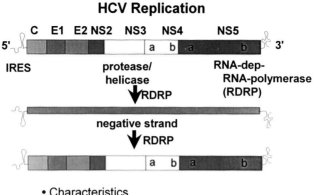

HCV Replication

- Characteristics
  - High nucleotide substitution rate
  - A heterogeneous virus

Fig. 1. The replication strategy of HCV. HCV virus produces a negative strand template (with the 5' end of RNA corresponding to the 3' end of the virus and vice versa). This template serves as the backbone for the production of more positive-strand RNA, the viral genome itself. The copying between RNA-positive and RNA-negative stranded RNAs occurs through the viral RNA-dependent RNA polymerase (RDRP). This type of enzyme, in general, lacks proofreading activity and, hence, HCV is genetically

clature of HCV-genotypes has been very confusing. At present, the system proposed by Simmonds et al. *(5)*, is the most accepted system. Different geographic regions have different patterns of genotype prevalence (*see* Fig. 2). In the United States, HCV genotype 1 is the most common, accounting for 70–80% of the infection, followed by type 2 (approx 10–15%) and type 3 (5–10%). Even within an infected patient, HCV exists as a spectrum of closely related genomes, known as quasispecies. The clinical impact of quasispecies heterogeneity is not yet well defined.

3. PATHOGENESIS

HCV is the major etiologic agent of blood-borne and sporadic community-acquired NANB hepatitis. The most striking feature of HCV-induced liver disease is its tendency towards chronicity and slowly progressive liver injury. The mechanism by which HCV persists in the host is unknown. The virus replicates at a very low level and may not trigger an adequate immune response for its elimination. The high nucleotide substitution rate may also allow HCV to escape immune surveillance. The pathogenetic mechanisms responsible for liver injury in acute and chronic HCV infection are not well understood. Both cellular immune effector arms mediated by CD4+ and CD8+ cells have been suggested to play a role in the host defense against HCV infection *(6–9)*. As a result of this defense process, liver is damaged. Repeated insults lead to chronic hepatitis and eventually cirrhosis. Antibodies to HCV have not been found to be protective against HCV infection. In chimpanzees who have recovered from experimental infection, rechallenge with the same or a new HCV strain resulted in HCV infection with the subsequent challenge virus *(10)*. More recent evidence suggests that neutralizing antibodies are present for at least a period of time after infection *(11)*. It was noticed that serum obtained 2 yr after the onset of primary infection was able to neutralize the inoculum, whereas serum obtained 11 yr after the infection was not protective. Currently, it is believed that the high nucleotide substitution rate within the envelope proteins, which translates into different amino acid sequences, provides a mechanism for HCV to escape antibody related immune-surveillance.

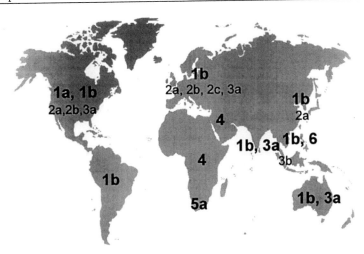

Fig. 2. The distribution of HCV genotypes worldwide. Bold types represent the major type in that geographic area.

4. EPIDEMIOLOGY

HCV infection is a common disease. Based on antibody to HCV as a marker, it was estimated that there are approx 100 million HCV carriers worldwide (*see* Fig. 3). In the United States, the Centers for Disease Control estimated that 1.8% of the entire population are chronic HCV carriers and every year there are approx 150,000 or more acute HCV infections. Hepatitis C is the most common cause of the nonalcoholic liver disease. Currently, only 6% of patients with acute hepatitis C have a history of transfusion in the 6 wk to 6 mo prior to the onset of their illness, whereas 46% report injection drug use, 1% are dialysis patients, 2% are health care workers with occupational exposure to blood, and 10% have a history of exposure to a sexual or household contact with someone who has had hepatitis, or exposure to multiple sexual partners *(12)*. Approximately 40% of infected individuals deny a known risk factor for hepatitis C. A low socioeconomic level is associated with a large portion of these patients. More than half have histories of some type of high-risk behavior or contact, including imprisonment, use of noninjection illegal drugs, and one or more sexually transmitted diseases. Saliva has been implicated as a vector of transmission. However, the existence of infectious virus in saliva is controversial. Sharing of hygiene items such as combs, razors, toothbrushes, and nail scissors has also been proposed as a possible means of transmission.

With the mandatory testing of blood donors for antibody to HCV in the United States since 1990, the risk of acquiring posttransfusion HCV infection has declined dramatically and is now less than 1%. Transfused recipients of blood and blood products are at particularly high risk of acquiring HCV infection, as are hemophiliacs who require factor concentrates prepared from pooled plasma from hundreds of individuals who, in many cases are paid donors. The seroprevalence of antibody to HCV ranges from 10–16% in paid donors compared to rates 10-fold less in volunteer donors *(13)*. The risk of sexual transmission is quite low compared to hepatitis B virus, human immunodeficiency virus and other sexually transmitted diseases *(14)*. HCV has not been identified in semen. However, epidemiological evidence has suggested that sexual transmission may account for up to 20% of cases who have no other identifiable risk factors *(15)*. Coinfection with HIV does not substantially enhance the transmission of HCV.

Perinatal transmission is known to occur with an average of 6% of the infants becoming infected, and ranges from 0–13%. Some studies have suggested that risk of perinatal transmission is related to the titer of HCV RNA in serum of mothers.

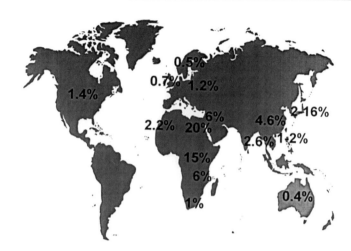

Fig. 3. The prevalence of HCV infection worldwide. Note the very high incidence in the Middle East and Central Africa.

HCV-related cirrhosis is a common indication for liver transplantation, an extremely expensive therapy. Adding together, health care costs for HCV related illness sums up to approx 1 billion dollars per year in the United States.

5. CLINICAL FEATURES

Many of the features of acute HCV hepatitis were demonstrated best in patients with transfusion-associated HCV infection. The mean incubation period is intermediate between those for acute hepatitis A and hepatitis B, with a peak onset at around 7–8 wk after infection. Eighty percent of cases occur between 5 and 12 wk, although the range is 1–26 wk *(16)*. The majority of cases of acute hepatitis C are asymptomatic. Fatigue is the most common symptom, but its onset is insidious and is usually mild. Compared to hepatitis B, the acute infection tends to be clinically mild. Jaundice is present in less than 25% cases. However, infection may be severe and clinically indistinguishable from severe cases of hepatitis A or B. Fulminant hepatitis is an unusual outcome of acute HCV infection. A common feature of HCV hepatitis is the episodic, fluctuating pattern of serum aminotransferase activity. Other patients may have persistently elevated serum aminotransferase activity or acute elevation that resolves completely. Because of fluctuating aminotransferase levels in these patients, it is difficult to evaluate convalescence accurately on the basis of few serum aminotransferase determinations, and prolonged follow-up is necessary. In fact, normalization of liver biochemistry after acute infection does not always represent resolution of infection *(17)*.

Despite its usual clinical silence, HCV is an insidiously progressive disease. Chronic hepatitis C evolves in 65–80% of patients who acquire acute infection. The natural history of chronic hepatitis C is known to be variable. The more common course is one of an insidiously progressive liver disease that often remains clinically silent for many years or even decades *(18–20)*. Spontaneous remission is extremely rare. The mean time from infection to recognition of chronic liver is usually 1–2 decades. Development of cirrhosis usually takes 1–3 decades *(20)*. Hepatic failure and other complications of cirrhosis, such as variceal hemorrhage, encephalopathy and ascites, eventually occur in 20% of cirrhotic patients, but usually take years to decades to develop. Chronic HCV now accounts for approx one quarter of adult patients referred for liver transplantation.

Table 1

HCV-Associated Extrahepatic Manifestations

Membranoproliferative glomerulonephritis
Mixed essential cryoglobulinemia
Porphyria cutanea tarda
Thyroiditis
Idiopathic thrombocytopenic purpura
Lichen planus
Mooren's corneal ulcers
Sjogren's syndrome
Autoimmune hepatitis, Type I and II
Polyarteritis nodosa
Aplastic anemia
Erythema multiforme

Various factors have been implicated in determining the progression from chronic hepatitis to cirrhosis. Among them, age at exposure, duration of infection and level of liver damage in initial liver biopsy have been found to correlate with progression of liver disease in a number of studies. Host immunity, alcohol intake, and concomitant infection with hepatitis B virus or hepatitis D virus and human immunodeficiency virus may also influence the course of histologic progression of chronic HCV infection.

A number of extrahepatic manifestations of this disease have been reported (*see* Table 1) (21). Essential mixed cryoglobulinemia was reported to be associated with approx 50% of patients positive for HCV. Membranoproliferative glomerulonephritis was reported to be associated with patients with HCV infection and cryoglobulinemia.

6. DIAGNOSTIC TESTS

Most subjects seropositive for antibody to HCV are also positive for HCV RNA in their serum. Hence, one can establish the diagnosis of HCV infection by either detecting the antibody to HCV in the host, or detecting the viral genome in the serum.

6.1. Testing for Antibody to HCV: Enzyme Immunoassays (EIAs)

The molecular cloning of HCV has provided an efficient way to produce large quantities of HCV polypeptides using recombinant technologies. These purified polypeptides were used to produce a capture assay for the detection of reactive antibody in sera from patients with HCV infection. The first generation EIA incorporated the c100-3 polypeptide. This assay detected nearly all cases of posttransfusion NANBH, and most of those with sporadic or community-acquired NANBH. However, the first generation EIA were plagued by the occasional false negatives and the frequent occurrence of false-positives, especially in patients with high serum globulin levels. This assay is no longer available.

The second generation EIA, which employed multiple HCV polypeptides to capture the reactive antibodies, was developed to overcome the problems of both low specificity and sensitivity that were observed with the first generation test. It contained two HCV polypeptides c200 (derived from NS3 and NS4) and c22 (derived from core) to enhance sensitivity and, at the same time, offer better specificity. The third generation EIA had another polypeptide derived from NS5 added to the existing two polypeptides in the second generation EIA to further improve sensitivity. In 1996, this version of EIA (referred to as EIA 3.0) was licensed by the Food and Drug Administration.

6.2. Recombinant Immunoblot Assay (RIBA)

The RIBA test is used to confirm the presence of anti-HCV as detected by the EIAs. This assay was developed in response to the problem of specificity seen in the first generation EIA. The test, briefly, consists of HCV polypeptide and a control coated as two bands in a strip. If the sample contains anti-HCV, it will bind to the HCV band which can then be detected with another antibody tracer. If the band coated with the control antigen is found to be positive, and the band coated with HCV polypeptide negative, the EIA positive result is considered to be false positive.

With the production of second and third generation EIAs, the RIBA test was also refined to its second and third generation versions. The second RIBA contains four bands coated with four different HCV polypeptides (c-22, c-100, 5-1-1, c33) together with a control polypeptide. If two or more bands are positive, the test is interpreted as positive. If only one band is positive, the test is considered as indeterminate. The third generation RIBA again contains four bands, formed by c22, c33, a combined band with c100 peptide and 5-1-1 peptide, and a NS5 polypeptide.

The immunoblot assay is, in general, slightly less sensitive, but more specific than the corresponding version of EIA tests. Hence, it should be used as a confirmatory test for the presence of anti-HCV. In 1996, the second generation RIBA was licensed by the Food and Drug Administration.

6.3. Hepatitis C Viral RNA Tests

The detection of HCV RNA confirms the diagnosis of active HCV infection. Advanced molecular biologic techniques, including reverse transcription and polymerase chain reaction (RT-PCR), provide a sensitive tool for the detection of viral RNA in serum and liver tissue. A positive HCV RNA test in serum indicates ongoing viremia. The blood specimens require special handling, including separating the serum from the clot and freezing within 2 h after the blood sample is drawn (22). There are two common types of HCV RNA tests available, RT-PCR and the branched DNA signal amplification (bDNA) assay (see Chapter 3).

The RT-PCR method requires primers constructed from a highly conserved region to exclude the possibility of missing viremia because of sequence heterogeneity. Most RT-PCR assays in use utilize primers derived from the conserved 5'-terminal noncoding region of the HCV genome (see Chapter 3). After RNA is extracted from serum, cDNA is produced by reverse transcription. The cDNA is then amplified by PCR. There are now commercial assays available for the detection of HCV RNA. Viremia can be detected using PCR assays within a few days of exposure to the virus, and weeks before the elevation of serum aminotransferases or appearance of viral antibody. The lower limit of detection for RT-PCR is dependent on efficiency of reverse transcription and usually no less than 500–2000 genomes equivalents/mL of serum can be detected. PCR is becoming an important tool for determining the response to antiviral therapy (23). PCR based assay has also been modified into a quantitative assay and is already available commercially for research purposes. The dynamic range of quantitation of this assay is between 4000–1,000,000 genome equivalents/mL. Samples with viremia level higher than the upper limit require dilution. The bDNA assay is a novel approach to the detection and quantitation of viral nucleic acids (see Chapter 3). The detection limit of the first generation assay is 350,000 viral genome equivalents/mL of serum and, for the second generation assay, the detection limit is 200,000 genome equivalents/mL. This assay has been modified to detect down to 500 genomes/mL for human immunodeficiency virus and it is expected that this assay can be further modified to increase its sensitivity.

One important issue of molecular detection of HCV RNA is the effect of genetic variation of HCV in relation to its detection using molecular tools. This issue has been addressed by the bDNA assay. The first generation was found to underestimate HCV RNA levels in patients with HCV types 2 and 3 infection by an average factor of 3 and 2, respectively. Quantitation of HCV RNA in types 1, 4, 5, and 6 was found to be accurate. This issue has been properly addressed with the bDNA version 2.0 assay. There is already evidence that similar problems in underestimation of HCV RNA genotypes other than type 1 are also present with PCR-based assays. It is expected that PCR-based assays also need to be adapted or modified to quantitate HCV RNA irrespective of HCV genotypes.

6.4. Clinical Utility

Because of its sensitivity, specificity, and low cost compared to molecular assays, testing anti-HCV by a late version EIA is sufficient to screen patients for possible HCV infection.

6.4.1. PATIENTS WITH LIVER DISEASES

Anti-HCV, as detected by the second and third generation EIAs, is positive in a majority of patients with chronic hepatitis C. This group of patients seldom have false positive results for anti-HCV. Hence, RIBA confirmation is usually not necessary. A RIBA test, however, should be obtained in patients positive for anti-HCV, suspected of having high globulin levels, features of autoimmune hepatitis or hypergammaglobulinemia. Most patients positive for anti-HCV and with elevated serum aminotransferases are also viremic. Hence, one should consider positivity of anti-HCV in a patient with elevated aminotransferase or with liver disease as evidence for chronic HCV infection until proven otherwise by molecular tools (e.g., reverse transcription polymerase chain reaction).

However, before considering interferon-alpha therapy, most clinicians prefer to have documentation of active viremia, and RT-PCR or bDNA assay can be used. The documentation of viremia level may have some value in providing prognostic information to the patients.

6.4.2. BLOOD DONORS

In healthy blood donors who are found to be positive for anti-HCV, the positivity should be confirmed by a recombinant immunoblot assay. For those patients with confirmed anti-HCV positivity, a large proportion are viremic.

For those blood donors with negative RIBA, most blood centers retest them for anti-HCV by EIA in 6 mo and, if this is negative, they are allowed to re-enter into the donor pool. For those blood donors with indeterminate results, they are retested in 6 mo with both EIA/RIBA tests before considering their eligibility as blood donors.

6.4.3. PATIENTS WITH SYSTEMIC ILLNESS/ON IMMUNOSUPPRESSION

False negative tests for anti-HCV are commonly seen in patients with major systemic illness or immunosuppressed patients with HCV infection. This is due to the poor production of antibody secondary to long-term illness or immunosuppression. In patients undergoing hemodialysis, up to 40% of the patients with HCV viremia may be negative for anti-HCV (24). Similarly, organ transplant recipients on long-term immunosuppressive therapy and with HCV infection may test negative for anti-HCV. In these patients, molecular assays should be used for the direct testing of HCV RNA in serum.

6.4.4. ACUTE HEPATITIS C

In acute hepatitis C, anti-HCV may be detected by the first generation enzyme immunoassay 10–12 wk after the exposure. With the improved sensitivity with the second and third EIAs, anti-HCV may be detected 4–6 wk after the exposure. However, it is important to remember that in patients with acute hepatitis, the possibility of HCV infection cannot be eliminated with a negative anti-HCV test within 6 wk of exposure. Patients should be retested for anti-HCV 6 wk after the initial exposure.

7. TREATMENT

Interferon is the only therapy proven to be effective in a proportion of patients with chronic HCV infection. The drug was approved for the treatment of chronic hepatitis C by the Food and Drug Administration in 1991. Neither corticosteroids, gamma interferon, nor acyclovir have been found to have any beneficial effects on HCV infection. Ribavirin has been shown to reduce serum aminotransferase levels in 40–50% of patients with chronic HCV infection, but it has no effect on HCV viremia. Long-term immunosuppressive therapy may be detrimental.

As of June 1996, all patients with positive anti-HCV with evidence of liver disease should be considered for interferon-alpha therapy.

7.1. Interferon-Alpha Therapy

Interferons are natural glycoproteins produced by cells in response to infection by viruses, including HCV. Interferons have many biological effects, including direct anti-viral and immunomodulatory activities. Currently, recombinant interferon alpha-2b is the only interferon approved for the treatment of chronic HCV infection in the United States. As this interferon preparation is produced by recombinant technology, there is no risk of transmitting infections. Other types of interferons such as alpha-2a or beta have not been studied as extensively in the United States for the treatment of chronic hepatitis B or C (although they have been approved in other parts of the world).

The usual recommended dose of interferon alpha-2b is 3 million units subcutaneously or intramuscularly 3 times per week for 6 mo. Presently, interferon therapy for chronic hepatitis C is approved for 6 mo, although a second 6-mo course is recommended for patients who respond initially and then relapse. The optimal dosage and duration are currently under investigation. Recent studies have suggested that longer treatment duration reduces relapse and, thereby, increases the longevity of response (25).

A biochemical response, in terms of normalization of serum aminotransferase levels, can be anticipated in approx 40% of treated patients. Nearly all patients who responded to interferon showed response within 12 wk. HCV RNA levels fall and become undetectable within 4–8 wk in most patients who subsequently normalized serum ALT levels (24,26–29). These biochemical and virologic changes are accompanied by histologic improvement (19,30).

Despite the prompt antiviral and biochemical responses to interferon treatment, biochemical relapse shortly after cessation of interferon therapy occurs in at least 50% of patients who showed a complete biochemical response to interferon. Even in those patients with sustained biochemical response, a proportion of them were still viremic, adding further confusion as to the best definition of response to interferon therapy. For those patients who responded initially, and relapsed after cessation of therapy, reinstitution of interferon treatment appeared to be almost universally effective in reinducing remission of disease (27,31). Whether these patients should be treated with long-term interferon is still being studied.

Approximately 50–60% of patients treated with interferon fail to respond to interferon. They usually have persistent elevation of serum aminotransferase levels even after 12 wk of interferon therapy. For these interferon nonresponders, increasing the dose of interferon does not appear to enhance the response significantly, but is associated with more side effects. Hence, from a clinical perspective, it is recommended that interferon may be terminated if the patient still has elevated serum aminotransferase levels at the end of 12 wk of interferon therapy.

Some patients who initially appear to respond to interferon by normalizing serum ALT levels will demonstrate a progressive rise in the serum ALT levels, despite continuation of interferon. Although the cause of this phenomenon is not clear, it is believed that some of these patients may have had the emergence of interferon resistant strains. Alternatively, these patients may have developed interferon toxicity or interferon-induced autoimmune hepatitis.

7.2. Patient Selection

Several factors have been reported to be associated with a greater likelihood of response to interferon therapy. They include absence of cirrhosis, female gender, younger age, shorter duration of disease, lower body weight, lower pretreatment viremia level, and HCV nongenotype 1 infection (in particular HCV genotypes 2 and 3). When multivariate analysis was performed, most studies showed that mild histology (or absence of fibrosis), low pretreatment viremia level, and HCV nongenotype 1 infection appeared to be independent favorable factors (32–34). It seems logical to select patients who are likely to respond to interferon to receive treatment. However, the predictive value of each of these parameters ranges from 60–80%. When this model was applied to an actual pool of patients, half of the patients who responded to interferon would be missed by the above criteria. Analysis of cost-effectiveness has shown that it is beneficial to treat patients with early disease as well as late disease, because the cost of management of liver cirrhosis is extremely expensive and carries significant morbidity (35).

In the author's view, any therapeutic guideline should only be applied to all patients if the predictive value is on the order of 95% or higher. Because of the desire not to miss patients who may benefit from interferon therapy, some institutions treat all patients with interferon. Clearly, parameters that are associated with better treatment response should be discussed with the patient to identify optimal therapeutic regimes.

7.3. Special Treatment Groups

Certain subgroups of patients have been excluded from both the clinical trials reported to date and current indications for the use of interferon. These groups include decompensated cirrhotic patients, solid organ transplant recipients, children, and patients with extrahepatic manifestations of infection. Recent reports suggest that interferon can be used safely and effectively in HIV-infected patients, and solid-organ transplant recipients. However, the response rate may be lower in these patients. In addition, in solid-organ transplant recipients, the immunomodulatory properties of interferon may make rejection a potential risk. Long-term studies with careful surveillance of the graft for evidence of rejection are necessary before interferon can be recommended in these patients. Interferon therapy appears to be effective in eliminating extrahepatic manifestations of HCV infection, such as essential mixed cryoglobulinemia.

7.4. Side-Effects of Interferon

Interferon therapy is generally well-tolerated. Most patients have flu-like side effects consisting of fever, myalgia, arthralgia, and headache during the first few days of treatment. Typically, these symptoms are ameliorated by pretreatment with acetaminophen and tachyphylaxis after the first few doses. Persistent fatigue, irritability, nausea, and depression may occasionally require dose reductions. Mild reversible alopecia (24%) and intermittent diarrhea (34%) occur late in the course of therapy. Mild leukopenia and thrombocytopenia are not uncommon, but do not usually become clinically significant in noncirrhotic patients without baseline cytopenia. In a United States multicenter study, 14% of treated patients required

ACKNOWLEDGMENTS

J. Y. N. Lau was supported in part by the American Liver Foundation Hans Popper Liver Scholar Award and a Public Health Service Award AI41219.

REFERENCES

1. Bradley DW, Maynard JE, Popper H. Post transfusion NANBH: physicochemical properties of two distinct agents. J Infect Dis 1983;148:254–265.
2. Bradley DW, McCaustland KA, Cook EH. Post-transfusion non-A, non-B hepatitis in chimpanzees: physico-chemical evidence that tubule-forming agent is a small, enveloped virus. Gastroenterology 1985;88:773–779.
3. Choo QL, Kuo G, Weiner AJ. Isolation of a cDNA clone derived from a blood borne non-A, non-B viral hepatitis genome. Science 1989;244:359–362.
4. Dusheiko G, Schmilovitz-Weiss H, Brown D. Hepatitis C virus genotypes: an investigation of type-specific differences in geographic origin and disease. Hepatology 1994;19:13–18.
5. Simmonds P, Alberti A, Alter HJ, Bonino F. A proposed system for the nomenclature of hepatitis viral genotypes (Letter). Hepatology 1994;19:1321–1324.
6. Koziel MJ, Dudley JD, Afdhal N. Hepatitis C virus-specific cytotoxic T lymphocytes recognize epitopes in the core and envelope proteins of HCV. J Virol 1993;67:7522–7533.
7. Shirai M, Akatsuka T, Pendleton CD. Induction of cytotoxic T cells to across-reactive epitope in the hepatitis C virus nonstructural RNA polymerase-like protein. J Virol 1992;66:4098–4106.
8. Koziel MJ, Dudley D, Wong J. Intrahepatic cytotoxic T lymphocytes specific for hepatitis C virus in persons with chronic hepatitis. J Immunol 1992;149:3339–3344.
9. Kita H, Moriyama T, Kaneko T. HLA B44-restricted cytotoxic T lymphocytes recognizing an epitope on hepatitis C virus nucleocapsid protein. Hepatology 1993;18:1039–1044.
10. Farci P, Alter HJ, Govindarajan S. Lack of protective immunity against reinfection with hepatitis C virus. Science 1992;258:135–140.
11. Farci P, Alter HJ, Wong DC. Prevention of hepatitis C virus infection in chimpanzees after antibody-mediated in vitro neutralization. Proc Natl Acad Sci USA 1994;91:7792–7796.
12. Alter MJ. Inapparent transmission of hepatitis C: footprints in the sand. Hepatology 1991;14:389–391.
13. Alter HJ, Purcell RH, Shih JW. Detection of antibody to hepatitis C virus in prospectively followed transfusion recipients with acute and chronic non-A, non-B hepatitis. N Engl J Med 1989;321:1494–1500.
14. Tor J, Llibre JM, Carbonell M. Sexual transmission of hepatitis C virus and its relation with hepatitis B virus and HIV. Br Med J 1990;301:1130–1133.
15. Alter MJ, Coleman PJ, Alexander WJ. Importance of heterosexual activity in the transmission of hepatitis B and non-A, non-B hepatitis. JAMA 1989;262:1201–1205.
16. Dienstag JL. Non-A, non-B hepatitis. I. Recognition, epidemiology and clinical features. Gastroenterology 1983;85:439–462.
17. Shibata M, Morishima T, Kudo T. Serum hepatitis C virus sequences in posttransfusion non-A, non-B hepatitis. Blood 1991;15:1157–1160.
18. Seeff LB, Buskell-Bales Z, Wright E. Long term mortality after transfusion associated non-A, non-B hepatitis. N Engl J Med 1992;327:1906–1911.
19. Davis GL, Balart LA, Schiff ER. Treatment of chronic hepatitis C with recombinant interferon alfa: a multicenter randomized controlled trial. N Engl J Med 1989;321:1501–1506.
20. Kiyosawa K, Sodeyama T, Tanaka E. Interrelationship of blood transfusion, non-A, non-B hepatitis and hepato-cellular carcinoma. Analysis by detection of antibody to hepatitis C virus. Hepatology 1990;12:671–675.
21. Gordon SC. Extrahepatic manifestations of hepatitis C. Dig Dis 1996;14:157–168.
22. Davis GL, Lau JYN, Urdea MS. Quantitative detection of hepatitis C virus RNA with a solid-phase signal amplification method: definition of optimal conditions for specimen collection and clinical application in interferon-treated patients. Hepatology 1994;19:1337–1341.
23. Bresters D, Mauser-Bunschoten EP, Cuypers HT. Disappearance of hepatitis C virus RNA in plasma during interferon alpha-2b treatment in hemophilia patients. Scand J Gastroenterol 1992;27:166–168.
24. Lau JYN, Davis GL, Brunson ME. Hepatitis C virus infection in renal transplant recipients. Hepatology 1993;18:1027–1031.
25. Poynard T, Bedossa P, Chevallier M. A comparison of three interferon alfa-2b regimens for the long term treatment of chronic non-A, non-B hepatitis. N Engl J Med 1995;332:1457–1462.
26. Hagiwara H, Hayashi N, Mita E. Detection of hepatitis C virus RNA in serum of patients with chronic hepatitis C treated with interferon alpha. Hepatology 1992;15:37–41.

27. Chayama K, Saitoh S, Arase Y. Effect of interferon administration on serum hepatitis C virus RNA in patients with chronic hepatitis C. Hepatology 1991;13:1040–1043.
28. Brillanti S, Garson JA, Tuke PW. Effect of alpha interferon therapy on hepatitis C viremia in community-acquired chronic non-A, non-B hepatitis: a quantitative polymerase chain reaction study. J Med Virol 1991;34:136–141.
29. Shindo M, Di Bisceglie AM, Cheung L. Decrease in serum hepatitis C viral RNA during alpha-interferon therapy for chronic hepatitis C. Ann Int Med 1991;115:700–704.
30. Schvarcz R, Glaumann H, Weiland O. Histological outcome in interferon-alpha-2b treated patients with chronic post-transfusion non-A, non-B hepatitis. Liver 1991;11:30.
31. Davis GL. Recombinant alpha interferon treatment of non-A, non-B (type C) hepatitis: review of studies and recommendations. J Hepatol 1990;11(Suppl 2):72–77.
32. Davis GL. Prediction of response to interferon treatment of chronic hepatitis C. J Hepatol 1994;20;1–3.
33. Martinot-Peignoux M, Marcellin P, Pouteau M. Pretreatment serum hepatitis C virus RNA levels and hepatitis C virus genotype are the main and independent prognostic factors of sustained response to interferon alfa therapy in chronic hepatitis C. Hepatology 1995;22:1050–1056.
34. Lau JYN, Davis GL, Kniffen J. Significance of serum hepatitis C virus RNA levels in chronic hepatitis. Lancet 1993;341:1501–1504.
35. Bennett WG, Inoue Y, Beck JR. Justification of a single 60-month course of interferon (IFN) for histologically mild chronic hepatitis C. Hepatology 1995;22:290A.
36. Feray C, Gigou M, Samuel D. The course of hepatitis C infection after liver transplantation. Hepatology 1994;20:1137–1143.
37. Chazouilleres O, Kim M, Combs C. Quantitation of hepatitis C virus RNA in liver transplant recipients. Gastroenrol 1994;106:994–999.
38. Simons JN, Pilot-Mattes TJ, Leary TP. Identification of two flavivirus-like genomes in the GB hepatitis agent. Proc Natl Acad Sci USA 1995;92:3401–405.
39. Simons JN, Leary TP, Dawson GP. Isolation of novel virus-like sequences associated with human hepatitis. Nat Med 1995;1:564–569.
40. Linnen J, Wages J Jr, Zhang-Keck ZY. Molecular cloning and disease association of hepatitis G virus; a new transfusion transmissible agent. Science 1996;271:505–508.

SUGGESTED READING

1. Schiff ER. The patient with chronic hepatitis C. Hosp Pract 1993;28:25–33.
2. Davis GL, Balart LA, Schiff ER. Treatment of chronic hepatitis C with recombinant interferon alfa: a multicenter randomized controlled trial. N Engl J Med 1989;321:1501–1506.
3. Davis GL, Lau JYN. Hepatitis C virus. In: Haubrich WS, Schaffner F, Berk JE, eds. Bockus's series of gastroenterology. Saunders, Philadelphia, 1994, pp. 2082–2114.
4. Alter MJ, Margolis HS, Krawczynski K. The natural history of community-acquired hepatitis C in the United States. N Engl J Med 1992;327:1899–1905.

11

Autoimmune Hepatitis

F. Wilson Jackson and Raymond A. Rubin

1. INTRODUCTION

Autoimmune hepatitis (AIH) is a progressive inflammatory liver disease which affects females four times as commonly as males. The disease predominantly affects women in their third through fifth decades. Presenting symptoms usually include fatigue, malaise, oligomenorrhea, and sometimes jaundice. AIH is characterized by persistent elevations in serum transaminases, increased serum IgG, and histologic evidence of piecemeal necrosis, often with predominant plasma cell infiltration of the portal tracts. Classically, patients with AIH display high titers of antinuclear antibody (ANA) and anti-smooth muscle antibody (ASMA).

The pathogenesis of AIH is incompletely understood. It is classified as an autoimmune disorder based on the presence of serum autoantibodies, the association with other autoimmune conditions, and the potential responsiveness to immunosuppressive therapy. Although relatively uncommon, it is important to recognize AIH because early treatment may prevent the development of cirrhosis and its attendant complications.

2. HISTORICAL PERSPECTIVE

Any current understanding of AIH begins with a historical perspective. Over the years, such terms as lupoid hepatitis, plasma cell hepatitis, idiopathic autoimmune chronic active hepatitis, and chronic active hepatitis have been devised for this clinical entity in an attempt to incorporate histologic findings and presumptive etiology into the nomenclature.

Waldenstrom provided an early description of what is now considered AIH (1). He characterized a syndrome of jaundice, amenorrhea, and hypergammaglobulinemia afflicting young

From: *Diseases of the Liver and Bile Ducts: Diagnosis and Treatment*
Edited by: G. Y. Wu and J. Israel © Humana Press Inc., Totowa, NJ

women. Mackey later coined the term lupoid hepatitis when he noted the presence of lupus erythematosus cells in the serum of patients with this syndrome *(2)*. This term has been discarded as it has been since observed that systemic lupus erythematosus is only rarely associated with substantial liver disease *(3)*. AIH is a distinct clinical entity from SLE.

For many years, the term chronic active autoimmune hepatitis was applied for this entity in an effort to differentiate it from other, primarily viral, causes of chronic hepatitis. Whereas hepatitis B viral infection is distinguishable based on serologic studies and unique histologic features, until more specific testing for hepatitis C virus (HCV) became available, "non A, non B" hepatitis was frequently confused with AIH. In fact, first generation ELISA testing for HCV-antibody was often falsely positive in patients with autoimmune disorders (including AIH) with elevated immunoglobulin levels *(4)*. Over the past few years, the ability to diagnose HCV specifically has improved dramatically. Since then, it has been argued that a small subset of patients with HCV also has an autoimmune hepatitis caused by cross reactivity between HCV and host antigens.

Recently, an international panel concluded that the name "autoimmune chronic active hepatitis" should be changed to "autoimmune hepatitis" because the designation "autoimmune" implies chronicity. The same panel also devised a scoring system to assess the likelihood of AIH based on clinical, serologic, and biochemical findings *(5)*. These more standardized criteria should facilitate future studies concerning the pathogenesis, natural history, and therapy of AIH.

3. PATHOGENESIS

There are several lines of evidence pointing to an immunologic origin for AIH. These include its frequent association with certain HLA haplotypes *(6–8)*, the typically elevated IgG levels, and the clinical response of AIH to immunosuppressive medications. Additionally, patients with AIH have a high prevalence of other autoimmune disorders, including thyroid disease, rheumatoid arthritis and Sjogren's syndrome *(7)*.

Both the cellular and humoral immune systems are abnormal in patients with AIH. Immunohistochemical studies have shown that the hepatic inflammation in this disease is mediated predominantly by CD8 cells. This may indicate a deficiency in T-cell suppressor function. The hypergammaglobulinemia seen in many patients with AIH also suggests a deranged humoral immune system. Whether this is of etiologic importance or secondary to an environmental or infectious stimulus is unknown.

Additional support for an immune origin for AIH is reflected in the high titers of serum autoantibodies found in affected patients. Whereas these antibodies are neither organ specific nor pathogenic, they can be used to classify patients with AIH into three main subgroups. Patients with "classical" or Type 1 AIH usually have high titers of ANA, ASMA, and perinuclear anti-nuclear cytoplasmic antibody (pANCA) *(9–11)*. The vast majority of American patients have Type 1 disease. The usual age of onset for Type 1 AIH is between the second and fourth decades, but there is a second, smaller peak of incidence in late middle age. In contrast, Type 2 is largely confined to children. Patients with Type 2 and Type 3 AIH do not display high titers of ANA or ASMA. However, they do mount antibodies against a liver-kidney microsome (LKM) antigen or a soluble liver antigen (SLA), respectively *(12–15)*, (*see* Table 1).

4. CLINICAL PRESENTATIONS

4.1. Cardinal Signs and Symptoms

4.1.1. Symptoms

For all types, AIH usually has an insidious onset characterized by nonspecific symptoms such as anorexia, fatigue, and malaise. In women, amenorrhea or oligomenorrhea are addi-

Table 1

Autoimmune Hepatitis Subtypes

	Type 1	Type 2	Type 3
Autoantibody (% positive)	ANA (50–80)	Anti-LKM (100)	Anti-SLA (100)
HLA association	A1, B8, DR3, DR4	DR-3, DR-7	
Median age of onset (yrs)	0–40	2–14	20–40
Gender (% female)	70	90	90
Hypergammaglobulinemia	+++	++	+++
Response to glucocorticoids	+++	++	+++

tional common symptoms *(11)*. Though generally considered a chronic disease, up to 20% of patients with AIH may present with signs and symptoms mimicking acute viral hepatitis. A small percentage of patients with AIH (especially in Type 2) may present with fulminant hepatic failure with encephalopathy developing within weeks of the onset of illness *(16)*. Thus, AIH is important to consider in young patients with acute liver disease and negative viral serologies. Patients with AIH in whom treatment is delayed or ineffective usually develop cirrhosis and its complications, including variceal bleeding, ascites, and hepatic encephalopathy.

4.1.2. PHYSICAL EXAMINATION

At presentation, 20–50% of patients with AIH are jaundiced. Tender hepatomegaly, spider nevi, and splenomegaly are also relatively common signs. Extrahepatic manifestations of AIH may include fever, arthropathy, acne, maculopapular rash, and, less commonly, cutaneous striae.

4.1.3. LABORATORY FINDINGS

Laboratory data in patients with AIH characteristically indicate hepatocellular inflammation. The serum aminotransferases are usually increased 2–10 times the normal range *(17)*. Marked elevations of the serum aminotransferases beyond 1000 IU/L usually reflect substantial hepatic necrosis. Normal or near-normal aminotransferases levels, however, do not necessarily indicate normal liver histology. This is especially true in patients on immunosuppressive therapy or those with established cirrhosis. Serum immunoglobulins are also typically elevated in patients with AIH *(18)*. Whereas IgM and IgA may be increased, polyclonal elevations of IgG are more commonly observed. Serum bilirubin and alkaline phosphatase levels are typically mildly increased in patients with AIH *(7)*. Substantial elevations of these markers of cholestasis should prompt consideration of alternative diagnoses. Abnormalities in markers of hepatic synthetic function such as prothrombin time and serum albumin are adverse prognostic signs. Other laboratory abnormalities frequently noted in patients with AIH include a mild normochromic, normocytic anemia and, in patients with splenomegaly or cirrhosis, thrombocytopenia.

5. DIAGNOSIS

As there are no pathognomonic clinical findings, the final diagnosis of AIH is based on a composite of the patient's presentation, laboratory data, and histology. In an effort to create uniform agreement, a scoring system has been proposed to help confirm the likelihood of the diagnosis of AIH *(11)*. Parameters such as gender, serum laboratory results, autoimmune markers, and response to treatment are used to estimate the probability of the diagnosis. Routine laboratory data and serologic studies help considerably to refine the differential diagnosis in patients with chronic hepatitis (*see* Fig. 1).

A liver biopsy should be performed in all patients suspected of having AIH in order to exclude other diseases and to assess the extent of inflammation and/or presence of cirrhosis.

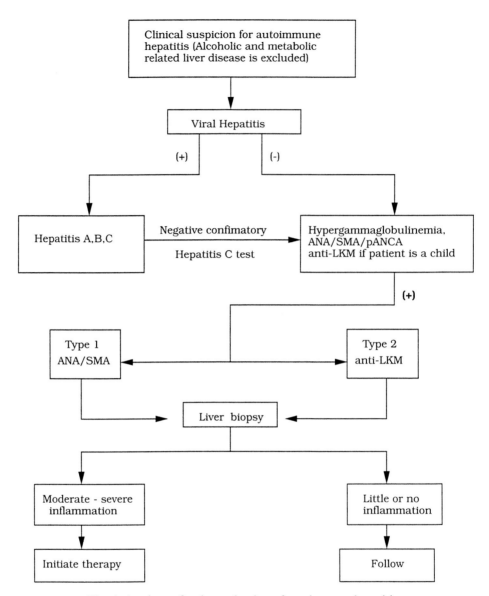

Fig. 1. A scheme for the evaluation of autoimmune hepatitis.

Liver biopsy specimens from patients with AIH are often difficult to distinguish from those of patients with other causes of chronic liver disease, especially chronic HCV infection. In these conditions, inflammation may extend beyond the limiting plate of the portal tracts ("piecemeal necrosis") and even to the central veins ("bridging necrosis"). Pathologic findings strongly suggestive of AIH include prominent plasma cell infiltration of portal tracts and grouping of hepatocytes into rosettes *(19)*. In patients with AIH, as with other chronic liver diseases, hepatic inflammation and necrosis frequently eventuate in macronodular cirrhosis. In fact, nearly one third of patients with AIH will already have cirrhosis when their liver disease is clinically recognized. The liver biopsy specimens from patients with cirrhosis secondary to AIH may be indistinguishable from those from other patients with other chronic liver diseases, especially if there is no ongoing active hepatic inflammation.

6. TREATMENT

As with many other autoimmune diseases, corticosteroids are the mainstay of therapy for AIH *(20)*. Improvement in symptoms, normalization or near normalization of serum aminotransferases, and decreases in serum immunoglobulins can be achieved in 70–80% of patients treated with daily prednisone (which requires hepatic metabolism for efficacy) or prednisolone *(21–24)*. The initial response to corticosteroids may be more limited in patients with established cirrhosis, although this issue is controversial. Patients without cirrhosis at the outset of treatment may still develop cirrhosis during therapy despite an apparent clinical response. This is especially true for individuals with severe acute disease and confluent necrosis on pretreatment biopsy.

The optimal initial corticosteroid dose for AIH is controversial. Depending on the extent of inflammation, most hepatologists recommend an initial daily prednisone dose of 40–60 mg. Older patients or those with milder disease are often started on a lower dose. The daily dose of corticosteroids is gradually tapered several months after achieving a biochemical response with the goal of using the minimal dose necessary to maintain remission. If corticosteroids are withdrawn completely, however, relapse occurs in a majority of patients *(21,24)*.

Although effective, corticosteroid therapy is limited by numerous adverse effects such as accelerated osteoporosis, cataracts, diabetes mellitus, infection, weight gain, and neuropsychiatric symptoms. Concurrent treatment with alternative immunosuppressive medications such as azathioprine (1–1.5 mg/kg/d) often permits substantial reduction of corticosteroid doses needed to maintain remission *(22–24,25)*. This "steroid sparing" effect, however, is delayed for 2–3 mo. After remission has been achieved, some patients may even be maintained on azathioprine monotherapy *(26)*. The incidence of important adverse effects, such as myelosuppression, opportunistic infection, neoplasm, and pancreatitis are relatively low with azathioprine. The goal for treating patients with AIH is administering the lowest dose of immunosupressive medication that safely maintains biochemical and histologic remission.

Alternative treatment regimens have been evaluated for their efficacy against AIH *(27,28)*. Alternate-day dosing of glucocorticoids has been found less effective than daily dosing. The role of high dose induction and lower dose maintenance azathioprine monotherapy (without induction corticosteroids), as well as treatment with cyclosporin, cyclophosphamide, and tacrolimus, are being investigated. Currently, these treatments are not considered the standard of care and their use should be restricted to investigational protocols.

Pregnancy does not appear to affect the course of AIH. Pregnant patients with AIH who are in remission should be maintained on their corticosteroid therapy. Whereas azathioprine has been used safely in some pregnant patients *(29)*, consultation with an experienced obstetrician is advised, given the questions regarding teratogenicity of this medication.

For patients who develop complications of cirrhosis despite therapy, liver transplantation remains an effective treatment option *(30)*. Graft and patient survival for patients with AIH is similar to that of patients transplanted for other indications. To date, there have been only scattered reports of recurrent AIH after transplantation *(31)*.

7. PROGNOSIS

The natural history for patients diagnosed with AIH is highly variable and somewhat unpredictable. Asymptomatic patients with normal serum liver tests and minimal inflammation on biopsy may never develop the complications of cirrhosis. Specific treatment is, therefore, not indicated for these patients. However, in patients with moderate to severe disease, spontaneous remission is rare. The majority of patients will inevitably develop cirrhosis unless they are treated with immunosupressive medications. Timely medical intervention has been shown not only to prolong survival *(11)*, but also to improve quality of life. Therapy may even obviate the need for more drastic interventions, such as liver transplantation. Prompt diagnosis and initiation of treatment is, therefore, a critical issue *(32)*. Spontaneous remission of moderate-severe AIH is rare *(33)*. Biochemical and histologic remission can be achieved in a majority of patients who are treated with corticosteroids alone or in combination with azathioprine. If immuno-supressive therapy is withdrawn completely, however, approximately 80% will relapse *(34)*. AIH is one of the few causes of fulminant hepatic failure that has a specific and effective therapy and, consequently, carries a favorable prognosis.

8. COMPLICATIONS

Untreated, patients with moderate-severe AIH have expected 3- and 10-yr survivals of 50 and 10%, respectively. The mortality is greatest within the first 6 mo after diagnosis *(24,33)*. Patients with marked elevations of serum aminotransferases and liver biopsy findings of confluent necrosis have the worst prognosis. Asymptomatic patients with AIH have a relatively low rate of progression to cirrhosis and, consequently, an improved expected survival *(33)*.

9. INDICATIONS FOR CONSULTING THE SUBSPECIALIST

The evaluation and management of patients with suspected AIH often presents a formidable challenge. The clinical and laboratory investigation of patients with chronic hepatitis (including AIH) is usually conducted by a primary care provider. An experienced hepatologist should be consulted to perform a liver biopsy, to interpret the histologic findings in the specific clinical context, and to initiate immunosupressive therapy when appropriate. For patients who do not respond to treatment or who have cirrhosis at the time of diagnosis, the specialist's input is helpful for managing the complications associated with portal hypertension, especially variceal bleeding, ascites and hydrothorax, and encephalopathy. For patients with advanced chronic disease, evaluating candidacy for liver transplantation requires specific expertise as well.

Patients with severe acute hepatitis or fulminant hepatic failure are at great risk for morbidity and mortality. Expeditious referral to an experienced hepatologist, preferentially at a transplantation center, is critical for optimizing a patient's clinical outcome.

SUMMARY

Autoimmune hepatitis (AIH) is a disease that primarily affects young to middle-aged women.

Laboratory studies reflect hepatocellular injury as indicated by elevation of serum aminotransferases. Hypergammaglobulinemia and serum autoantibodies are usually present.

Liver biopsy findings are not pathognomonic of AIH although plasma cell infiltration of the portal tracts is strongly suggestive. A substantial proportion of patients with AIH already have cirrhosis at presentation.

Recommended therapy usually consists of glucocorticoids and azathioprine. Treatment may prevent the development of cirrhosis. Liver transplantation is an option for patients with refractory or progressive disease.

REFERENCES

1. Waldenstrom J, Leber B. Bluproteine und Nahrungseiweiss. Deutsche Gesellschaft Zeitschrift für Verdaungs - und Staffwechselkrankheiten, 1950;15:113–119.
2. Mackay JR, Taft LI, Cowling DC. Lupoid hepatitis. Lancet 1956;2:1323–1326.
3. Soloway RD, Summerskill WHJ, Baggenstoss AH, et. al. "Lupoid" hepatitis, a nonentity in the spectrum of chronic active liver disease. Gastroenterology 1972;63:458.
4. Lenzi M, Ballordini G, Fusconi M. Type 2 autoimmune hepatitis and hepatitis C virus infection. Lancet 1990;355:258–259.
5. Johnson PJ, McFarlance IG. Meeting report: International Autoimmune Hepatitis Group. Hepatology 1993;18:998–1005.

6. Donaldson PT, Doherty DG, Hayllar KM, McFarlane IG, Johnson PJ, Williams R. Susceptibility to autoimmune chronic active hepatitis: human leukocyte antigens DR-4 and A1-B8-DR-3 are independent risk factors. Hepatology 1991;13:701–706.
7. Czaja AJ, Davis GL, Ludwig J. Autoimmune features as determinants of prognosis in steroid-treated chronic active hepatitis of uncertain etiology. Gastroenterology 1983;85:713.
8. Donaldson P, Daherty D, Underhill J, Williams R. The molecular genetics of autoimmune liver disease. Hepatology 1994;20:225–239.
9. Lidman K, Biberfield G, Fagraeus A. Anti-actin specificity of human smooth muscle antibodies in chronic active hepatitis. Clin Exp Immunol 1976;24:266–272.
10. Targan SR, Landers C, Vidrich A, Czaja AJ. High titer antineutrophil cytoplasmic antibodies in Type 1 autoimmune hepatitis. Gastroenterology 1995;108:1159–11-66.
11. Czaja AJ. Natural history, clinical features, and treatment of autoimmune hepatitis. Sem Liver Dis 1984;4:1–12.
12. Czaja AJ, Manns MP, Homburger HA. Frequency and significance of antibodies to liver/kidney microsomes type 1 in adults with chronic active hepatitis. Gastroenterology 1992;103:160–165.
13. Homberg JC, Abuaf N, Bernard O. Chronic active hepatitis associated with anti liver/kidney microsome antibody type 1: a second type of "autoimmune" hepatitis. Hepatology 1987;7:1333–39.
14. Manns MP, Griffin KJ, Sullivan KF, Johnson EF. LKM-1 autoantibodies recognize a short linear sequence in P450IID6, a cytochrome P-450 monooxygenase. J Clin Invest 1991;88:1370–1378.
15. Manns M, Gerkin G, Kyriatsoulis. Characteristics of a new subgroup of autoimmune chronic active hepatitis by autoantibodies against a soluble liver antigen. Lancet 1987;1:62.
16. Porta G, DaCosta Gayotto LC, Alvarez F. Anti-liver-kidney microsome antibody-positive autoimmune hepatitis presenting as fulminant liver failure. J Ped Gastroenterol Nutr 1990;11:138.
17. Davis GL, Czaja AJ, Baggenstoss AH. Prognostic and therapeutic implications of extreme serum aminotransferase elevation in chronic active hepatitis. Mayo Clin Proc 1982;57:303.
18. Kenny RP, Czaja AJ, Ludwig. Frequency and significance of antimitichondrial antibodies in severe chronic active hepatitis. Dig Dis Sci 1986;31:705.
19. Bach N, Thung SN, Schaffner F. The histological features of chronic hepatitis C and autoimmune hepatitis: a comparative analysis. Hepatology 1992;15:572–577.
20. Summerskill WHJ. Chronic active liver disease reexamined: prognosis hopeful. Gastroenterology 1974;66:450–464.
21. Czaja AJ. Treatment strategies in chronic active hepatitis. In: Czaja AJ, Dickson ER, eds. Chronic active hepatitis: the Mayo Clinic experience. Marcel Dekker, New York, 1986, pp. 247–267,269–283.
22. Cook AG, Mulligan R, Sherlock S. Controlled prospective trial of corticosteroid therapy in chronic active hepatitis. Q J Med 1971;158:159–185.
23. Murray-Lyon IM, Stren RB, Williams, R. Controlled trial of prednisone and azathioprine in active chronic hepatitis. Lancet 1973;1:735–737.
24. Soloway RD, Summerskill WHJ, Baggenstoss AH. Clinical, biochemical, and histological remission of severe chronic active liver disease: a controlled study of treatments and early prognosis. Gastroenterology 1972;63:820–833.
25. Summerskill WHJ, Korman MG, Ammon HV. Prednisone for chronic active liver disease: dose titration, standard dose, and combination with azathioprine compared. Gut 1975;16:876.
26. Johnson PJ, McFarlane IG, Williams R. Azathioprine for the long-term maintenance of remission in autoimmune hepatitis. N Engl J Med, 1995;333:958–963.
27. Person JL, McHutchenson JG, Fong TL, Redeker AG. A case of cyclosporin-sensitive, steroid-resistant, autoimmune chronic active hepatitis. J Clin Gastroenterol 1993;17:317–320.
28. Hyams JS, Ballow M, Leichtner AM. Cyclosporin treatment of autoimmune chronic active hepatitis. Gastroenterology 1987;93:890–893.
29. Alstead EM, Ritchie JK, Lennard-Jones. Safety of azathioprine in pregnancy in inflammatory bowel disease. Gastroenterology 1990;99:443–446.
30. Sanchez-Urdazpal L, Czaja AJ, van Hoek B. Prognostic features and role of liver transplantation in severe corticosteroid-treated autoimmune chronic active hepatitis. Hepatology 1992;15:215.
31. Neuberger J, Portman B, Calne R. Recurrence of autoimmune chronic active hepatitis following orthotopic liver grafting. Transplantation 1984;37:363.
32. Burroughs AK, Bassendine MF, Thomas HC, Sherlock S. Primary liver cancer in autoimmune chronic liver disease. Brit Med J 1981;282:273.
33. Kemeny MJ, O'Hanlon G, Gregory PB. Asymptomatic chronic active hepatitis–prognosis and treatment. (Abstract) Gastroenterology 1984;86:1325.
34. Czaja AJ, Davis GL, Ludwig J. Complete resolution of inflammatory activity following corticosteroid treatment of HBsAg-negative chronic active hepatitis. Hepatology 1984;4:622.

12
Hepatocellular Carcinoma

Thomas J. Devers

CONTENTS

1. INTRODUCTION

Hepatocellular carcinoma (HCC) is one of the most common malignancies on a global scale, with an incidence of 20–150 cases per 100,000 population per year in some areas of Asia and Africa. It occurs much less frequently in Western Europe and the United States (1–5 cases per 100,000 population per year) *(1)*. In a prospective study from Japan, liver cirrhosis, and viral hepatitis were implicated as risk factors for HCC, each carrying a 3-yr cumulative risk of 12.5 and 3.8%, respectively. The risk of HCC was increased almost sevenfold in patients with hepatitis B surface antigen *(2)* and fourfold in patients with hepatitis C antibody *(3)*. Studies from Western Europe have confirmed a yearly incidence of 3–5% for HCC in patients with cirrhosis *(4)*. HCC is the seventh most common form of cancer in men and the ninth most common in women worldwide *(5)*. Each year there are 1 million new cases globally. The male prevalence is 3 times greater than female.

There are marked variations in the development of HCC in cirrhotic livers. The worldwide rate of cirrhosis associated with HCC is 60% *(6)*. However, 30% of patients in Africa and the United Kingdom do not have cirrhosis. Ninety percent of patients with HCC in the United States are between the ages of 60 and 80, and 90% have cirrhosis. These variations can be explained by the presence of cofactors that alter the risk of HCC in different populations. These cofactors include hepatitis viruses B and C, histologic type of cirrhosis, etiology of cirrhosis, and environmental exposure to aflatoxin. They may be present alone or in combination and make huge differences in risk of HCC. Understanding these variations is crucial to the development of a rational approach to the diagnosis and treatment of HCC.

From: *Diseases of the Liver and Bile Ducts: Diagnosis and Treatment*
Edited by: G. Y. Wu and J. Israel © Humana Press Inc., Totowa, NJ

Fibrolamellar HCC has a much better prognosis with a surgical resection or liver transplant yielding 5-yr survivals of 60%. This variant HCC is rare and occurs in young (5–35 yr) patients of both sexes, and is not associated with cirrhosis (7).

2. PATHOGENESIS

2.1. Cirrhosis

As mentioned above, cirrhosis is closely associated with the development of HCC. In some circumstances, HCC may be the inevitable consequence of cirrhosis, time, and cofactors. For instance, patients with iron overload (hemochromatosis) who are positive for hepatitis C or B or alcoholics are 150 times more likely to develop HCC than cirrhotics without either factor. Hemochromatosis in Australia is complicated by HCC in 30% of all cases. Excessive alcohol ingestion is a frequent cofactor in the development of HCC in patients with hemochromatosis. In genetic hemochromatosis without cirrhosis there is a very low risk of HCC (see Chapter 18). The presence of the hepatitis B virus increases the risk of HCC in hemochromatosis by 4.9-fold. Age above 55 yr increases the risk of HCC in hemochromatosis by 13.3-fold. If cirrhosis is present in hemochromatosis, removal of iron by phlebotomy does not reduce the risk of HCC. However, starting phlebotomy in the precirrhotic stage leads to a normal life expectancy (8).

2.2. Hepatitis Viruses

The rate of hepatitis C in patients with HCC is very high worldwide, averaging 53% in Miami, 58% in Paris, 73% in Japan, 75% in Spain, 76% in Sicily, and 65% in northern Italy (6). In a prospective study of 795 patients with viral and alcoholic cirrhosis in Japan, 221 developed HCC. The rates were 19.4%, 44.3%, and 58.2% at the end of the fifth, tenth, and fifteenth years, respectively. The risk of HCC in this study was much greater for hepatitis C than hepatitis B-induced cirrhosis. Of 349 patients with hepatitis C, 75.2% developed HCC over 15 yr. Of 180 patients with hepatitis B, only 27.2% developed HCC over the same time period (9). Most HCC-associated with hepatitis B developed in patients infected through perinatal transmission and occurred at an average age that was 10 yr younger than hepatitis C (62 vs 52 yr). Also, the hepatitis B virus was strongly associated with HCC in younger patients who were noncirrhotic, accounting for 100% of children under 17 yr in one study. In contrast, HCC associated with hepatitis C was almost always in cirrhotics and in an older age group. Hepatitis C virus has never been reported to cause HCC in infants (10). Integrated hepatitis B DNA is found in most HCC associated with hepatitis B (6). Both viruses may be present simultaneously in HCC.

2.3. Alcohol

Figure 1 illustrates the large increase in risk of the combination of hepatitis C and alcoholism in the development of HCC in cirrhotics (11).

2.4. Miscellaneous Diseases Associated with HCC

HCC is a rare complication of autoimmune hepatitis, and is most often associated with concomitant hepatitis C infection (12). Evidence of hepatitis C was found in 6 of 8 such cases reported from King's College Hospital. HCC is rare in Wilson's disease and primary biliary cirrhosis. It is common in type 1 glycogen storage disease and porphyria cutanea tarda. The Budd-Chiari syndrome may be chronic and in South Africa HCC developed in 48 of 101 of such cases.

2.5. Medications

Oral contraceptives are associated with hepatic adenomas, but there is no clear evidence of progression to HCC in such patients. Most cases of HCC in women under age 40 are, in fact,

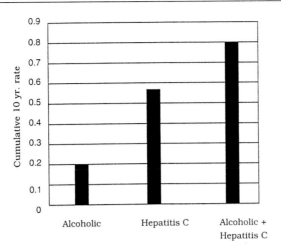

Fig. 1. Hepatocellular carcinoma in cirrhosis.

fibrolamellar carcinoma, and are not due to oral contraceptives *(6)*. Anabolic steroids have been associated with HCC in males.

2.6. Environmental Contaminants

Aflatoxin is produced from *Aspergillus flavus*, which is a contaminant of food stored in tropical conditions. It is highly carcinogenic to animal species, including monkeys. In Africa, there is a linear correlation between aflatoxin ingestion, and development of HCC, especially in Mozambique. In Taiwan, the highest incidence of HCC is in the Penghu Islets where a recent study revealed that more than one third of the peanuts in Penghu were heavily contaminated with aflatoxin. Sixty-five percent of 20 HCC patients had evidence of aflatoxin in serum samples *(13)*.

3. CARDINAL SIGNS AND SYMPTOMS

3.1. Symptoms

Most patients are asymptomatic until the tumors are large. The most common presenting symptoms of HCC are abdominal pain and weight loss (*see* Table 1). The pain is usually a dull ache in the right upper quadrant of the abdomen, sometimes radiating to the right shoulder. A sudden increase in pain can be seen with intratumor hemorrhage. That is a not an uncommon complication. Weight loss is frequently accompanied by early satiety. The diagnosis of HCC should be considered when a patient with stable cirrhosis undergoes an unexplained deterioration, especially if hemoperitoneum is noted on diagnostic paracentesis. The development of obstructive jaundice, obstruction of the hepatic or portal veins, and tumor emboli to the lungs are more unusual manifestations. Paraneoplastic phenomena such as hypercalcemia, polycythemia, hypoglycemia, or hypercholesterolemia should increase the index of suspicion for HCC. The frequency of such paraneoplastic features depends on the patient population. For example, up to 38% of sub-Saharan African patients with HCC demonstrated hypercholesterolemia *(14,15)*.

3.2. Physical Examination

Hepatomegaly is the most common physical finding (*see* Table 2). Ascites, sometimes bloody, may be present. An arterial bruit over the tumor is helpful when present, but is often absent. Jaundice and splenomegaly are common findings. Other stigmata of chronic liver disease may be present as a consequence of accompanying cirrhosis.

Table 1

Symptoms of Primary Hepatocellular Carcinoma

Symptom	Frequency (%)
Abdominal pain	91
Weight loss	35
Weakness	31
Anorexia	27
Abdominal distension	43
Jaundice	7
Vomiting	8

Adapted from: Kew MC, Geddes EW. Hepato-cellular carcinoma in rural southern African blacks. Medicine 1982;61:98.

Table 2

Physical Findings in Patients with Hepatocellular Carcinoma

Physical sign	Frequency (%)
Hepatomegaly	89
Hepatic arterial bruit	28
Ascites	52
Splenomegaly	54
Jaundice	41
Cahexia	15
Fever	38

Adapted from: Kew MC, Geddes EW. Hepatocellular carcinoma in rural southern African blacks. Medicine 1982;61:98.

4. SCREENING

A prospective study of 447 patients from Italy found the incidence of HCC to be 3%/yr. These patients were followed from 1985 through 1990 with alpha-fetoprotein and real time ultrasound every 3 mo. Fifty-nine cases of HCC were discovered, but only 17 patients were surgical candidates. The percentage of operable tumors found by the screening was less than at enrollment (4 of 29 vs 13 of 30). The 1-yr surgical survival was 67%, and there was a 60% tumor recurrence rate. The five patients who refused surgery had an equivalent outcome (3).

In contrast, a prospective study from China done in 432 patients with chronic hepatitis B found eight cases of HCC using ultrasound and serum alpha fetoprotein screening. Six underwent surgery and, of these, 50% did not have cirrhosis (16).

The two commonly employed screening tools for detection of HCC are alpha-fetoprotein (AFP) and ultrasound. AFP is a normal protein of fetal serum that disappears in the perinatal period. Elevations may also be found in embryonal cell carcinoma and teratocarcinoma of the testis. Slight increases may be present in acute hepatitis, chronic hepatitis, and cirrhosis, especially in hepatitis B. Levels above 400 ng/mL are strongly suggestive of HCC, and above 1000 ng/mL are diagnostic. Forty percent of HCC found by screening have normal AFP (<20 ng/mL). In HCC less than 3 cm in diameter reported from Japan, 21 of 22 cases had

AFP <400 ng/mL. Twenty-eight percent of cases screened can be expected to have tumors of this size. Rapidly increasing AFP level indicates a rapidly growing tumor. Unfortunately, AFP is of little value in the detection of the most potentially curable tumors (17).

Ultrasound is the next accepted screening method for HCC. In the study of 447 patients from Italy, ultrasound alone detected 59% of the tumors. Seventy-one percent (40/56) had unifocal tumors and 16/56 (28%) had multifocal disease. When CT scan was added to ultrasound, the yield rose to 93%. The addition of hepatic angiography increased the yield another 7% (9). The ultrasound image typically shows a hypoechoic lesion, but small HCC with fatty change may appear hyper-echoic, and are frequently mistaken for hemangiomas.

If the above study is used as a guide, the cost of ultrasound screening would be $15,000/yr per case detected.

5. DIAGNOSIS

Serum markers of HCC include AFP and des-gamma-carboxy prothrombin, an abnormal prothrombin which may be present in 90% of cases of HCC. Sixty-seven percent of HCC have elevations in the range of 300 ng/mL. Lower levels are seen in metastatic liver disease and chronic hepatitis. The value as a screening tool is unknown (18).

Serum ferritin is often elevated in HCC, but is also elevated in active hepatocellular disease and, therefore, is not useful in screening. Circulating messenger RNA for the human albumin gene can be used to detect circulating HCC cells. It may be useful as a preoperative test for transplant or surgical resection candidates.

Due to its sensitivity (50–90%) for detecting tumors as small as 2 cm in diameter, its low cost relative to other imaging modalities, and the lack of exposure to ionizing radiation, ultrasonography (US) is the standard imaging modality for the screening of large populations at risk for HCC (19,20). In one study, for tumors <3 cm in size, US had a sensitivity of 91.3%, compared with 63.2% for computerized tomography (CT) scan, and 81.8% for angiography. For tumors 3–5 cm in size, US was 92.9% sensitive vs 81.8% and 89.3% for CT scan and angiography, respectively (21). In another study, CT scan and US were equivalent (56 vs 50% sensitivities, respectively), whereas angiography, including infusion hepatic angiography, was superior to both (94% sensitivity), and was deemed to be essential for diagnosis of lesions <2 cm in diameter (22).

When the superior mesenteric arterial catheter is left in place following conventional angiography, CT with arterial portography (CTAP) may be performed, which has been shown to be superior to conventional contrast-enhanced CT, US, and angiography in detection of liver metastases in patients with colon cancer (84 vs 63, 58, and 50% sensitivities, respectively) (23). In a small prospective study that included patients with both primary and secondary liver tumors, CTAP was superior to magnetic resonance imaging (MRI), delayed CT, and contrast-enhanced CT (81 vs 57, 52, and 38% sensitivities, respectively), and was far superior in detecting lesions <1 cm in diameter (61 vs 17, 0, and 0% sensitivities, respectively) (24). Another adjunct to CT is Lipiodol (iodized oil) enhancement. Lipiodol injected into the main hepatic artery is cleared from normal hepatic tissue, but accumulates in HCC (25). This method may pick up HCC as small as 3 mm. It is also positive in focal nodular hyperplasia, a benign condition, but the Lipiodol is cleared within 3 wk. A CT scan performed 10–14 d later will show a dense lesion. This is useful in disease staging, as it may confirm that a small lesion is solitary and can localize the segmental site of the tumor (26). The more invasive modalities, angiography, CTAP, and Lipiodol-enhanced CT, are not considered as screening procedures, but are utilized as part of the preoperative evaluation.

For detection of hepatic tumors, conventional MRI of the liver may offer an advantage, compared to US and contrast-enhanced CT scan, particularly for discriminating hepatic angiomas and metastases *(27)*, and some success has been reported using MRI to identify HCC *(28)*. Another diagnostic imaging modality, which has gained widespread acceptance as an adjunct to hepatic resection of HCC, is intraoperative ultrasonography (IOUS), which has been reported to detect 25–35% of additional lesions, compared to preoperative US and CT *(29)*. In a recent study of IOUS, 14 nodular lesions were found incidentally in 10 of 33 patients (30.3%), 11 (78.6%) of which were HCC *(30)*. In addition to its identification of previously undetected lesions, IOUS can be used to localize the proximity of lesions to critical vascular structures, and may alter the operative plan in a significant number of cases. Laparoscopic ultrasound may prove useful in this regard in the future, but rather as a preoperative procedure.

Histologic confirmation is the gold standard for the diagnosis of HCC. The best results are with ultrasound or CT guidance using a fine needle aspiration cytology technique. This will detect poorly or moderately differentiated HCC. Well-differentiated HCC tends to occur in nodules smaller than 2 cm and may appear to be normal hepatocytes on biopsy. Progression likely involves hyperplastic nodules in cirrhosis becoming dysplastic and eventually malignant. Multiple nodules undergoing this sequence of events can explain the high rate of multicentricity in HCC *(6)*.

6. TREATMENT

6.1. Curative Procedures

There are multiple treatment options available for HCC patients. Some of these are potentially curative, such as transplantation or hepatic lobectomy. Palliative options abound and can be divided into invasive and noninvasive methods. The natural history of untreated HCC must be examined in order to put these options in proper perspective.

Thirty-nine asymptomatic cases of HCC in cirrhosis were followed with an observation period of 90–962 d. Three different growth patterns were observed: slow (doubling time >200 d) 10 cases (37%); tumors with declining growth over time, nine cases (33.4%); and tumors with a constant growth rate, eight cases (29.6%). All tumors were <5 cm initially. The survival statistics were 81% at 1 yr, 55.7% at 2 yr, and 21% at 3 yr. A discriminant analysis using albumin, alcohol intake, number of nodules, echo pattern, and histologic type was used to identify a group with a long tumor doubling time. Child's class A cases had a 2-yr survival of 82%. In Child's B and C cases, survival was 35.6% at 2 yr, and zero at 3 yr *(31)*. The severity of the liver disease is the major factor in the survival of patients with HCC. The effectiveness of any current therapy has to be established in studies over 3 yr in length.

Surgery for HCC is either hepatic resection or transplantation. The hepatic resection experience from Memorial Sloan-Kettering in New York involved 106 cases. Thirty-three percent had cirrhosis and 95% were Child's class A. Survivals were 41% at 5 yr and 32% at 10 yr. Early cirrhosis (Child's A) did not adversely affect survival *(32)*.

In general, the 5-yr survival rarely exceeds 30% in the West, although better results have been reported from Japan. The major problems with surgery are tumor recurrence and hepatic failure. Prior to surgery, measurement of the hepatic venous pressure gradient should be done. High pressures (13.9 vs 7.4) predict postoperative hepatic failure *(33)*. Polyprenoic acid, an antioxidant retinoid, has been shown to reduce tumor recurrence and second primary HCC following surgery or percutaneous alcohol injection. In a prospective study of 89 patients, polyprenoic acid (600 mg/d) effectively prevented recurrent or second primary tumors (27% treatment group vs 49% placebo group) *(19)*. The factors that influence tumor recurrence are listed in Table 3 *(20,34,35)*.

Hepatic transplantation is another surgical option. The Pittsburgh Transplant Institute described experience with 105 patients. The 5-yr survival was 36%, but this was closely

Table 3

Factors that Predict Tumor Recurrence

1. Tumor size >5 cm.
2. Absence of a capsule.
3. Satellite nodules.
4. Vascular invasion.
5. Positive lymph nodes.
6. Hepatitis B.
7. AFP >1000 ng/mL.
8. DNA flow cytometry indicating aneuploid tumor with more than one G0/G1 peak.
9. Circulating mRNA for human albumin gene.

correlated with the pathologic stage: I- 75%, II- 68%, III- 52.1%, and IVA-11% *(36)*. The failure rate was due to tumor recurrence. Any improvement in these figures will likely require improved ability to detect micrometastasis at the time of surgery.

Patients with hepatitis C should abstain from drinking alcohol.

6.2. Palliative Therapy

This type of therapy can be divided into invasive and noninvasive. The first principle of palliative therapy is that there is no benefit in the asymptomatic patient.

6.2.1. INVASIVE METHODS

1. Percutaneous ethanol injection *(37)*.
2. Chemoembolization.
3. Laparoscopic cryoablation.
4. Laparoscopic microwave coagulation.

These methods are available at most regional medical centers. There are no controlled trials to demonstrate their role in the general population of HCC patients, but those methods may be useful in individual cases.

6.2.2. NONINVASIVE PALLIATION

Sex hormones have been tested in the therapy of HCC. A controlled trial in 85 patients with unresectable HCC has demonstrated that Tamoxifen 10 mg three times daily plus 3.75 mg of Triptolin had a significantly longer survival than placebo (282 vs 127 d). The tumor doubling time was also longer in the treatment group *(38)*.

Pravastatin, an HMG-CoA reductase inhibitor, has been demonstrated in a controlled trial to prolong survival in HCC. Fifty patients with nonresectable HCC received 40 mg of Pravastatin per day or placebo. The Pravastatin group survived 26 mo in contrast to 10 mo in the placebo group *(39)*.

7. COMPLICATIONS

Rupture of HCC resulting in hemoperitoneum is an acute catastrophic complication with high mortality. Severe pain or infection are recognized complications of chemoembolization and injection techniques.

8. PREVENTION

The following have been mentioned as having a potential to decrease the incidence of HCC in the future. However, studies have yet to confirm their value for this purpose.

1. Interferon therapy of hepatitis C *(40)*.
2. Hepatitis B vaccine.
3. Phlebotomy treatment in precirrhotic hemochromatosis.
4. Alcohol abstinence in patients with hepatitis C.
5. Reduction of aflatoxin contamination of food.

9. INDICATIONS FOR CONSULTING THE SUBSPECIALIST

The major reason for seeking consultation by a subspecialist is for help in deciding among the wide variety of treatment options available to patients with HCC. On a worldwide basis, the diagnosis of HCC should and will be made by the primary care physician, either by screening or by serendipity. The next steps are crucial to the patient diagnosed with HCC:

1. Is a biopsy necessary or will it change the possible surgical outcome?
2. Is the patient a surgical candidate, either transplantation or resection?
3. What preoperative tests help determine surgical options and the possibility of long-term survival?
4. If surgery is not a possibility, what methods of palliation are best?
5. If surgery is a possibility, who should do it and where should it be done? (HMOs should not be the major determinant here.)

These questions and others which may arise are best answered in consultation with a qualified specialist. The major goal should be optimization of diagnostic protocols for early detection of HCC, and utilizing the surgical options to enhance long-term survival.

SUMMARY

Cirrhosis is the basic risk factor for hepatocellular carcinoma (HCC).

Hepatitis B and C are the most important cofactors in developing HCC.

Hepatitis B vaccine will reduce the incidence of HCC worldwide.

Treating some forms of liver reduces the risk of developing HCC.

Ultrasound is the most practical screening imaging test for HCC.

Surgical resection or transplantation is the only chance for cure, but only a few are surgical candidates and few of those survive.

Invasive methods of palliation in asymptomatic patients is not indicated. Tamoxifen or Pravastatin may prolong survival.

Prevention is best achieved by early treatment of underlying liver disease.

REFERENCES

1. Sherlock S, Dooley J. Diseases of the Liver and Biliary System. Blackwell Scientific Publications, Oxford, 1993, p. 503.
2. Okuda K. Hepatocellular carcinoma: recent progress. Hepatology 1992;15:948-963.
3. Fargion S, Fracanzani AL, Piperno A. Prognostic factors for hepatocellular carcinoma in genetic hemachromatosis. Hepatology 1994;20:1426.
4. Ikeda K, Saitoh S, Koida I. A multivariate analysis of risk factors for hepatocellular carcinogenesis: a prospective observation of 795 patients with viral and alcoholic cirrhosis. Hepatology 1993;18:47–53.
5. Di Bisceglie. AM. Hepatitis c and hepatocellular carcinoma. Sem Liver Dis 1995;15:64–69.
6. Okuda K. Hepatocellular carcinomas associated with Hepatitis B and C virus infections: are they different? Hepatology 1995;22:1883–1885.
7. Ryder SD, Koskinas J, Rizzi PM. Hepatocellular carcinoma complicating autoimmune hepatitis: role of hepatitis C virus. Hepatology 1995;22:718–722.
8. Chen CJ, Wang LY, Lu SN. Elevated aflatoxin exposure and increased risk of hepatocellular carcinoma. Hepatology 1996;24:38–42.
9. Colombo M, DeFranchis R, Del Ninno E. Hepatocellular carcinoma in cirrhosis. N Engl J Med 1991;325:675–680.

Name of Drug	Reaction Type	Data	Mortality
CALAN (verapamil)	C	+	
Calcium carbimide	C/CH	++	
CAPOTEN (captopril)	C/CH	++	
CAPOZIDE	See captopril		
	(and hydrochlorothiazide)		
Captopril	C/CH	++	
Carbamazepine	CH	+++	
Carbimazole	CH	+++	
Carbutamide	C	+	+
CARDIZEM (diltiazem)	CH	+++	
Ceftriaxone	Biliary sludge	+	
Cephalosporins	C/CH/rare	+	
Chloramphenicol	C/rare	+	
Chlordiazepoxide	CH	+	
Chloromycetin (chloramphenicol)	C/rare	+	
Chlorothiazide	C/CH	+	
Chlorozotocin	C	+	
Chlorpromazine	CH	+++	+
Chlorpropamide	CH	+++	
Chlorthalidone	CH	+	
Chlorzoxazone	CH	+++	
Chromoglycate (cromolyn)	CH	++	
Cimetidine	C/CH/rare	+++	
Cisplatin	C	+++	
Clavulanate	See augmentin and timentin		
Clavulanic acid (clavulanate)	See augmentin and timentin		
CLIMARA	See estrogens		
CLINORIL (sulindac)	C/CH	+++	
Clofibrate	C	+	
Clorazepate	CH	+	
Cloxacillin	CH/rare	++	
Clozapine	CH	+++	
Clozaril (clozapine)	CH	+++	
Co-trimoxazole	See sulfonamides (and trimethoprim)		
COLBENEMID	See probenecid (and colchicine)		
COMBIPRES	See chlorthalidone (and clonidine)		
COMPAZINE (prochlorperazine)	CH	++	
Conjugated estrogens	See estrogens		
CORDARONE (amiodarone)	CH	+	
COUMADIN (warfarin)	C	++	
Cromolyn	CH	++	
CUPRIMINE (penicillamine)	CH	++	
Cyclosporin A	C/CH/HB	++	
PALA (N-phosphonoacetyl-L-aspartate)	HB/C	+	
N-phosphonoacetyl-L-aspartate	HB/C	+	
Cyproheptadine	C	++	
Cyproterone	C	++	
CYTADREN (aminoglutethamide)	CH	+++	
Cytarabine	C	+++	
CYTOSAR-U (cytarabine)	C	+++	
Cytosine arabinoside (cytarabine)	C	+++	
DALMANE (flurazepam)	C	+	
Danazol	See anabolic steroids		
DANOCRINE (danazol)	See anabolic steroids		

(continued)

Table 1 (continued)

Name of Drug	Reaction Type	Data	Mortality
DANTRIUM (dantrolene)	C	+++	
Dantrolene	C	+++	
Dapsone	ch	+++	
DEMI-HYGROTON	*See* chlorthalidone (and reserpine)		
DEMI-REGROTON	*See* chlorthalidone (and reserpine)		
DEMULEN	*See* estrogens and progestins		
DEPEN (penicillamine)	CH	++	
Desipramine	*See* tricyclic antidepressants		
DESOGEN	*See* estrogens and progestins		
DESYREL (trazodone)	C	++	
Dextropropoxyphene	CH	+++	
DIABENESE (chlorpropamide)	CH	+++	
DIABETA (glyburide)	C	++	
Diazepam	CH	+	
Dicloxacillin	CH/rare	++	
Diethylstilbestrol	C	+	
DIFLUCAN (fluconazole)	C	+++	
Diflunisal	CH/rare	++	
DILACOR XR (diltiazem)	CH	+++	
DILANTIN (phenytoin)	CH	+++	
Diltiazem	CH	+++	
Disopyramide	CH	++	
DIUPRES	*See* chlorothiazide (and reserpine)		
DIURIL (chlorothiazide)	C/CH	+	
DIZAC (diazepam)	ch	+	
DOLOBID (diflunisal)	CH/rare	++	
E-MYCIN	[erythromycin base]		
E.E.S. (erythromycin ethylsuccinate)	CH	+++	
EC-NAPROSYN (naproxen)	C/CH	+++	
ELAVIL (amitriptyline)	CH	+++	
EMGEL	(Erythromycin)		
Enalapril	CH	++	
ERY-TAB	[Erythromycin base]		
ERYC	[Erythromycin base]		
ERYCETTE	[Erythromycin base]		
ERYGEL	[Erythromycin]		
ERYMAX	[Erythromycin]		
ERYPED (erythromycin ethylsuccinate)	CH	+++	
ERYTHRA-DERM	[Erythromycin base]		
Erthrocin stearate (erythromycin stearate)	CH	+	
Erythromycin estolate	CH	+++	
Erythromycin ethylsuccinate	CH	+++	
Erythromycin propionate	CH	+++	
Erythromycin	*See* specific agent		
Erythromycin stearate	CH	+	
ERYZOLE (erythromycin ethylsuccinate)	CH	+++	
ESTRACE	*See* estrogens		
ESTRADERM	*See* estrogens		
ESTRATAB (estrogens)	*See* estrogens		
ESTRATEST	*See* estrogens and methyltestosterone		
Estrogens	C/CH	+++	

Name of Drug	Reaction Type	Data	Mortality
Estropipate	*See* estrogens		
Ethambutol	CH/rare	+++	
ETRAFON	*See* amitriptyline and perphenazine		
Etretinate	CH	++	
EULEXIN (flutamide)	C	+++	
Exifone	CH	++	
FELDENE (piroxicam)	C/CH	++	
Fenoprofen	CH	+++	
Floxacillin	CH	++	
Floxuridine (FUDR)	C	++	
Flucloxacillin	C/CH/rare	+++	
Fluconazole	C	+++	
Fluorodeoxyuridine	C	++	
Fluphenazine	C	+?	
Flurazepam	C	+	
Flutamide	C	+++	
FUDR	C	++	
FULVICIN P/G (griseofulvin)	C	+	
Furazolidone	CH	+++	
FUROXONE (furazolidone)	CH	+++	
Fusidic acid	C	++	
GANTANOL (sulfamethoxazole)	*See* sulfonamides		
GASTROCROM (cromolyn)	CH	++	
GEN-XENE (clorazepate)	CH	+	
GLIBENCLAMIDE (glyburide)	C	++	
Glyburide	C	++	
GLYNASE (glyburide)	C	++	
Gold salts	CH	+++	
GRIFULVIN V (griseofulvin)	C	+	
GRIS-PEG (griseofulvin)	C	+	
GRISACTIN (griseofulvin)	C	+	
Griseofulvin	C	+	
H2-blockers	CH/rare	+++	
HALCION (triazolam)	C	++	
HALDOL (haloperidol)	CH	++	
Haloperidol	CH	++	
HCTZ [hydrochlorothiazide]	(No documented cholestasis)		
HYDRA-ZIDE	*See* hydralazine (and HCTZ)		
Hydralazine	C	+++	
Hydrochlorothiazide	(No documented cholestasis)		
HYGROTON (chlorthalidone)	CH	+	
IBU TABLETS (ibuprofen)	C/H	+++	
IBU-TAB (ibuprofen)	C/CH	+++	
Ibuprofen	C/CH	+++	
Il-2 (interleukin-2)	C	+++	
ILOSONE (erythromycin estolate)	CH	+++	
ILOTYCIN glucceptate	[Erythromycin glucceptate]		
ILOTYCIN ophthalmic	[Erythromycin base]		
Imipenem/cilastatin	C	++	
Imipramine	CH	+++	
IMURAN (azathioprine)	C/CH/rare	+++	
INDOCIN (indomethacin)	CH	+	
Indomethacin	CH	+	
INTAL (cromolyn)	CH	++	

(continued)

Table 1 *(continued)*

Name of Drug	Reaction Type	Data	Mortality
Interleukin-2	C	+++	
Iprindole	C	+++	
ISOPTIN (verapamil)	C	+	
Isoxicam	CH	+	
Itraconazole	C	++	
Ketoconazole	C	+++	
Labetolol	CH	++	+?
LEVIEN	*See* estrogens and progestins		
LIBRAX	*See* chlordiazepoxide (and clidinium)		
LIBRITABS (chlordiazepoxide)	CH	+	
LIBRIUM (chlordiazepoxide)	CH	+	
LIMBITROL	*See* amitriptyline and chlordiazepoxide		
LO/OVRAL	*See* estrogens and progestins		
LUDIOMIL (maprotiline)	CH	+	
MACRODANTIN (nitrofurantoin)	C/CH	+++	
Macrolide antibiotics	*See* erythromycins and troleandomycin		
Maprotiline	CH	+	
MELLARIL (thioridazine)	CH	++	
Menest	*See* estrogens		
MENRIUM	*See* chlordiazepoxide and estrogen		
Mercaptopurine-6	CH	+++	
Metahexamide	CH	+++	
Metandienone	*See* anabolic steroids		
Metaprine	C	+	
Metenolone	*See* anabolic steroids		
Methimazole	C	+++	
Methyldopa	CH	++	
Methylenedianiline	CH	++	
Methyltestosterone	C/CH	+++	+
MICRONASE (glyburide)	C	++	
MICRONOR	*See* progestins		
MINTEZOL (thiabendazole)	C/CH	+++	+
MODICON	*See* estrogens and progestins		
MOTRIN (ibuprofen)	C/CH	+++	
Moxisylyte	CH	+++	
MP-6 (6-mercaptopurine)	CH	+++	
MUCOMYST (n-acetylcysteine)	C	+++	
MYAMBUTOL (ethambutol)	CH/rare	+++	
MYLERAN (busulfan)	C	+	
MYOCHRYSINE (gold salts)	CH	+++	
N-Acetylcysteine	CHA	+++	
N-Phosphonoacetyl-L-aspartate	C	++	
NALFON (fenoprofen)	CH	+++	
NAPRELAN (naproxen)	C/CH	+++	
NAPROSYN (naproxen)	C/CH	+++	
Naproxen	C/CH	+++	
NASALCROM (cromolyn)	CH	++	
NECON	*See* estrogens and progestins		
NELOVA	*See* estrogens and progestins		
NEORAL (cyclosporin A)	C/CH/HB	++	
Niacin (nicotinic acid)	C	+++	

Name of Drug	Reaction Type	Data	Mortality
NIACIN-TIME (nicotinic acid)	C	+++	
Niclofan	CH		++
NICOBID (nicotinic acid)	C	+++	
NICOLAR (nicotinic acid)	C	+++	
Nicotinamide	*See* nicotinic acid		
Nicorinic acid	C	+++	
Nifedipine	C	+	
Nitrazepam	CH	+	
Nitrofurantoin	C/CH	+++	
Nitropropane-2	C	++	
NIZORIL (ketoconazole)	C	+++	
NOLVADEX (tamoxifen)	C	+++	
NOR-QD	*See* progestins		
Norandrostenolone cyclohexylpropionate	C	++	
Nordette	*See* estrogens and progestins		
Norethandrolone 17-alpha-ethinyl-19-nortestosterone	C	++	
NORETHIN	*See* estrogens and progestins		
Norethisterone	*See* progestins		
Norethynodrel	*See* progestins		
NORINYL	*See* estrogens and progestins		
NORMODYNE (labetolol)	CH	++	+
NORPACE (disopyramide)	CH	++	
NORPRAMIN (desipramine)	*See* tricyclic antidepressants		
Novobiocin	C	+	
NSAIDS	*See* specific agent		
OGEN	*See* estrogens		
OMNIPEN (ampicillin)	CH	+	
OPTICROM (cromolyn)	CH	++	
Oral contraceptive	*See* estrogen and progestins		
ORETON (methyltestosterone)	C/CH	+++	+
ORTHO-CEPT	*See* estrogens and progestins		
ORTHO-CYCLEN	*See* estrogens and progestins		
ORTHO-EST	*See* estrogens		
ORTHO-NOVUM	*See* estrogens and progestins		
ORTHO-TRI-CYCLEN	*See* estrogens and progestins		
OVRON	*See* estrogens and progestins		
OVRAL	*See* estrogens and progestins		
Oxacillin	CH/rare	++	
Oxandrolone	*See* anabolic steroids		
Oxazepam	CH	+	
Oxymetholone	*See* anabolic steroids		
Para-aminobenzoic acid	C	++	
Paracetamol	CH	+++	
PARAFLEX (chlorzoxazone)	CH	+++	
PARAFON FORTE (chlorzoxazone)	CH	+++	
Paraquat	C/CH	+++	
PARNATE (tranylcypromine)	CH	+	
PCE	(Erythromycin base)		
Pecazine	C	+	
PEDIAZOLE (erythromycin ethylsuccinate)	CH *See* erythromycin ethylsuccinate and sulfonamides	+++	

(continued)

Table 1 *(continued)*

Name of Drug	Reaction Type	Data	Mortality
Penicillamine	CH	++	
Penicillins	C/rare	+	
Pentazocine	C	+	
PERIACTIN (cyproheptadine)	C	++	
Perphenazine	CH	+	
Phenindione	C	++	+
Phenobarbitone	*See* barbiturates		
Phenothiazines	C/CH	++	
Phenylbutazone	CH	+++	
Phenytoin	CH	+++	
Piperazine	CH	+++	
Piroxicam	C/CH	++	
Pizotifen	C	++	
PLATINOL (cisplatin)	C	+++	
PMB 200/400	*See* estrogens (and meprobamate)		
POLYCILLIN (ampicillin)	CH	+	
Prajmalium	H	+++	
PREMARIN	*See* estrogens		
PREMPHASE	*See* estrogens and medroxyprogesterone		
PREMPRO	*See* estrogens and medroxyprogesterone		
PRIMAXIN (imipenem/cilastatin)	C	++	
Probenecid	C/HB	++	
Procainamide	C	+++	
PROCAN SR (procainamide)	C	+++	
PROCARDIA (nifedipine)	C	+	
Prochlorperazine	CH	++	
Progestins	C	+	
PROLIXIN (fluphenazine)	C	+?	
Promazine	C	+	
Propafenone	C	+	
Propylthiouracil	CH	+++	
PROVERA	*See* progestins		
PTU (propylthiouracil)	CH	+++	
PURINETHOL (mercaptopurine)	CH	+++	
Pyritinol	CH	+++	
Ranitidine	CH/rare	+++	
REGROTON (chlorthalidone)	CH	+	
REMULAR (chlorzoxazone)	CH	+++	
RESTORIL (temazepam)	CH	+	
RETROVIR (zidovudine)	CH	+++	
RHYMOLE (propafenone)	C	+	
Rifampicin	CH	+	
ROCEPHIN (ceftriaxone)	biliary sludge	+	
SANDIMMUNE (cyclosporin A)	C/CH/HB	++	
Saramycin	C	+	
SECTRAL (acebutolol)	CH	+++	
SEPTRA	*See* sulfonamides (and trimethoprim)		
SER-AP-ES	*See* hydralazine (and HCTZ and reserpine)		
SERAX (oxazepam)	CH	+	
SINE-AID IB	*See* ibuprofen (and pseudoephedrine)		
SLO-NIACIN (nicotinic acid)	C	+++	

Name of Drug	Reaction Type	Data	Mortality
Spiramycin	CH	++	
SPORANOX (itraconazole)	C	++	
STANOZOLOL	*See* anabolic steroids		
STELAZINE (trifluoperazine)	C	+	
STILPHOSTROL (diethylstilbestrol)	C	+	
Sulfamethoxazole	*See* sulfonamides		
Sulfasalazine	C	++	+
Sulindac	C/CH	+++	
SULFATRIM	*See* sulfonamides (and trimethoprim)		
Sulfonamides	C/CH	+++	
T-STAT	[Erythromycin base]		
TAGAMET (cimetidine)	C/CH/rare	+++	
TALACEN	*See* pentazocine (and acetaminophen)		
TALWIN (pentazocine)	C	+	
Tamoxifen	C	+++	
TAO CAPSULES (troleandomycin)	CH	+++	
TAPAZOLE (methimazole)	C	+++	
TEGISON (etretinate)	CH	++	
TEGRETOL (carbamazepine)	CH		+++
Temazepam	CH	+	
TENORETIC	*See* atenolol and chlorthalidone		
TENORMIN (atenolol)	C	++	
TESTRED (methyltestosterone)	C/CH	+++	+
THALITONE (chlorthalidone)	CH	+	
THERAMYCIN Z	(Erythromycin base)		
Thiabendazole	C/CH	+++	+
Thiazide diuretics	*See* specific agent		
Thioguanine-6	C	+	
Thiola (tiopronin)	C	+	
Thioridazine	CH	++	
Thioxanthenes	C	+	
THORAZINE (chlorpromazine)	CH	+++	
Tiaprofenic	CH	+++	
TIAZAC (diltiazem)	CH	+++	
Ticarcillin/clavulanate	CH	++	
TICLID (ticlopidine)	C	++	
Ticlopidine	C	++	
TIMENTIN (ticarcillin/clavulanate)	CH	++	
Tiopronin	C	+	
TMP-SMX	*See* sulfonamides (and trimethoprim)		
TOFRANIL (imipramine)	CH	+++	
TOFRANIL-PM (imipramine)	CH	+++	
Tolazemide	C/CH	++	
Tolbutamide	CH	+++	+
Total parental nutrition (TPN)	C	++	
TRANSDATE (labetolol)	CH	++	
TRANXENE (clorazepate)	CH	+	
Tranylcypromine	CH	+	
Trazodone	C	++	
TRI-LEVLEN	*See* estrogens and progestins		
TRI-NORUNYL	*See* estrogens and progestins		
Triacetyloleandomycin (troleandomycin)	CH	+++	

(continued)

Table 1 (continued)

Name of Drug	Reaction Type	Data	Mortality
TRIAVIL	See amitriptyline and perphenazine		
Triazolam	C	++	
Tricyclic antidepressants	C/CH	++	
Trifluoperazine	C	+	
TRILAFON (perphenazine)	CH	+	
Trimethoprim/sulfamethoxazole	See sulfonamides (and trimethoprim)		
TRIPHASIL	See estrogens and progestins		
Troleandomycin	CH	+++	
UNASYN (ampicillin)	CH	+	
VALIUM (diazepam)	CH	+	
VALRELEASE (diazepam)	CH	+	
VASERETIC	See enalapril (and hydrochlorothiazide)		
Vasotec (enalapril)	CH	++	
Verapamil	C	+	
VERELAN (verapamil)	C	+	
VIRILON (methyltestosterone)	C/CH	+++	+
Warfarin	C	++	
WINSTROL (stanozolol)	See anabolic steroids		
XANAX (alprazolam)	C	++/+	
Xenalamine	C/CH	++	
ZANTAC (ranitidine)	CH/rare	+++	
Zidovudine	C		

United States Trade Names as listed in the 1997 Physicians' Desk Reference are listed in capitals.

(**Generic**) The generic name of the suspected component has been included immediately after the trade name in parentheses. A '+' sign indicates other ingredients in formulation present, but not known to cause drug reaction.

[**Generic**] are drugs not known to cause cholestasis, but are included because reactions noted in similar drugs.

Note: All drugs known to cause cholestasis or cholestatic hepatitis as of the publication date are listed in this table. The drug families included in this table summarize what has been seen with the entire class, but may not be true for a particular drug. Drugs known to be withdrawn from the world market were excluded from this table. This table only contains drugs associated with cholestasis and cholestatic hepatitis. Drug combinations only list component known to cause cholestasis.

Types of reaction: BD = bile duct injury, inflammation or destruction documented; C = cholestatic; CH = cholestatic hepatitis; RARE = cholestasis rarely seen but documented in commonly used drug; HB = hyperbilirubinemia.

Data: + = anecdotal or not well described; ++ = good temporal relationship; +++ = confirmed by rechallenge.

Note: Confirmation does not imply greater frequency and most clinicians regard ++ and +++ to suggest reasonable proof. Frequency of cholestasis is difficult to estimate except with the most commonly used drugs and usually cannot be accurately obtained from the medical literature.

Mortality = "+" indicates mortality associated with medication.

? = causality unclear or only single case documented.

See reference to drug group implies characteristic believed to be generalizable to drug class. Reference to specific drug indicates cholestasis only documented in drug indicated.

Table 2

Hepatotoxicity of Some Nonprescription Drugs

Agent	Injury
Chaparral leaf/creosote bush	Hepatocellular
Jin Bu Huan/germander	Hepatocellular
Pyrrolizidine alkaloids/bush tea	Veno-occlusive disease
Vitamin A (>10,000 IU/d)	Hepatocellular/cirrhosis
Saccharin	Hepatocellular

Table 3

Medications Associated with Predominantly Hepatocellular Injury

Name of drug	Reaction type	Data	Mortality
Acebutolol	H	+++	
Acitretin	H	++	
Albendazole	H	+++	
Allopurinol	H	+++	FH
Acetaminophen	TOX	+++	M
Amieptine	H	+++	
Amiodarone	H	++	
Amiodiaquine	H/TOX	++/+++	FH
Amitriptyline	H	+++	FH
Amoxicillin/Clavulanic Acid	H	++	
Amoxicillin	H	+	
Ampicillin	H	+	
Aprindine	H	+++	
Aspirin	H	+++	
Azapropazone	H	++	
Azathioprine	H	+++	
BCG	H	++	
Benzarone	H	+++	
Captopril	H	+++	FH
Carbamazepine	H	+++	
Carbimazole	H	+++	
Carbutamide	H	+	
Cephalexin	H	+	
Cephalosporins	*See* specific agent		
Chlordiazepoxide	H	+	
Chlormezonone	H	++	FH
Chlorothiazide	H	+	
Chlorpromazine	H	+	FH
Chlorpropamide	H	+	
Chlorzoxazone	H	+++	
Cimetidine	H	+++	FH
Clindamycin	H	++	
Clofibrate	H	+	
Clometacin	H	+++	
Clomipramine	H	++	
Clonazepam	H	+++	
Clotrizepam	H	++	FH
Cocaine	H	++	
Copper Salts	TOX	+++	
Co-trimoxazole	*See* sulfonamides (and trimethoprim)		
Dantrolene	H	+++	FH
Dapsone	H	++	
Desipramine	H	+	
Diazepam	H	+	FH
Diclofenac	H	+++	FH
Difenamizole	H	+	

(continued)

Table 3 *(continued)*

Name of drug	Reaction type	Data	Mortality
Diflunisal	H	++	
Diltiazem	H	+	
Disulfiram	H	+++	
Dothiepim	H	++	
Doxorubicin	CAH	+	
Enalapril	H	++	
Enflurane	H	+++	FH
Ethionamide	TOX	+++	
Acetaminophen	TOX	+++	FH
Aspirin	H/TOX	++	
Etretinate	H	+++	
Exifone	H	++	FH
Fenbufen	H	+++	
Fenfibrate	H	+	
Fenfluramine	H	+	
Fipexidine	H	++	FH
Flucloxacillin	H	+	
Flucytosine	H	++	
5-Fluorouracil	LFT	+	
Flutamide	H	+++	
Glafenine	H	+++	
Glyburide	H	++	
Gold Salts	H	+++	FH
Halothane	H	+++	FH
Heparin	LFT	++	
Hycanthone	TOX	+++	
Hydralazine	H	+++	
Ibuprofen	H	+++	
Idarubicin	H	++	FH
Indocine N-oxide	H	++	FH
Indomethacin	H	+	FH
Iodipamide meglumine	H	++	
Iron	TOX	+++	
Isocarboxazide	H	++	
Isoniazid	H	+++	
Kanamycin	H	+	
Ketoconazole	H	+++	FH
Labetalol	H	+++	FH
Lergotrile	H	++	
Lisinopril	H	++	FH
Mebendazole	H	+++	
Meclofenamate	H	+	
Mercaptopurine-6	H/TOX	+++	
Mesalazine	H	++	
Metahexamide	H	+++	FH
Methimazole	H	+++	
Methotrexate	TOX	+++	
Methoxyflurane	H	+++	FH
N-Methylcarbamate	H	+	
Methyldopa	H	+++	FH
Metoprolol	H	++	

Name of drug	Reaction type	Data	Mortality
MINOCYCLINE	H	+++	M
Mistletoe	H	+++	
Monochlorobenzene	TOX	+++	
Moxisylyte	H	+++	
Naproxen	H	+++	
Nicotinic Acid	TOX	+++	
Niacin (Nicotinic Acid)	TOX	+++	
Nifedipine	H	++	
Niflumic Acid	H	++	
Nitrofurantoin	H	+++	FH
Norfloxacin	H	++	
Omeprazole	H	+	M
Oxacillin	H	++	
Oxyphenbutazone	H	+	
Para-aminosalicylic Acid	TOX	+++	
Paracetamol	H	+++	
Paraquat	TOX	+++	
Pemoline	H	++	FH
Penicillin	H	+	
Pennyroyal oil	H	++	
Perhexiline	H	++	
Phencyclidine	H	+	
Pheniprazine	H	+	
Phenoxyproperazine	H	+	
Phenozopyridine	H	+	
Phenylbutazone	H	+++	
Phenytoin	H	+++	FH
Phosphorus	TOX	+++	
Piperazine	H	+++	
Pirprofen	H	+++	FH
Piroxicam	H	++	FH
Probenecid	H	++	
Procainamide	H	+++	
Procarbazine	H	++	
Prochlorperazine	H	++	
Progabide	H	++	
Propylthiouracil	H	+++	
Pyrazinamide	H	+++	FH
Pyricarbate	H	+++	
Quinidine	H	+++	
Quinine	H	+++	
Ranitidine	H	+++	
SEATONE	H	++	
Simvastatin	H	++	
Spironolactone	H	+++	
Sulfadioxine-pyrimethamine	H	++	FH
Sulfasalazine	H	+++	
Sulfonamides	H	+++	FH
Tetrachloroethane	TOX	+++	
Tetrahydroaminoacridine	H	+++	
Tocainide	H	+	

(continued)

Table 3 *(continued)*

Name of drug	Reaction type	Data	Mortality
Tolbutamide	H	+	
Toloxatone	H	++	FH
Tolrestat	H	++	
Tranylcypromine	H	+	
Trazodone	H	++	
Trichlormethiazide	H	+	
Trimethobenzamide	H	++	
Trimethoprim	H/Rare	+++	
Trinitrotoluene (TNT)	H	++	
Valproic Acid	H	++	
Verapamil	H	+++	
Vinyl Chloride	H	++	
Zidovudine (AZT)	H	+	
Zimelidine	H	+++	

Generic: are in uppercase. US tadenames are in lowercase (as indicated in 1996 Physician's Desk Reference).

(Generic): The generic name of the suspected component has been included immediately after the tradename in parenthesis. A '+' sign indicates other ingredients in formulation present but not known to cause drug reaction.

[Generic]: are drugs not known to case hepatits, but are included because of reactions noted in similar drugs.

Note: All drugs known to cause hepatitis as of 1997 are listed in this table. The drug families included in this table summarize what has been seen with the entire class, but may not be true for a particular drug. Drugs known to be withdrawn from the world market were excluded from this table. This table contains only drugs associated with hepatitis. Drug combinations only list component known to cause hepatitis.

Types of reaction: H = hepatitis (aminotransferase elevations or biopsy); TOX = hepatotoxic (unspecified); H/Tox = mixed hepatitis/toxic; LFT = serum liver test abnormality (unspecified); RARE = hepatocellular reaction rarely seen.

Data: + = anecdotal or not well described; ++ = good temporal relationship; +++ = confirmed by rechallenge.

Note: Confirmation does not imply greater frequency and most clinicians regard ++ and +++ to suggest reasonable proof. Frequency of hepatitis is difficult to estimate except with the most commonly used drugs and usually cannot be accurately obtained from the medical literature.

Mortality: M = mortality associated with medication; ? = causality unclear or only single case documented; FH = fulminant hepatitis.

See reference to drug group implies characteristic believed to be generalizable to drug class.

Table 4

Medications Associated with Tumors and other Liver Pathology

Name of drug	Reaction type
Aflatoxin	C, HCC
Allopurinol	GH
Amiodarone	GH
Amoxacillin	GH
Ampicillin	GH
Androgens	P, A, HCC, AS
Arsenic	As, HCC, C, P
Aspirin	GH
Azapropazone	GH
Azathioprine	P
BCG	GH
Beryillium	GH
Calcium carbamide	C
Carbamazepine	GH
Carbon tetrachloride	C, HCC
Carbutamide	GH
Cephalexin	GH
Chlorothiazide	GH
Chlorpromazine	GH
Chlorpropamide	GH
Clofibrate	GH
Clometacin	C, GH
Co-trimoxazole	GH
Copper salts	Gh, AS
Danazol	P, A, HCC
Dapsone	GH
Diazepam	GH
Diethylnitrosamine	C, HCC
Diethylstilbestrol	P, HCC
Diltiazem	GH
Estrogens	GH, A, AS, CHA, Others
Fenfluramine	GH
Flucloxacillin	GH
Glyburide	GH
Gold salts	GH
Halothane	GH
Hydralazine	GH
Hydroxyurea	P
Isoniazid	C, GH
Labetalol	C
Medroxyprogesterone	P
Methotrexate	C, HCC
Methyldopa	GH, C, CHA
Metolazone	GH
Nitrofurantoin	GH
Oxacillin	GH
Oxyphenbutazone	GH

(continued)

Table 4 *(continued)*

Name of drug	Reaction type
Oxyphenisatin	C
Papaverine	GH, C
Penicillin	GH
Perhexiline	GH
Phenelzine	HCC, C
Phenylbutazone	GH
Phenytoin	GH
Polychlorinated biphenyls (PCB)	C
Procainamide	GH
Procarbazine	GH
Pyrrolizidine alkaloids	C, HCC
Quinidine	GH
Quinine	GH
Ranitidine	GH
SEATONE (herbal extract)	GH
Silica	GH
Stilbestrol	AS
Sulfadioxine-pyrimethamine	GH
Sulfasalazine	GH
Sulfonamides	GH
Talc	GH
Tamoxifen	P
Testosterone	P, A
Tetrachloroethane	F
Tetrahydroaminoacridine	GH
Thioguanine-6	P
Thorium dioxide	AS, P, CHA, HCC
Thorotrast (Thorium dioxide)	AS,P, CHA, HCC
Tocainide	GH
Tolbutamide	GH, HCC
Trichlormethiazide	GH
Trinitrotoluene (TNT)	C
Vinyl chloride	F, AS, P, C, Others
Vitamin A	C, P
Zimelidine	GH

A = Adenoma; AS = Angiosarcoma; C = Cirrhosis; CHA = Cholangiocarcinoma; GH = Granulomatous Hepatitis; HCC = Hepatocellular Carcinoma; P = Peliosis.

TABLE 5

Medication Associated with Vascular Disease

Name of drug	Reaction type
Actinomycin-D	VOD, PH
Adriamycin (doxorubicin)	VOD
Aflatoxin	VOD
Arsenic	PH, VOD
Azathioprine	PH, VOD
BCNU	VOD
Busulfan	VOD
Carboplatin	VOD
Copper salts	PH
Cyclophosphamide	VOD
Cysteamine	VOD
Cytosine arabinoside	VOD
Dacarbazine	VOD, BC
Dactinomycin (actinomycin-D)	VOD, PH
Dimethylnitrosamine	VOD
Doxorubicin	VOD
Estrogens	BC
Indocine N-oxide	VOD
Medroxyprogesterone	BC
Methotrexate	PH
Mitomycin C	VOD
Nitrogen mustard	VOD
Progestin (medroxyprogesterone)	BC
Pyrrolizidine alkaloids	VOD
Thioguanine- 6	VOD, PH
Vincristine	VOD
Vitamin E (iv form only)	VOD

BC = Budd-Chari Syndrome; PH = Portal Hypertension (Non-cirrhotic); VOD = Veno-occlusive disease.

TABLE 6

Chemical Classes of NSAIDS

Salicylic acid derivatives
• Diflunisal
Pyrazolon derivatives
• Phenylbutazone
• Oxyphenbutazone
• Ketobutazone
• Azopropazone
• Feprazone
• Phenazone
Para-aminophenol derivatives
• Phenacetin
• Acetaminophen
Acetic acid derivatives
• Indomethacin
• Sulindac
• Tolmentin
• Floctafenine
• Etodolec
Anthranilic acid derivatives
• Mefenamic acid
• Meclofenamic acid
• Diclofenac
Proprionic acid derivatives
• Ibuprofen
• Naproxen
• Flubiprofen
• Fenoprofen
• Ketoprofen
Oxicam derivatives
• Piroxicam

With permission: Rabinovitz M. Hepatotoxicity of nonsteroidal anti-inflammatory drugs. Am J Gastro 1992;87:1696–1704.

TABLE 7

Hepatotoxic Drugs Requiring Chronic Monitoring

Amiodarone (Cordarone): Periodic serum liver enzyme levels should be obtained in patients on chronic therapy, especially with high daily dosage, although effectiveness in preventing liver disease is unclear.

Anabolic steroids, androgens: Periodic serum liver enzyme levels should be obtained. If suspicion of peliosis hepatis or other tumor is suspected, the patient should be carefully evaluated.

Dantrolene (Dantrium): Hepatocellular toxicity is increased in females and patients over 35 y, serum liver enzyme levels should be obtained at intervals. The medication should be discontinued if not clear.

Doxorubicin (Adriamycin, Rubex): Dosage reduction in patients is necessary with impaired hepatic function.

Table 7 *(continued)*

Erythromycin estolate (Ilosone): Hepatic dysfunction has occurred, primarily in adults and is contraindicated in patients with pre-existing liver disease.

Etretinate (Tegison): Monitor AST, ALT and LDH at baseline, at 1–2 wk intervals for 1–2 mo, and then every 1–3 mo thereafter. Serum liver enzyme level abnormalities are common, but if fibrosis, necrosis, or cirrhosis is suspected, the medication should be discontinued and the patient should be evaluated.

Felbamate (Felbatol): Hepatic failure is definitely associated with use, but details of risk factors is limited because drug use is limited to refractory epilepsy. Serum liver enzyme levels are recommended at baseline and every 1–2 wk thereafter, with immediate withdrawal if abnormalities develop.

HMG-CoA enzyme reductase inhibitors, fluvastatin, lovastatin, simvastatin (Lescol, Mevacor, Zocor): Aminotransferase elevations >3X normal should prompt discontinuation of therapy. Serum liver enzyme levels should be taken at baseline, 6 wk, 12 wk, and periodically from the initiation of therapy and with any increase in dose.

Interferon alfa (Roferon-A, Intron A): Periodic serum liver enzyme levels are recommended may be more useful to determine effectiveness of therapy rather than monitor for hepatic failure. "Flares" with aminotransferase elevations <3X normal are common early in therapy and usually only requires monitoring.

Isoniazid (Nydrazid, Rifamate, Rifater): Risk of fatal hepatitis, (generally increased age increases risk) and is increased with daily alcohol consumption. Late reactions (after several months) can be seen. Asymptomatic, mild transient serum liver enzyme level abnormalities are common and can be followed. Clinical symptoms of hepatitis should prompt immediate withdrawal of drug with consideration of an alternative medication for TB.

Metformin (Glucophage): Lactic acidosis occurs primarily in patients with renal impairment, but patients with evidence of hepatic impairment should avoid this medication because of potential impairment in clearing lactic acid.

Methotrexate (Rheumatrex): Hepatotoxicity with fibrosis and cirrhosis can occur with prolonged therapy and are often not preceded by symptoms or abnormal serum liver enzyme levels. Hepatotoxicity can only be monitored with liver biopsies. Although the frequency of liver biopsies is controversial, a reasonable approach is a baseline liver biopsy followed by biopsies every additional 1.0–1.5 g, although the exact interval, or need for every patient is controversial. Alcohol use, renal impairment, pre-existing liver disease, daily therapy, and higher total weekly dose, diabetes, obesity, and age may increase the risk of hepatic injury. Transient, asymptomatic serum liver enzyme level abnormalities do not predict or indicate methotrexate-induced liver disease. Periodic serum liver enzyme levels and serum albumin is recommended, but there is no consensus in terms of frequency.

Recommendations for high dose therapy for malignancies are not reviewed here.

Methyldopa, methyldopate (Aldoclor, Aldomet, methyldopate): Fatal hepatic necrosis has been reported and mimics many hepatocellular and biliary processes. Periodic serum liver enzyme levels should be drawn especially during the first 6–12 wk of therapy. If a hypersensitivity pattern is seen, patients should not be rechallenged.

Minocycline (Minocine, Dynacin, Vectrin): Serum sickness, a systemic lupus erythematosus-like syndrome, and autoimmune hepatitis, the latter sometimes severe with mortality has been reported with oral administration for the treatment of acne. ANA and aminotransferases should be drawn as a baseline and followed periodically during treatment.

Tacrine (Cognex): ALT should be monitored every other week for 16 wk, then monthly for another 8 wk, and every 3 mo thereafter. Refer to package insert for adjustment of dose and monitoring if ALT is elevated.

Jaundiced patients with total bili >3 mg/dL should be discontinued and not rechallenged.

Valproic acid, divalproex (Depakene, Depakote): Risk of hepatic failure. Monitor serum liver enzyme levels at baseline, and frequently thereafter, especially first 6 mo. Extreme caution in patients under 2 yr of age.

3.6. Diuretics

Hepatotoxicity is rarely seen with diuretics. Jaundice and an increased incidence of acute cholecystitis has been associated with thiazide diuretics.

3.7. Antiepileptics

3.7.1. CARBAMAZEPINE

Asymptomatic aminotransferase elevations are common. Carbamazepine may induce a granulomatous hepatitis that has a classic presentation 1–16 wk after starting the medication. Fever, chills, night sweats, anorexia, and malaise are seen. Symptoms may mimic cholangitis.

3.7.2. BARBITURATES

Although hepatotoxicity is rare, barbiturate-induced hepatitis is often severe and can be fatal.

3.7.3. PHENYTOIN

Phenytoin induces elevations in GGT, which alone is not considered evidence of hepatotoxicity. Toxicity is not dose dependent. Systemic symptoms, particularly fever and rash, are common. Typically a hepatitis picture occurs, but a pseudo-mononucleosis or pseudo-lymphoma syndrome has been documented. Recovery is rapid upon withdrawal. Severe hypersensitivity reactions have been reported with rechallenges.

3.8. Antituberculosis Agents

Streptomycin, ethambutol, rifampin, and isoniazid (INH) are agents generally used in combination for treatment of tuberculosis. Streptomycin and ethambutol appear to have relatively little hepatotoxicity (1). Hepatotoxicity associated with rifampin has been seen mainly in patients taking it in combination with INH, but has also been documented to cause toxicity alone (2). INH is the most widely used and important of the antituberculous drugs. The mechanism of INH hepatotoxicity is not entirely clear. Oxidation of acetylated isoniazid derivatives probably plays a role. These products have been reported to bind covalently to intracellular macromolecules producing injury (3). Mild elevations in aminotransferases (less than 2 times normal) are common, occurring in 10–20% of cases. Generally, these elevations are not of clinical significance, and will resolve spontaneously (4,5). In approx 1% of all individuals exposed, clinical hepatitis may develop. This percentage is higher in older persons, and is rare in individuals under the age of 35 (3). Alcohol appears to increase the risk of hepatitis, and certain other subgroups such as black females, postpartum women, and possibly Asian men may also be at higher risk to develop INH-induced hepatitis (3,6,7). It was also initially considered that rapid acetylators of isoniazid were at increased risk for developing INH hepatitis. However, this has not been supported by more recent studies (8). There is significant potential for fulminant hepatic failure. Patients with acute INH hepatitis have up to a 10% mortality. This is much higher than that associated with viral hepatitis. INH hepatitis is rare in those who have been treated with the drug for more than 6 mo without becoming ill (3). Because there is also no close correlation between aminotransferase elevations and the development of clinical hepatitis, the issue of monitoring these levels is controversial. Monitoring of aminotransferase levels is not recommended for individuals under the age of 35. This younger group of patients should be instructed, however, to report immediately any symptoms out of the ordinary, such as fatigue, flu-like symptoms, or gastrointestinal complaints. It should be noted that serious hepatoxicity may occur in the absence of complaints. In patients over the age of 35, monitoring of aminotransferases levels is recommended. It has been suggested that minor elevations <100 IU/L can be followed closely, particularly if they return to normal. If levels exceed 100 IU/L, discontinuation has been suggested (9). If there are any clinical symptoms or signs of hepatitis, the drug should be discontinued unless it is needed for life-threatening tuberculosis. Guidelines for the use of isoniazid should be strictly followed *(3,10)*. The treatment of isoniazid toxicity is supportive care.

3.9. Nonsteroidal Anti-Inflammatory Drugs (NSAIDS)

Whereas all these agents function similarly, they are chemically different and can be grouped based on their chemical structure as shown in Table 1. The mechanism of hepatic injury for most of the NSAIDS is felt to be an idiosyncratic reaction, that is generally reversible with discontinuation of the drug. The two notable exceptions are aspirin and acetaminophen. These drugs have intrinsic hepatotoxicity and cause injury in a dose-dependent manner. Salicylate toxicity is usually associated with blood levels exceeding 15–25 mg/dL. NSAIDS generally cause hepatocellular injury, but cholestatic hepatitis has been reported with diflunisal, naproxen, and sulindac *(11)*.

3.9.1. SALICYLATES

Salicylates also deserve separate mention in relation to Reye's syndrome. Reye's syndrome is seen mainly in children who have taken salicylates for fever, and results in acute fatty degeneration of the liver. The mechanism is not understood. Reye's syndrome has been rarely reported in adults. A low serum salicylate level and high serum ammonia are characteristic, but not pathognomic of Reye's syndrome.

For patients taking NSAIDS for a short period of time, monitoring is not needed. However, for patients with chronic inflammatory diseases, who will potentially be on the medication for a long period of time, monitoring may be considered, but this is controversial because hepatotoxicity is not a common problem. Most hepatotoxic reactions will occur in the first few months and only very rarely after 6 months of no ill effects. A reasonable approach would be to check a baseline ALT and then monthly for 6 mo. If the patient develops ALT abnormalities, changing to an alternative agent in a different chemical class (*see* Table 1) would be prudent because cross reactivity between classes has not been demonstrated. If the drug is working well for the patient and he does not want to discontinue it, the patient could be followed clinically and with serial ALTs on a weekly basis. If the levels do not increase more than 2–3 times normal or decrease, it is probably safe to continue the drug. If the ALT continues to increase, or the patient develops any clinical symptoms of hepatotoxicity, the drug must be stopped *(11–13)*.

3.9.2. ACETAMINOPHEN

Acetaminophen, or paracetamol, deserves special mention, because it is a very commonly used analgesic that may cause acute hepatitis and hepatic failure when taken in large doses. Most cases with severe liver injury involve doses greater than 15 g, but single doses of 6 g have been reported to produce severe liver injury *(14)*. The best predictor of the potential severity of an ingested dose of acetaminophen is the blood level of the drug when measured 4–12 h after ingestion. Persons with acetaminophen levels less than about 150 μg/dL at 4 h are unlikely to develop any significant toxicity. Levels greater than 300 μg/dL at 4 h predict a high likelihood of severe hepatitis.

3.9.2.1. Mechanism of Injury. Acetaminophen is primarily metabolized by conjugation to glucuronate and sulfate. A small amount is oxidized to other metabolites, one of which is N-acetyl-p-benzoquinone (NAPQI). NAPQI is considered to be the hepatotoxic intermediate. Small amounts of NAPQI are detoxified by binding to glutathione. Hepatotoxicity results when the amount of NAPQI exceeds the amount of glutathione present in the liver. This occurs when large doses of acetaminophen are ingested or when increased levels of NAPQI are produced secondary to increased activity of specific cytochrome P450 enzymes. Alcohol and other drugs such as anticonvulsants and omeprazole are known to induce these enzymes and may result in hepatotoxicity at lower doses. Alcohol abusers with chronic liver injury may additionally be at risk from lower levels of glutathione *(15)*.

3.9.2.2. Treatment. Acetaminophen overdoses are treated with the glutathione precursor N-acetylcysteine. When taken within 16 h of a large dose of acetaminophen, it will prevent most of the significant liver toxicity. The preparation is given orally in the United States. Treatment starts with a loading dose of 140 mg/kg and then 70 mg/kg every 4 h for a total of 17 doses. If the patient cannot drink, a nasogastric tube should be placed. In Europe an iv preparation is available. In the patient that presents with a suspected acetaminophen overdose, the timing of the ingestion should be determined, blood levels should be drawn prior to treatment (4–12 h after ingestion), and treatment started immediately with acetylcysteine. If blood levels show acetaminophen in the low toxic range, the acetylcysteine can be discontinued. If borderline or higher levels, are found, the treatment should be continued and the patient's aminotransferases, bilirubin and protime monitored. The patient should be carefully followed for any signs of encephalopathy. Hepatic failure will generally occur 3–5 d following ingestion of the drug. Treatment with acetylcysteine is most effective when begun early in the course of an acetaminophen overdose. There is good data to support treatment up to 16 h following ingestion. Beyond 16 h, there is controversy regarding its efficacy, but it may be beneficial up to 24 h postoverdose. Beyond 24 h, there is little data to support its use *(12,15–17)*. Recommended treatment for hepatotoxicity due to a single dose of acetaminophen does not apply to individuals who have ingested multiple doses of the drug or those chronically consuming alcohol or other drugs that induce the cytochrome P450 system.

Liver transplantation has been used successfully in patients with severe hepatotoxicity due to acetaminophen. As a general rule, if the patient shows no signs of encephalopathy, and the prothrombin time is not increasing significantly, transplantation will not be necessary. Because most acetaminophen toxicity is the result of a suicide attempt, psychiatric consultation should be obtained immediately. A patient considered to be at high risk for a repeat attempt at suicide may be refused consideration for liver transplantation.

3.10. Psychiatric Agents

3.10.1. Chlorpromazine/Phenothiazines

A cholestatic or mixed picture is commonly seen with chlorpromazine and is not dose-related. Jaundice is seen in nearly 1% of patients and is commonly preceded by a prodromal influenza-like or gastrointestinal syndrome. Response to withdrawal is rapid, but prolonged courses are not uncommon. Cholestatic hepatitis is not rare (1%) and not dose related. Cross-reactivity with other phenothiazines is documented but rare. Cholestasis occurs less commonly with other phenothiazines. It is unclear if chlorpromazine-induced cholestasis is immunoallergic or metabolic.

3.10.2. Antidepressants

3.10.2.1. MAO Inhibitors. Iproniazid is associated with greater hepatotoxicity than other MAO inhibitors, but is not available in the United States. Hepatotoxicity is variable among MAO inhibitors. The relative incidence is difficult to ascertain since these drugs are less commonly used.

3.10.2.2. Tricyclic Antidepressants. Liver toxicity with tricyclics is rare, but is most commonly cholestatic when it does occur. Amineptine may be more hepatotoxic than other tricyclics. The mechanism in this class may be a combination of individual metabolic susceptibility with a hypersensitivity reaction.

3.10.2.3. Serotonin Reuptake Inhibitors. Liver enzyme abnormalities have been reported with SRIs, but this is a relatively new medication, and incidence of hepatotoxicity is still difficult to assess.

3.10.2.4. Benzodiazepines. Hepatotoxicity is considered rare, with the exception of clotiazepam (not available in the United States). Hepatocellular injury usually responds to withdrawal and injury from rechallenge has not yet been reported. Cholestasis may be prolonged.

3.11. Lipid-Lowering Agents

3.11.1. HMG-CoA Reductase Inhibitors

HMG-CoA reductase inhibitors may commonly produce mild aminotransferase elevations, but the incidence of true hepatotoxicity is unclear. Monitoring serum liver enzymes is recommended to detect early signs of fulminant rhabdomyolysis that may be seen with the drug alone, but more commonly when used in combination with gemfibrozil. If serum liver enzymes are more than mildly abnormal, discontinuation of the drug is recommended.

3.11.2. Nicotinic Acid

Aminotransferase elevations are common with high-dose (3 g/d) nicotinic acid, but severe hepatotoxicity is rare. Jaundice is seen in up to 5% of patients. Hepatotoxicity can be delayed and has been reported up to 1 yr after starting high-dose nicotinic acid. Sustained release forms have been associated with an increased incidence of hepatotoxicity even at doses as low as 500 mg/d. Some patients who developed hepatotoxicity on sustained release nicotinic acid were subsequently able to tolerate the standard (nonsustained release) form.

3.12. Antibiotics

3.12.1. Nitrofurantoin

Nitrofurantoin is associated with chronic active hepatitis and is most commonly seen in older patients and females. This may be biased by its common use in treating chronic or recurrent urinary tract infections. Symptoms within 6 mo of initial exposure are uncommon. Hypoalbuminemia, hypergammaglobulinemia, and a positive antinuclear antibody (ANA) may often develop. A hypersensitivity reaction is suspected. Reaction to rechallenge is rapid, and intentional rechallenges are not recommended. Fulminant hepatitis and cirrhosis can occur if the medication is continued or readministered.

3.12.2. Tetracycline

Tetracycline is a renally excreted hepatotoxin causing steatosis, especially when given in high doses and intravenously. The maximum daily doses should generally not exceed 1 g intravenously or 2 g orally. Pancreatitis and renal failure are common complications. Jaundice was a poor prognostic sign with up to 50% mortality.

3.12.3. Beta-Lactam Antibiotics (Penicillins/Cephalosporins)

Although hypersensitivity is common with the penicillins, hepatotoxicity is rare. Oxacillin has a greater, but still rare, propensity to cause hepatocellular injury. Other oxypenicillins may have an increased likelihood of cholestatic hepatitis such as cloxacillin, dicloxacillin, and flucloxacillin. Amoxacillin-clavulanic acid is associated with a cholestatic hepatitis. Cephalosporins are a rare cause of hepatotoxicity. Ceftriaxone has been associated with ceftriaxone-calcium microcalculi or gall stone formation that can sometimes become symptomatic, but will usually resolve when the medication is discontinued. This has mainly been reported in children.

3.12.4. Macrolides

Erythromycin and other macrolide antibiotics can cause a cholestatic hepatitis. Typically there are hyperbilirubinemia and elevations in alkaline phosphatase or GGT. Recovery is rapid upon withdrawal, and recurrence can be dramatic with rechallenge. The estolate form is mostly associated with hepatotoxicity and is age dependent. Rechallenges with other erythromycin forms are generally safe.

3.13. Synthetic Hormones

Synthetic estrogens can cause a bland cholestasis or cholestatic hepatitis. The cholestasis has both genetic and dose-dependent components. Estrogens predictably decrease bile flow, although the predominant mechanism is not clear. The onset of jaundice may be delayed and may present with an initial elevation in aminotransferases that subsequently resolves. Hyperbilirubinemia is characteristic with mildly elevated alkaline phosphatase and GGT that may remain normal throughout. Prolonged cholestasis has been documented. Sinusoidal dilatation is a common histological finding, but frank peliosis hepatis is uncommon (18). Development of hepatocellular adenoma can occur, and is related to the duration of use. It may regress on discontinuation of the medication (19).

Androgens are also associated with bland cholestasis and cholestatic hepatitis. These syndromes are dose-dependent and seen more frequently than with estrogens. Hepatotoxicity responds to withdrawal of the drug. Hepatocellular carcinoma occurs more commonly in patients using androgens than in age-matched controls (20).

3.14. Agents for Suppression of Gastric Acid Production

3.14.1. H2-blockers

Idiosyncratic hepatitis and cholestasis have been reported with H2-receptor blockers, but are considered very rare. Liver enzyme abnormalities may be seen.

3.14.2. Proton Pump Inhibitors

No significant hepatoxicity has been reported with proton pump inhibitors such as omeprazole or lansoprazole.

3.15. Antihyperuricemic Agents

3.15.1. Allopurinol

Side effects with this medication are common, but severe drug reactions are rare. Acute hepatitis can be seen and may often accompany the acute systemic hypersensitivity syndrome seen with this agent. Mortality is high in these patients (15%). The patient may continue to deteriorate after discontinuing the medication, and recovery can be delayed. Granulomas and eosinophilia are commonly seen on liver biopsies. Steroids may be beneficial in severely ill patients.

3.16. Antiproliferative Agents

3.16.1. Methotrexate

In addition to its use as an antineoplastic agent, methotrexate is commonly used in the treatment of rheumatoid arthritis and psoriasis at low doses. This drug has been implicated in the development of hepatic fibrosis and cirrhosis. Toxicity is related to the total dose of the drug and also probably to the dosing interval (daily vs weekly). Toxicity appears to be more common in patients with psoriasis than rheumatoid arthritis. Liver enzymes are of little value in monitoring for toxicity. Whereas there is controversy regarding monitoring, baseline liver biopsy in patients who will be receiving long-term methotrexate is probably warranted. A cumulative dose of 1.5 g is associated with an increased risk of developing cirrhosis. It is prudent to obtain a liver biopsy when this total dose is reached. If the postmethotrexate biopsy shows increased fibrosis, (above grade 2), it is recommended that the medication be discontinued. If there is no increase in fibrosis, a repeat biopsy after each additional gram of drug is prudent *(21,22)*.

3.17. Sulfur Containing Agents

Although sulfonamide-induced hypersensitivity is common, hepatotoxicity is rare. Mortality is typically associated with extrahepatic hypersensitivity, but fulminant hepatitis has been reported.

3.18. Oral Hypoglycemic Agents

Hepatotoxicity with oral hypoglycemic agents is not related to the sulfa group and is uncommon. Glyburide can cause a pure cholestasis.

3.19. Anticoagulants

3.19.1. WARFARIN

Cholestasis has been reported with this agent, but is extremely rare.

3.20. Vitamins

3.20.1. VITAMIN A

Massive intake of vitamin A can cause acute hepatotoxicity. Chronic use of vitamin A has been associated with aminotransferase abnormalities, cirrhosis, and death. Liver toxicity has been seen typically in patients taking >40,000 IU/d *(12)*. However, it has been reported with doses as low as 25,000 IU/d over several years *(23)*.

3.20.2. NICOTINAMIDE (*SEE* SECTION 3.11., LIPID-LOWERING DRUGS)

3.21. Nontraditional Therapies

Nontraditional therapies using alternative drugs is increasing in popularity today. Whereas most of these agents taken in small doses are safe, it is important to realize that some of these medications have been associated with significant hepatotoxicity and patients should be questioned about these during the medical history. Table 2 contains a list of some herbal and over-the-counter medications to be considered in the patient with hepatotoxicity.

SUMMARY

Drug-induced hepatotoxicity can mimic any form of acute or chronic liver disease and should always be considered in evaluating patients with liver disease.

Drug-induced liver disease is a clinical diagnosis generally made by excluding other causes.

Idiosyncratic hypersensitivity reactions are the most common type of drug-induced hepatotoxicity.

Treatment generally involves withdrawal of the medication, monitoring for improvement, and supportive care.

REFERENCES

1. Zimmerman, HJ. Hepatotoxicity: the adverse effects of drugs and other chemicals on the liver. Appleton-Century-Crofts, New York, 1978.
2. Scheuer PJ. Rifampicin hepatitis: a clinical and histological study. Lancet 1974;1:421–425.
3. Mitchell JR. Isoniazid liver injury: clinical spectrum, pathology, and pathogenesis. Ann Int Med 1976;84:181–192.
4. Baily WC. The effect of isoniazid on transaminases levels. Ann Int Med 1974;81:200–202.

5. Mitchell JR. Acetylation rates and monthly liver function tests during one year of isoniazid preventive therapy. Chest 1975;68:181–190.
6. Kopanoff DE. Isoniazid-related hepatitis. A U.S. Public Health Service Cooperative Surveillance Study. Am Rev Respir Dis 1978;991–1001.
7. Snider DE. Isoniazid-associated hepatitis deaths: a review of available information. Am Rev Respir Dis 1992;145:494–497.
8. Gurumurthy P. Lack of relationship between hepatic toxicity and acetylator phenotype in three thousand South Indian patients during treatment with isoniazid for tuberculosis. Am Rev Respir Dis 1984;129:58–61.
9. Rigas B, Spiro HM. Clinical gastroenterology companion handbook, 4th ed. McGraw-Hill, New York, 1995, p. 574.
10. American Thoracic Society. Control of tuberculosis in the United States. Am Rev Respir Dis 1992;146:1623–1633.
11. Rabinovits M. Hepatotoxicity of non-steroidal anti-inflammatory drugs. Am J Gastro 1992;87:1696–1704.
12. Zimmerman HJ, Maddrey WC. Toxic and drug-induced hepatitis. In: Schiff L, Schiff ER, eds. Diseases of the liver. JB Lippincott, Philadelphia, 1993, pp. 707–783.
13. Schiff E, Maddrey W. Can we prevent nonsteroidal anti-inflammatory drug-induced hepatic failure? Gastrointest Dis Today 1994;3:7–13.
14. Hamlyn AN. The spectrum of paracetamol acetaminophen overdose: clinical and epidemiologic studies. Postgrad Med 1978;54:400–404.
15. Heathcote J. Hepatotoxicity: newer aspects of pathogenesis and treatment. Gastroenterologist 1995;3:119–29.
16. Smilkstein MJ. Efficacy of oral N-acetylcysteine in the treatment of acetaminophen overdose. N Engl J Med 1988;319:1557–1562.
17. Cheung L. Acetaminophen treatment nomogram. N Engl J Med 1994;330:1907,1908.
18. Stricker NJ, Spoelstra P. Drug-induced hepatic injury: a comprehensive survey of the literature on adverse drug reactions up to January, 1985. Elsevier, Amsterdam, 1985, p. 240.
19. Stricker BH. Drug-induced hepatic injury, 2nd ed. Elsevier, Amsterdam, 1992, p. 241.
20. Farrell, GC. Drug Induced Liver Disease. Churchill Livingstone, New York, 1994, p. 502.
21. Roenigk HH, Auerbach R, Maibach HI. Methotrexate in psoriasis: revised guidelines. J Am Acad Dermatol 1988;19:145–156.
22. Kremer JM. Methotrexate for rheumatoid arthritis: suggested guidelines for monitoring liver toxicity. Arth Rheum 1994;37:316–328.
23. Kowalski TE, Falestiny M, Furth E, Malet PF. Vitamin A hepatotoxicity: a cautionary note regarding 25,000 IU supplements. Am J Med 1994;97:523–552.

14 Bilirubin Metabolism and Hyperbilirubinemia

Yaron Ilan, Namita Roy Chowdhury, and Jayanta Roy Chowdhury

CONTENTS

INTRODUCTION
DISORDERS OF BILIRUBIN METABOLISM
REFERENCES

1. INTRODUCTION

As a physical sign and a biochemical marker, jaundice and hyperbilirubinemia are among the most frequently used "liver function tests." The clinical significance of jaundice varies according to the underlying disease. Knowledge of the pathophysiology of bilirubin metabolism is required for its interpretation. Acquired causes of hyperbilirubinemia, which usually indicate liver disease or biliary obstruction, need to be differentiated from inborn errors of bilirubin metabolism. In acute hepatitis, jaundice is common and usually transient, whereas in alcoholic hepatitis and alcoholic or nonalcoholic liver cirrhosis, jaundice has a dismal prognosis *(1)*. In the intensive care unit, in septic or multitrauma patients, it is associated with a higher mortality rate. In primary biliary cirrhosis, it is a major prognostic indicator predicting survival *(1)*. Impairment of bile flow due to obstruction of the intrahepatic or extrahepatic biliary tract leads to accumulation of conjugated bilirubin in the blood and jaundice, and is an indication for surgical or endoscopic relief of the obstruction.

1.1. Formation of Bilirubin

In normal human adults, 250–400 mg of bilirubin is produced daily from the breakdown of heme. Eighty percent is derived from hemoglobin; the remaining 20% comes from other hemoproteins, such as tissue cytochromes, myoglobin, catalase, and peroxidase, and from a small pool of free heme *(2)*. Breakdown and disposition of heme released by senescent erythrocytes are required for the synthesis of new heme.

Heme consists of a ring of four pyrroles joined by carbon bridges and a central iron atom (ferroprotoporphyrin IX) *(see* Fig. 1). Two groups of enzymes are required in the formation of bilirubin: microsomal heme oxygenases, which mediate the oxidation of heme specifically at the α-carbon bridge producing the green pigment, biliverdin IXa; and cytosolic biliverdin

From: *Diseases of the Liver and Bile Ducts: Diagnosis and Treatment*
Edited by: G. Y. Wu and J. Israel © Humana Press Inc., Totowa, NJ

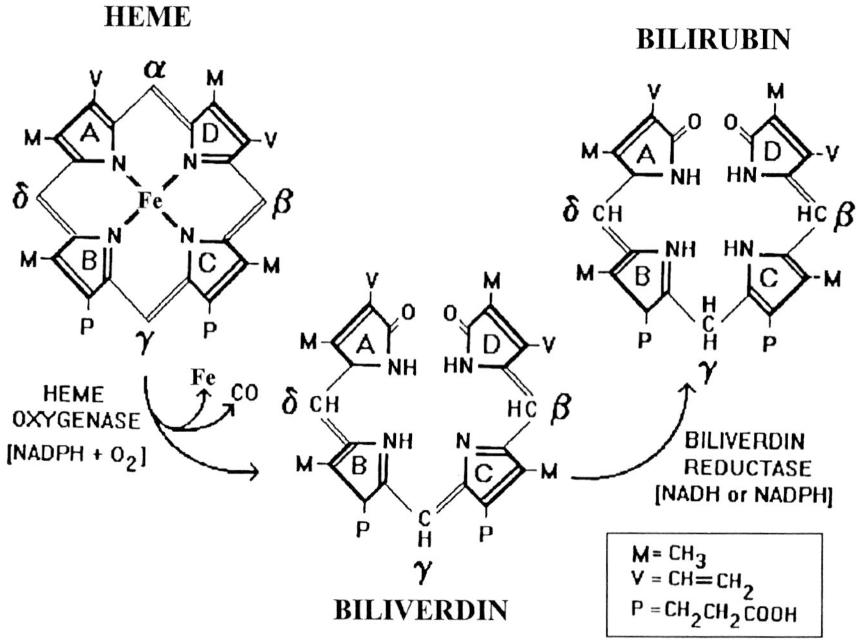

Fig. 1. Bilirubin production: Specific cleavage of the I-carbon bridge, mediated by heme-oxygenase, is rate-limiting in bilirubin production. The reaction requires molecular oxygen and a reducing agent, such as NADPH. The I-bridge carbon is eliminated as CO and Fe^{++} are released.

reductases, which convert biliverdin to bilirubin *(3)*. Heme oxygenase is concentrated in the reticuloendothelial cells of the spleen, the principal site of red cell breakdown, and is induced by heme. Its activity appears to be the rate-limiting step in bilirubin production *(3)*. Inhibition of heme oxygenase by tin-protoporphyrin or tin-mesoporphyrin reduces bilirubin production, and can be useful in temporary reduction of serum unconjugated bilirubin levels. Breakdown of heme releases an equimolar amount of CO. Therefore, measurement of CO production can be used clinically to estimate total bilirubin formation *(3,4)*.

1.2. Clinical Chemistry of Bilirubin

1.2.1. Solubility in Water

All of the polar groups of the molecule are engaged by internal hydrogen bonding. For this reason, bilirubin-IXα is insoluble in water. To be efficiently excreted, the molecule must be made water soluble. Physiologically, the most important mechanism by which this is accomplished in vivo, is the conjugation of the propionic acid side chains of bilirubin with glucuronic acid. Bilirubin glucuronides are water-soluble and are readily excreted in bile *(4)*.

Alternatively, isomerization by exposure to light can make bilirubin water soluble. Blue-green light disrupts the internal hydrogen bonds by inducing photoisomerization of bilirubin-XIα. The resulting geometric or structural isomers are more polar and can be excreted into bile without conjugation *(5)*.

1.2.2. Carriage in Circulation

Unconjugated bilirubin is insoluble in water, and circulates in plasma tightly, but reversibly bound to albumin *(6)*. Because albumin is normally present in molar excess, it serves as a buffer during sudden fluctuations of bilirubin production. Albumin binding inhibits bilirubin deposition in extrahepatic tissues, thereby protecting sensitive tissues, such as the brain *(6)*. Because

bilirubin, resulting in the sequential green and yellow discoloration of the skin overlying a hematoma.

2.1.3. Intravascular Hemolysis

As opposed to extravascular hemolysis, the major sites of intravascular hemolysis are liver and kidney. Hemoglobin released in the circulation is bound to haptoglobin, and then internalized and degraded by hepatocytes. In massive hemolysis, circulating haptoglobin is reduced. In these cases, unbound hemoglobin is converted to methemoglobin, from which the heme moiety is transferred to hemopexin or to albumin forming methemalbumin. Heme-hemopexin and methemalbumin are internalized by hepatocytes, in which heme is degraded to bilirubin. A fraction of free methemoglobin is filtered by renal glomeruli, and the heme moiety of filtered. Methemoglobin is largely degraded to bilirubin by tubular epithelial cells (1,3).

The normal hepatic excretory capacity for bilirubin exceeds the normal daily bilirubin load. But under maximal stress, erythropoiesis can increase by 10-fold, and the bilirubin production may exceed the excretory capacity. In dyserythropoietic syndromes, such as megaloblastic and sideroblastic anemias, severe iron-deficiency anemia, erythropoietic porphyria, erythroleukemia, and lead poisoning, a large fraction of hemoglobin heme is degraded without incorporation into erythrocytes. In these conditions, bilirubin synthesis greatly exceeds the production of red cells. Even in the presence of marked increase in bilirubin production, in the presence of normal liver function, plasma bilirubin concentrations do not usually exceed 4 mg/dL. The extra bilirubin load is excreted in bile, resulting in increased urobilinogen excretion in stool and urine. However, in the presence of abnormalities of liver function, hemolysis may result in marked hyperbilirubinemia (1–4).

Increased bile pigment excretion over a long time may result in the precipitation of monoconjugated and unconjugated bile pigments, leading to the formation of brown or black pigment stones (10,12). Black pigment stones generally form in the gallbladder and may contain polymerized bile pigments. Brown stones often form in bile ducts in the presence of infection.

2.1.4. Inherited Disorders of Glucuronidation

Three degrees of inherited defect of bilirubin conjugation are known in humans. In order of severity, these are Crigler-Najjar syndrome, type I, Crigler-Najjar syndrome, type II (Arias syndrome) and Gilbert's syndrome (16) (see Table 2). Crigler-Najjar syndromes type I and II are discussed in detail in Chapter 23, and only a short summary is provided here.

2.1.4.1. Crigler-Najjar Syndrome Type I. Crigler-Najjar syndrome type I is characterized by severe life-long unconjugated hyperbilirubinemia (17) with undetectable hepatic UDP-glucuronosyltransferase activity towards bilirubin. The syndrome occurs in all ethnic groups, and is inherited as an autosomal recessive characteristic. There is a high incidence of consanguinity in the families of these patients. Unless vigorously treated, most of these patients die by 15 mo of life. The others remain icteric until puberty when they often succumb to kernicterus precipitated by unknown causes. With advances in the management of hyperbilirubinemia, more subjects are surviving to adulthood (16,18).

1. Laboratory tests: Hepatic bilirubin-UGT activity is undetectable (1,3). Abnormalities of serum biochemical parameters are limited to unconjugated hyperbilirubinemia. Serum bilirubin concentrations are usually between 20–26 mg/dL, but may be as high as 50 mg/dL. There is no conjugated bilirubin in serum. All other liver function tests, including serum bile acid levels, are normal and there is no bilirubinuria. Biliary excretion of organic anions that do not require glucuronidation for canalicular transport are normal. Thus, the gallbladder is visualized by oral cholecystography, despite very high bilirubin levels. The liver histology is normal (2).

Table 2

Differential Diagnosis of Inherited Disorder Associated with Unconjugated Hyperbilirubinemia

	Crigler-Najjar syndrome, type I	Crigler-Najjar syndrome, type II	Gilbert's Syndrome
Prevalence	Rare	Rare	2–7% of the population have hyperbilirubin emia; up to 15% have the genotype
Plasma bilirubin	20–26 mg/dL	7–20 mg/dL	1–5 mg/dL
Hepatic bilirubin-UGT activity	Undetectable	Low	50% of normal
Pigments in bile	Only trace amounts of bilirubin glucuronides	Decreased proportion of bilirubin diglucuronide	Decreased proportion of bilirubin diglucuronide
Plasma BSP retention	Normal	Normal	Normal
Effect of phenobarbital on serum bilirubin levels	None	Reduction by over 25%	Jaundice disappears
Treatment	Phototherapy, liver transplantation	Phenobarbital	None
Inheritance	Autosomal recessive	Autosomal recessive	Probably autosomal recessive (autosomal dominant inheritance is also suggested)
Prognosis	Kernicterus, unless treated vigorously	Usually benign; rarely causes kernicterus	Benign

2. Bile biochemistry: The bile is pale yellow due to the presence of a small amount of unconjugated bilirubin (18). The absence of significant amounts of unconjugated bilirubin in bile readily distinguishes this syndrome from Crigler-Najjar syndrome, type II (see Section 2.1.4.2.).

3. Genetic basis and molecular diagnosis: Crigler-Najjar syndrome type I results from genetic lesions of any of the five exons of the UGT1 gene that encode bilirubin-UGT (19–22). These mutations may cause a lack of synthesis of the protein, premature truncation, a frame-shift, or a single amino acid substitution. In all cases, the structural abnormality of the enzyme reduces the bilirubin-UGT activity to physiologically insignificant levels. Identification of heterozygous carriers is now possible by genetic analysis. In several cases, prenatal diagnosis has been performed in families with previous children with Crigler-Najjar syndrome by genetic analysis of amniotic cells or chorionic villus sample (1,3).

4. Conventional treatment of Crigler-Najjar syndrome type I: The major aim is to reduce serum bilirubin concentration. This can be accomplished by phototherapy, which promotes the formation of photoisomers of bilirubin IXα that lack internal hydrogen bonds, and are excreted in bile without conjugation (1,3). In cases of impending kernicterus, bilirubin can be removed rapidly by plasmapheresis. Following plasmapheresis, bilirubin is mobilized from tissue deposits to plasma. Orthotopic liver transplantation is currently the only curative treatment for Crigler-Najjar syndrome, type I (23). Auxiliary transplantation of a hepatic lobe has also been performed in several patients.

5. Experimental methods of treatment: Passage of blood through albumin-agarose columns extracorporeally has resulted in removal of bilirubin and amelioration of hyperbilirubinemia

in Gunn rats, the animal model for Crigler-Najjar disease. Transplantation of normal liver cells into the peritoneal cavity of congeneic Gunn rats, resulted in excretion of conjugated bilirubin in bile, and progressive decrease in serum bilirubin levels *(24)*. Agents that induce UGT activity are ineffective in patients with Crigler-Najjar syndrome, type I. However, induction of a specific group of cytochromes have been reported to result in the reduction of serum bilirubin level. Another approach involves reducing bilirubin production by the administration of tin-protoporphyrin or tin-mesoporphyrin, potent inhibitors of heme-oxygenase. Although the effect is temporary, it may be useful in reversal of crises.

2.1.4.2. Crigler-Najjar Syndrome, Type II (Arias Syndrome). These patients have high levels of unconjugated hyperbilirubinemia, but unlike patients with Crigler-Najjar syndrome, type I, have residual bilirubin-UGT activity *(25)*. Therefore, induction of the enzyme activity by phenobarbital therapy significantly reduces serum bilirubin concentrations in most cases. As in Crigler-Najjar syndrome, type I, the liver histology, erythrocyte life span and serum liver enzyme tests are normal. These patients run a more benign course than do those patients with Crigler-Najjar type I. Serum bilirubin levels usually fluctuate between 7 and 20 mg/dL, but may go up as high as 20 mg/dL with fasting or systemic infections *(1,3)*. Kernicterus has been reported in several cases, especially under stressful situations, or when phenobarbital is withdrawn. Neurological abnormalities range from slight intention tremor, nonspecific electro-encephalographic abnormality, perceptual deficit, and subnormal intelligence to death from full-blown kernicterus. Hepatic bilirubin-UGT activity is greatly reduced, and often undetectable. The bilirubin monoglucuronide exceeds 30% of the pigments excreted in bile.

As in Crigler-Najjar syndrome, type I, the genetic lesion consists of mutations that cause structural abnormalities of bilirubin-UGT. However, in the case of Crigler-Najjar syndrome, type II, all the mutations cause a single amino acid substitution that markedly reduces, but does not abolish the catalytic activity of the enzyme *(26)*.

The main condition that needs clinical differentiation is Crigler-Najjar syndrome, type I. This can be accomplished by bile analysis, which shows a significant amount of conjugated bilirubin excretion in the type II syndrome *(27)*. Phenobarbital therapy is not completely reliable as a diagnostic test. Liver biopsy is usually not necessary for diagnosis, and may not always differentiate between the two types of Crigler-Najjar syndrome.

1. Treatment: Phenobarbital may work by inducing residual bilirubin-UGT1 activity, thus ameliorating the jaundice in these patients. In some patients, discontinuation of phenobarbital therapy resulted in rapid increase of serum bilirubin levels, and in irreversible brain damage.

2.1.4.3. Gilbert's Syndrome. This is the mildest and most common form of inherited nonhemolytic unconjugated hyperbilirubinemia affecting 2–7% of the population *(28)*. Serum bilirubin concentrations are generally 1–5 mg/dL, and fluctuate with time, increasing during intercurrent illness, emotional stress, fasting, and in relation to the menstrual cycle. Apart from icterus, the physical examination is normal.

1. Laboratory tests: Unconjugated hyperbilirubinemia is the only serum biochemical abnormality; other liver function tests including serum alkaline phosphatase, and aminotransferase activities, bile salt levels, and oral cholecystography are normal. Liver biopsy is not required for diagnosis; the liver is histologically normal *(1,3)*. Hepatic bilirubin-UGT activity is decreased to 30–50% of normal. The reduced bilirubin-UGT activity is reflected by an increased proportion of bilirubin monoconjugates in bile. In addition to the conjugation defect that is consistently found in Gilbert's syndrome, approx 30% of the patients have reduced organic anion uptake by the liver. The relation between this abnormality and the bilirubin-UGT defect is unknown *(3,16)*.

2. Diagnosis: Gilbert's syndrome is conventionally diagnosed in individuals with mild unconjugated hyperbilirubinemia without evidence of hemolysis or structural liver disease. Gilbert's syndrome is more commonly diagnosed in males after puberty than in females. This sex difference may be due to higher daily serum bilirubin production in males, which makes the effect of reduction of the enzyme activity clinically recognizable. Although hemolysis is not a part of the syndrome, some patients have concomitant hemolysis; the combination of increased bilirubin production and Gilbert's syndrome results in more clinically apparent hyperbilirubinemia. In people with a minimal elevation of serum bilirubin levels, differentiation from normal may be difficult. For these people, two provocative tests, e.g., caloric deprivation (400 calorie diet for 24–48 h) and nicotinic acid administration may be used (1,2). Fasting-induced hyperbilirubinemia appears to result from increased hepatic bilirubin production. However, serum bilirubin levels also increase upon fasting in normal people, and in individuals with other hepatobiliary disorders. The effect of nicotinic acid is probably mediated by enhanced bilirubin formation in the spleen by increasing erythrocyte fragility and enhanced splenic heme oxygenase activity. Intravenous nicotinic acid administration also does not clearly separate patients with Gilbert's syndrome from normal people or those with hepatobiliary disease. Serum unconjugated bilirubin levels of 5–8 mg/dL may occur in both Gilbert's syndrome and Arias syndrome. In both disorders, serum bilirubin levels decrease in response to phenobarbital therapy (1). Hepatic UDP-glucuronosyltransferase activity, and biliary bilirubin monoconjugate contents may also overlap, making the differentiation between these two disorders difficult. However, serum bilirubin levels in this range are not associated with brain toxicity, and, therefore, the differential diagnosis is not critical clinically.

3. Genetic basis and molecular diagnosis: Although Gilbert's syndrome is inherited as an autosomal disorder, many subjects with Gilbert's syndrome do not have a family history of the disorder. Recently, an abnormality in the promotor region of the UGT1 gene was reported to be present in all cases of Gilbert's syndrome, although all subjects homozygous for this abnormality do not exhibit significant hyperbilirubinemia (29).

4. Management: Subjects with Gilbert's syndrome have normal life expectancy and health. Once the diagnosis is made, only reassurance is necessary. Increased hepatic toxicity to acetaminophen has been reported in Gilbert's syndrome.

2.2. Predominantly Conjugated Hyperbilirubinemia

2.2.1. Acquired Disorders of Canalicular Excretion

2.2.1.1. Bile Duct Obstruction. Obstruction of bile ducts may occur outside the liver, within the liver or both (10). Diseases causing extrahepatic obstruction of bile ducts, such as calculi, strictures, or neoplasm, are often amenable to surgical treatment. Chronic obstruction of extrahepatic and/or intrahepatic portions of the bile ducts may be apparent in the neonates due to congenital biliary atresia, and in adults who develop primary sclerosing cholangitis (12). In hepatobiliary obstruction, conjugated bile pigments, and other contents of bile, such as bile salts and alkaline phosphatase regurgitate into the circulation through the junctions of hepatocyte plasma membranes. Obstruction to outflow may cause some retention of conjugated bilirubin within hepatocytes, where they may undergo reversal of glucuronidation. Thus, unconjugated bilirubin also leaks into the plasma, and both unconjugated and conjugated bilirubin accumulate in serum.

2.2.1.2. Intrahepatic Cholestasis. Disorders primarily affecting bile canaliculi cause decreased bile flow, and reduced elimination of bile pigments and bile. During the neonatal period, various hepatitic syndromes predominantly manifest as cholestasis. Some of these disorders, such as Byler's syndrome, hereditary cholestasis with lymphedema and cholestasis of North American Indians, run in families and are associated with giant cell formation (12). Cholestasis is the predominant manifestation of primary biliary cirrhosis. Some drugs, including alkylated steroids (e.g., methyl testosterone and ethynyl estradiol), cause cholestasis in a dose-related fashion. Other drugs, such as chlorpromazine, cause cholestasis as an idiosyncratic reaction (*see* Chapter 13). Patients undergoing liver transplantation may develop cholestasis as a manifestation of chronic rejection, veno-occlusive disease or biliary strictures.

2.2.1.3. Hepatocellular Injury. In contrast to cholestatic syndromes, disorders associated with general hepatocellular injury result in the regurgitation of intracellular proteins and other small molecules into the plasma. Thus, not only conjugated and unconjugated bilirubin and bile salts, but also intrahepatocellular proteins, such as aspartate aminotransferase (AST), alanine aminotransferase (ALT), gamma-glutamyltranspeptidase (GGT), alkaline phosphatase, and glutathione-S-transferases (GST), accumulate in plasma *(2)*.

2.2.1.4. Benign Recurrent Intrahepatic Cholestasis. This is a rare disorder characterized by recurrent attacks of cholestasis, usually in adolescents and young adults. Following a 2–4 wk prodromal period during which patients experience malaise, anorexia, and pruritus, jaundice develops and the liver may become enlarged and tender *(30)*. The differential diagnosis includes biliary obstruction, which may lead to unnecessary surgical procedures. Typically, episodes of cholestasis last from a few weeks to several months, and intervals between attacks may range from several months to years. Symptoms and duration during the episodes are similar in individual patients. Between attacks, patients are clinically normal. The disease does not affect longevity. Although the disorder runs in families, the mode of inheritance is not known *(30)*.

During a cholestatic episode, serum bile acids, alkaline phosphatase activity and conjugated bilirubin concentration increase to abnormal levels. Serum aminotransferases may be mildly elevated, and the prothrombin time may be elevated because of malabsorption of vitamin K. Plasma disappearance of unconjugated bilirubin is normal, but conjugated bilirubin level increases as it refluxes from the liver. Liver biopsy shows characteristic features of intrahepatic cholestasis. Electron microscopy shows marked distortion and reduction in the number of bile canalicular microvilli, almost complete disappearance of nucleotide phosphatase activity, and reduction in the number of acid phosphatase-rich lysosomes. These changes are not specific for this disorder and may be seen in other forms of cholestasis. Between attacks, liver histology returns to normal *(1,30)*.

The pathogenesis is unknown and no effective treatment for preventing or shortening the cholestatic episodes exist.

2.2.2. INHERITED DISORDERS RESULTING IN THE ACCUMULATION OF CONJUGATED BILIRUBIN

In acquired cholestasis, the canalicular excretion of all organic anions, including bile salts, is reduced. In contrast, inherited disorders of canalicular organic anion excretion do not affect bile salt excretion. Other liver function tests are normal *(1,2)*. As the accumulation of conjugated bilirubin in plasma usually suggests acquired liver disease, ascertaining the correct diagnosis of these benign disorders is important (*see* Table 3).

2.2.2.1. Dubin-Johnson Syndrome. This syndrome is characterized by mild, conjugated hyperbilirubinemia and a black liver *(31)*. Patients are usually asymptomatic. Occasionally, patients complain of mild, vague abdominal pain and weakness, but pruritus is absent. The syndrome is detected usually after puberty, although cases have been reported in neonates. It may be initially diagnosed during intercurrent illness, pregnancy, or use of oral contraceptives, which increase the mild hyperbilirubinemia to a level at which jaundice becomes apparent. Except for jaundice, physical examination is normal. Dubin-Johnson syndrome has been described in both sexes in virtually all races. It is frequent (1:1300) in Persian Jews in whom it is associated with clotting factor VII deficiency. The disorder is familial and is inherited as an autosomal trait *(31–33)*.

Table 3

Differential Diagnosis of Inherited Disorders Associated with Conjugated Hyperbilirubinemia

	Dubin-Johnson Syndrome	*Rotor Syndrome*
Prevalence	Rare	Rare
Plasma bilirubin	2–23 mg/dL	2—5 mg/dL
Plasma BSP retention	Initial clearance is normal, but a second peak appears at 90 min	Increased retention at 45 min, no secondary rise
Oral cholecystogram	No visualization	Usually visualizes
Urinary coproporphyrin	Total coproporphyrin excretion is normal, but approx 90% is isomer I	Total excretion is increased; approx 65% isomer I
Treatment	None required	None required
Inheritance	Autosomal recessive	Autosomal recessive
Prognosis	Harmless	Harmless

1. Laboratory tests: Serum bilirubin usually is 2–5 mg/dL, but can be as high as 20–25 mg/dL. As 50% or more of total serum bilirubin is conjugated, bilirubinuria is frequent. Bilirubin diglucuronide is the major conjugated bile pigment in serum in contrast to other hepatobiliary disorders where it is predominantly bilirubin monoglucuronide. Similar to normal subjects, bilirubin diglucuronide is also the predominant pigment excreted in the bile. Hematological parameters, serum liver tests, and serum bile salt concentrations are normal. Because Dubin-Johnson syndrome affects canalicular excretion of most organic anions except bile salts, oral cholecystography, even using a "double dose" of contrast material, may not visualize the gallbladder. Serum bile salt levels are normal, which helps to distinguish this syndrome from acquired liver diseases *(33)*.

   Following iv administration of 5 mg/kg body weight sulfobromophthalein (BSP), the initial plasma disappearance is normal at 45 min, indicating normal uptake and hepatic storage. However, a secondary increase of plasma BSP level occurs at 90 min because of the reflux of conjugated BSP from the liver cell into the circulation *(11,33)*. Such biphasic BSP clearance curves are highly characteristic of Dubin-Johnson syndrome, but not pathognomonic, as it may be found in other hepatobiliary disorders *(1,33)*.

   Normally, daily biliary coproporphyrin excretion is approximately three times that of daily urine excretion. In normal bile, coproporphyrin isomer I constitutes approx two thirds of the total, whereas 75% of coproporphyrins excreted in urine is isomer III *(32,33)*. In most hepatobiliary disorders, including cholestasis, total urinary coproporphyrin excretion increases, but the proportion of isomer I in urine remains less than 65%. Dubin-Johnson syndrome is unique in that total urinary coproporphyrin is normal, but the proportion of isomer I exceeds 80%. Although neonates normally have elevated urinary content of coproporphyrin I as compared to adults, levels are not as high as seen in Dubin-Johnson syndrome, and urinary porphyrin analysis can be useful in the diagnosis of Dubin-Johnson syndrome in neonates.
2. Liver morphology: Macroscopically, the liver is black. Light microscopy reveals normal histology except for accumulation of a pigment, which on electron microscopy, appears as electron-dense granules contained within lysosomes. During attacks of coincidental diseases, such as acute viral hepatitis, the pigment is cleared from the liver, and reaccumulates slowly after recovery.
3. Organic anion transport.

2.2.2.2. Rotor Syndrome. This syndrome is also characterized by chronic, mild, predominantly conjugated hyperbilirubinemia, and the physical examination is normal, except for jaundice. Rotor syndrome has been described in several nationalities and races. It is rare and inherited as an autosomal recessive characteristic. Apart from the hyperbilirubinemia, serum liver tests are normal. In contrast to the findings in Dubin-Johnson syndrome, the liver is not hyperpigmented (34,35).

Compared to Dubin-Johnson syndrome, there is excessive plasma retention (over 25%) of BSP at 45 min after iv injection, and there is no secondary rise. The gallbladder is usually visualized during oral cholecystography. An important difference between Dubin-Johnson and Rotor syndrome is that storage capacity is normal in Dubin-Johnson syndrome, whereas the transport is markedly reduced. In Rotor syndrome, hepatic storage capacity is reduced to 10–25% of normal, and the maximum transport is reduced by half (34).

In contrast to the findings in Dubin-Johnson syndrome, total urinary coproporphyrin is increased by 250–500% in Rotor syndrome, and the proportion of coproporphyrin I in urine is approx 65% of total. Phenotypically normal obligate heterozygotes have coproporphyrin excretory pattern, which is intermediate between that of normal people and patients with Rotor syndrome. Both syndromes are harmless and do not require any treatment aside from reassurance (33).

SUMMARY

Unconjugated bilirubin is insoluble in water because of internal hydrogen bonding. It circulates in plasma bound to albumin.

Bilirubin conjugation by the enzyme, bilirubin-UDP-glucuronosyltransferase (bilirubin-UGT), is required for its excretion in bile.

Normally, serum bilirubin is predominantly unconjugated. Unconjugated bilirubin levels can increase because of overproduction of bilirubin, reduced hepatic bilirubin uptake, or disorders of bilirubin glucuronidation.

Inherited deficiency of bilirubin-UGT can result in three grades of unconjugated hyperbilirubinemia: Crigler-Najjar syndrome type I (complete bilirubin-UGT deficiency), Crigler-Najjar syndrome type II (severe, but partial deficiency of bilirubin-UGT), and Gilbert's syndrome (mild reduction of bilirubin-UGT).

Hepatocellular disorders, abnormalities of canalicular excretion, and biliary obstruction result in the accumulation of both conjugated and unconjugated bilirubin in the plasma.

The presence of bilirubin in the urine indicates high conjugated bilirubin in the plasma, resulting from liver disease, biliary obstruction, or inherited disorders of canalicular excretion of organic anions.

Phototherapy promotes the formation of isomers of bilirubin that are polar and can be excreted in bile without conjugation. Phototherapy is the routine treatment for Crigler-Najjar syndrome type I.

Induction of the residual bilirubin-UGT activity by phenobarbital reduces serum bilirubin concentrations in most cases of Crigler-Najjar syndrome type II.

Gilbert's syndrome is the mildest and most common form of nonhemolytic unconjugated hyperbilirubinemia.

Benign recurrent intrahepatic cholestasis is a rare disorder characterized by recurrent transient attacks of cholestasis.

Dubin-Johnson syndrome results from an inherited abnormality of canalicular excretion of organic anions other than bile salts, and results in the accumulation of a black pigment in the liver and conjugated bilirubin in plasma, but serum bile salt levels are normal.

In Rotor syndrome, hepatic storage capacity is reduced and conjugated bilirubin accumulates in the plasma. There is no pigmentation of the liver.

ACKNOWLEDGMENTS

This work was supported in part by the following NIH grants: RO1-DK 46057 (to JRC); RO1-DK 39137 (to NRC). Y.I. was supported by an NIH Hepatology Training Grant T32-DK-07218 and the APF fellowship grant. The authors acknowledge the help of Indrajit Roy Chowdhury in preparing the manuscript.

REFERENCES

1. Roy Chowdhury J, Jansen PLM. Metabolism of bilirubin. In: Zakim D, Boyer TD, eds. Hepatology: a Textbook of Liver Disease. 3rd ed. WB Saunders, Philadelphia, 1996, pp. 323–347.
2. Roy Chowdhury J, Roy Chowdhury N, Arias IM. Hereditary jaundice and disorders of bilirubin metabolism. In: Sciver CR, Boudet AL, Sly WS, Valle D, eds. The Metabolic and Molecular Bases of Inherited Disease. 7th ed. McGraw Hill, New York, 1995; pp. 2161–2208.
3. Roy Chowdhury J, Roy Chowdhury N, Arias IM. Heme and bile pigment metabolism. In: Arias IM, Jakoby WB, Schachter D, Shafritz DA, eds. The Liver: Biology and Pathobiology. 3rd ed. Raven, New York, 1994, pp. 505–527.
4. Bissel DM. Heme catabolism and bilirubin formation. In: Ostrow JD, ed. Bile Pigments and Jaundice. Marcel Dekker, New York, 1986; pp. 133–156.
5. Lightner D. Structure, photochemistry and organic chemistry of bilirubin. In: Heirwegh KPM, Brown S, ed. Bilirubin, vol. I. CRC, Boca Raton, 1982; pp. 1–58.
6. Brodersen R. Aqueous solubility, albumin-binding and tissue distribution of bilirubin. In: Ostrow JD, ed. Bile Pigments and Jaundice. Marcel Dekker, New York, 1986; pp. 157–181.
7. Weiss JS, Gautam A, Lauff JJ. The clinical importance of a protein-bound fraction of serum bilirubin in patients with hyperbilirubinemia. New Engl J Med 1983;309:147–150.
8. Sorrentino D, Berk PD. Mechanistic aspects of hepatic bilirubin uptake. Sem Liver Dis 1988;8:119–136.
9. Roy Chowdhury J, Roy Chowdhury N, Falany CW, Tephly TW, Arias IM. Isolation and characterization of multiple forms of rat liver UDP-glucuronate glucuronosyltransferase. Biochem J 1986;233:827–837.
10. Boyer JL. Bile secretion- models, mechanisms and malfunctions. A perspective on the development of modern cellular and molecular concepts of bile secretion and cholestasis. J Gastroenterol 1996;31:475.
11. Wolpert E, Pascasio FM, Wolkoff AW, Arias IM. Abnormal sulfobromophthalein metabolism in Rotor's syndrom and obligate heterozygotes. N Eng J Med 1997;296:1099.
12. Reichen J, Simon FR. Cholestasis. In: Arias IM, Boyer JL, Fausto N, Jakoby WB, Schachter D, Shafritz DA, eds. The Liver: Biology and Patholphysiology. Raven, New York, 1994; 1291–1326.
13. Billing BH. Intestinal and renal handling of bilirubin including enterohepatic circulation. In: Ostrow JD, ed. Bile Pigments and Jaundice. Marcel Dekker, New York, 1986; pp. 255–69.
14. Arthur LJH, Bevan BR, Holton JB. Neonatal hyperbilirubinemia and breast feeding. Dev Med Child Neurol 1966;8:279.
15. Harding JB, Peeples MO. Serum bilirubin levels in newborn infants. distributions and associations with neurological abnormalities during the first year of life. Johns Hopkins Med J 1971;128:265.
16. Roy Chowdhury J, Roy Chowdhury N. Unveiling the mysteries of inherited disorders of bilirubin glucuronidation. Gastroenterology 1993;105:288–293.
17. Crigler JF, Najjar VA. Congenital familial non-hemolytic jaundice with kernicterus. Pediatrics 1952;10:169.
18. Wolkoff AW, Roy Chowdhury J. Crigler-Najjar syndrome (Type 1) in an adult male. Gastroenterology 1979;76:840–848.
19. Ritter J, Yeatman MT, Ferreira P, Owens IS. Identification of a genetic alteration in the code for bilirubin UDP-glucuronosyltransferase in the UGT_1 gene complex of a Crigler Najjar type 1 patient. J Clin Invest 1992;90:150–155.
20. Bosma PJ, Roy Chowdhury N, Goldhoorn BG, Hofker MH, Oude Elferink RPJ, Jansen PLM, Roy Chowdhury J. Sequence of exons and the flanking regions of human bilirubin-UDP-glucuronosyltransferase gene complex and identification of a genetic mutation in a patient with Crigler-Najjar syndrome, Type I. Hepatology 1992;15:941.
21. Bosma PJ, Roy Chowdhury J, Huang TJ, Lahiri P, Oude Elferink RPJ, Van es HHG, Lederstein M, Whitington PF, Jansen PLM, Roy Chowdhury N. Mechanism of inherited deficiencies of multiple UDP-glucuronosyl-transferase isoforms in two patients with Crigler-Najjar syndrome, Type I. FASEB J 1992;6:2859.
22. Bosma PJ, Seppen J, Goldhoorn B, Bakker C, Oude Elferink RPJ, Roy Chowdhury J, Roy Chowdhury N, Jansen PLM. Bilirubin UDP-glucuronosyltransferase 1 is the only relevant bilirubin glucuronidating isoform in man. J Biol Chem 1994;269:17960.
23. Kaufman SS, Wood RP, Shaw BW, et. al. Orthotopic liver transplantation for type I Crigler-Najjar syndrome. Hepatology 1986;6:1259.

24. Demetriou AA, Levenson SM, Whiting J, Feldman D, Moscioni AD, Kram M, Roy Chowdhury N, Roy Chowdhury J. Replacement of hepatic functions in rats by transplantation of microcarrier-attached hepatocytes. Science 1986;233:1190–1192.

25. Arias IM, Gartner LM, Cohen M, Benezzer J, Levi AJ. Chronic nonhemolytic unconjugated hyperbilirubinemia with glucuronyl transferase deficiency: clinical, biochemical, pharmacologic, and genetic evidence for heterogeneity. Am J Med 1969;47:395.

26. Jansen PLM, Bosma PJ, Roy Chowdhury J. Molecular biology of bilirubin metabolism. Prog Liver Dis 1995;13:125–150.

27. Roy Chowdhury J, Arias IM. Disorders of bilirubin conjugation. In: Ostrow JD, ed. Bile Pigments and Jaundice. Marcel Dekker, New York, 1986; pp. 317–32.

28. Gilberts A, Lereboullet P. La cholemie simple familiale. Sem Med 1901;21:241.

29. Bosma PJ, Roy Chowdhury J, Bakker C. A sequence abnormality in the promoter region results in reduced expression of bilirubin-UDP-glucuronosyltransferase-1 in Gilbert's syndrome. N Engl J Med 1995;1171–1175.

30. Summerskill WJH. The syndrome of benign recurrent cholestasis. Am J Med 1965;38:298.

31. Dubin IN, Johnson FB. Chronic idiopathic jaundice with unidentified pigment in liver cells: a new clinocopathologic entity with a report of 12 cases. Medicine (Baltimore) 1954;33:155.

32. Kondo T, Kuchiba K, Shimizu Y. Coproporphyrin isomers in Dubin-Johnson syndrome. Gastroenterology 1976;70:1117–1120.

33. Wolkoff AW. Inherited disorders manifested by conjugated hyperbilirubinemia. Sem Liver Dis 1983;3:65–72.

34. Wolkoff AW, Wolpert E, Pascasio FN. Rotor's syndrome, a distinct inheritable pathophysiological entity. Am J Med 1976;60:173–179.

35. Rotor AB, Manahan L, Florentin A. Famillial nonhemolytic jaundice with direct van den Bergh reaction. Acta Med Phi. 1948;5:37.

V Biliary Diseases

15

Primary Biliary Cirrhosis and Primary Sclerosing Cholangitis

Edward P. Toffolon

1. INTRODUCTION

Cholestasis (literally the stoppage of bile) has a variety of operational definitions. To the clinician, it is the jaundiced patient with marked elevations of alkaline phosphatase and minimally elevated aminotransferases. To the physiologist, it is the measurable decrease in hepatic secretion of water and solutes. To the histopathologist, it is the identification of bile pigment in the canaliculi, bile ducts or hepatocytes. Cholestasis results from an interference in normal bile flow. This interference may occur at any point from the canalicular membrane of the hepatocyte to the ampulla of Vater in the duodenal wall. Clinical manifestations of cholestasis range from asymptomatic abnormalities in liver function tests to fatigue, pruritus, jaundice, and right upper quadrant pain.

In this chapter we will focus on two disorders of bile ducts that result in cholestasis: one involving only intrahepatic bile ducts, i.e., primary biliary cirrhosis; and one that may involve intrahepatic bile ducts, extrahepatic bile ducts, or most frequently both, i.e., primary sclerosing cholangitis.

2. PRIMARY BILIARY CIRRHOSIS (PBC)

2.1. Pathogenesis

Primary biliary cirrhosis is an accurate description only of the last stages of this disease entity. In its early stages, there is only inflammation of, and damage to, the interlobular and interseptal bile ducts. This inflammatory process has also been referred to by the rather cumbersome, but accurate name of chronic nonsuppurative destructive cholangitis.

From: *Diseases of the Liver and Bile Ducts: Diagnosis and Treatment*
Edited by: G. Y. Wu and J. Israel © Humana Press Inc., Totowa, NJ

The etiology of PBC is unknown, but felt to be autoimmune in nature because of its association with numerous abnormalities of the immune system. For example, abnormal circulating antibodies such as AMA (antimitochondrial antibody) occur in almost every case of PBC. Other autoantibodies such as rheumatoid factor, SMA (smooth muscle antibody) and ANA (antinuclear antibody) may also be present. In addition, there is an increased association with other immune-mediated diseases such as the Sjogren's syndrome, scleroderma/CREST variants, and thyroiditis (1).

Once bile duct damage occurs, there is an accumulation of bile acids in the canaliculi and in the hepatocyte. The resulting cholestasis has two general effects that result in disease. First, the increased concentration of bile acids injures the lipid membranes of the hepatocyte, compounding the injury caused by the obstructed bile ducts (2). Second, the decreased flow of bile into the small intestine results in malabsorption of fat due to the decrease in bile acids necessary to form micelles. Although the malabsorption can, but is usually not sufficient to, result in weight loss, malabsorption of fat-soluble vitamins is a frequent problem. Night blindness from deficiency of vitamin A, osteopenia, and pathological fractures due to malabsorption of vitamin D, and bleeding diathesis due to deficiency of vitamin K are the most common.

2.2. Cardinal Symptoms and Signs

Many patients are diagnosed while asymptomatic (presymptomatic). These patients have abnormal liver chemistries in which there are elevations of alkaline phosphatase and GGT out of proportion to elevations of aminotransferases (cholestatic pattern of abnormal serum liver enzymes) (see Chapter 1). As the disease progresses, elevations of bilirubin, gamma globulin, and cholesterol also develop.

2.2.1. SYMPTOMS

When symptoms do appear, they most frequently are nonspecific, such as fatigue and pruritus. Occasionally specific symptoms, such as night blindness, and bone fractures resulting from fat soluble vitamin deficiencies can appear.

2.2.2. PHYSICAL EXAMINATION

The physical findings of jaundice, hepatosplenomegaly, and xanthomas develop as the disease progresses. Excoriations of the skin can frequently be seen due to scratching in an effort to relieve the pruritus. Signs of portal hypertension such as dilatation of superficial abdominal vessels, hemorrhoids, ascites, and encephalopathy can appear in the late stages when cirrhosis has developed.

2.3. Diagnosis

The diagnosis should be suspected when cholestatic serum liver enzyme levels are found to be elevated, especially in females of middle age (see Fig. 1). Antimitochondrial antibody (AMA) levels will be elevated in almost every case, making the diagnosis suspect in their absence. An abdominal ultrasound should be performed to determine whether an extrahepatic biliary obstruction exists. If an ultrasound fails to reveal dilated intrahepatic and extrahepatic ducts, the patient should have a liver biopsy to confirm the diagnosis (see Fig. 1, Chapter 1). Classical features of a liver biopsy include lymphocytic infiltration surrounding the bile ducts with ductular proliferation, and in late stages, disappearance of bile ducts, and replacement with fibrosis. Granulomas can be seen, and are helpful in making the diagnosis, if present. If the histological picture of the liver biopsy is not classical, or if the diagnosis is entertained in a male, other diagnostic tests may be necessary. An ERCP should be performed to determine whether PSC or other mechanical causes of a biliary obstruction are present. A serological test,

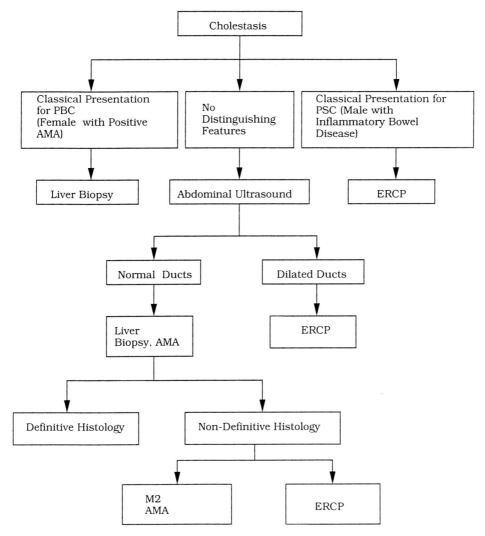

Fig. 1. A scheme for the evaluation of patients with possible PBC or PSC.

the anti M-2 antibody, is a selective AMA directed at antigens on the inner membrane of the mitochondria, and is very specific for PBC. This is can be very helpful in confirming the diagnosis *(3)*.

2.4. Treatment

There is no cure for the disease. However, there is general agreement that administration of ursodeoxycholic acid (UDCA) will improve liver function tests, may slightly improve the histology, and prolong the course of patients with PBC. This is especially true if treatment is started before the development of cirrhosis. It is presumed that hydrophilic bile acids such as UDCA are less injurious to the lipid membranes of the liver cell than the naturally occurring lipophilic bile acids. The dose is 13–15 mg/kg of body wt/day *(2,4)*.

Methotrexate has also been shown to be effective, not only in improving liver function, but in decreasing the inflammatory response around bile ducts. Unfortunately, the toxicity of the drug (predominantly interstitial pneumonia) has prevented its widespread use *(5)*. Colchicine also has been studied, is quite safe, but is only minimally effective in improving the symptoms, liver serum enzyme levels, and histology of PBC *(1)*.

If the presentation and imaging studies are insufficient to make the diagnosis, a liver biopsy may be helpful. Although not always seen, histologic findings of periportal fibrosis and obliteration of interlobular bile ducts support the diagnosis of PSC.

3.4. Treatment

The medical therapy of PSC in many respects is similar to that of PBC. UDCA will improve biochemical abnormalities, and may decrease the necroinflammatory changes seen on liver biopsy *(13)*. There is as yet no convincing data that UDCA prolongs survival *(13)*. Methotrexate initially appeared promising, but failed to improve most liver tests or decrease the rate of referral for transplantation in a recent prospective controlled trial *(14)*. In the selected patient with a stricture in an extrahepatic bile duct, dilatation and/or stenting may produce rapid symptomatic and biochemical improvement *(15)*. Care must be taken to brush this stricture for cells to eliminate the possibility of carcinoma. Surgical therapy of strictured ducts may be effective to relieve obstruction, but may make liver transplant technically more difficult. Ultimately, a liver transplant may be the best option for patients with progressive liver failure.

3.5. Potential Complications

Complications of PSC that are distinct from those mentioned for PBC include cholangitis, cholangiocarcinoma, and varices of the ileostomy when panproctocolectomy is necessary for the treatment of associated ulcerative colitis.

3.6. Prognosis

The prognosis depends on the stage of the disease at the time of diagnosis. Patients with early disease can expect to live 10–15 yr before complications develop *(16)*. Colectomy for underlying ulcerative colitis does not alter the course of the liver disease. When complications develop or liver decompensation occurs, liver transplant may be life saving and survival is excellent.

3.7. Indications for Consulting the Subspecialist

When the diagnosis of PSC is entertained, a subspecialist may be helpful with the differential diagnosis and to perform ERCP. If the cholangitis worsens, hepatic decompensation occurs, or there is concern about a superimposed cholangiocarcinoma, the subspecialist should be sought.

SUMMARY

PSC is a disease of young men, the majority of whom have ulcerative colitis.
The etiology is unknown and presumed to be autoimmune.
Ursodeoxycholic acid is the current medical therapy of choice.
Dilatation of dominant extrahepatic biliary strictures may benefit selected patients.
Liver transplantation is an effective therapy for patients with hepatic decompensation.

REFERENCES

1. Kaplan NM. Primary biliary cirrhosis. N Engl J Med 1987;316:521–528.
2. Poupon RE, Poupon R, Balhau B. Ursodiol for the long-term treatment of primary biliary cirrhosis. N Engl J Med 1994;330:1342–1347.
3. Bassendine MF, Yeaman SJ. Serologic markers of primary biliary cirrhosis: diagnosis, prognosis and subsets. Hepatology 1992;3:545–547.
4. Rubin RA, Kowalski TE, Khandelival M, Malet PF. Ursodiol for hepatobiliary disorders. Am Inter Med 1994;121:207–218.

5. Kaplan NM, Knox TA. Treatment of primary biliary cirrhosis with low-dose weekly methotrexate. Gastroenterology 1991;101:1332–1338.
6. Luketic VAC, Sanyal AJ. Medical therapy of pruritis of cholestasis. Gastroenterologist 1995;3:257–260.
7. Crippen JS, Jorgensen RA, Dickson ER, Lindor KD. Hepatic osteodystrophy in primary biliary cirrhosis: effects of medical treatment. Am J Gastroenterol 1994;89:47–50.
8. Markus BH, Dickson ER. Efficacy of liver transplantation in patients with primary biliary cirrhosis. N Engl J Med 1989;320:1709–1713.
9. Cello JP. Acquired immunodeficiency syndrome cholangiopathy: spectrum of disease. Am J Med 1989;86:539–546.
10. Shea WJ, Demos BE, Goldberg HJ. Sclerosing cholangitis associated with hepatic arterial RUDR chemotherapy: radiologic-histologic correlation. Am J Roentgenol 1986;146:717–776.
11. Cangemi JR, Weisner RH, Beaver SJ. Effect of proctocolectomy for chronic ulcerative colitis on the natural history of primary sclerosing cholangitis. Gastroenterology 1989;96:790–794.
12. Chapman RW, Arbough BA, Rhodes JM. Primary sclerosing cholangitis: a review of its clinical features, cholangiography, and hepatic histology. Gut 1980;21:870–877.
13. Bevers U, Spengler U, Krus W. Ursodeoxycholic acid for treatment of primary sclerosing cholangitis: a placebo-controlled trial. Hepatology 1992;16:707–714.
14. Knox TA, Kaplan NM. A double-blind controlled trial of oral-pulse methotrexate in the treatment of primary sclerosing cholangitis. Gastroenterology 1994;106:494–499.
15. May GR, Bender CE, LaRusso NF, Wiesner RH. Nonoperative dilatation of dominant strictures in primary sclerosing cholangitis. Am J Roentgenol 1985;145:1061–1064.
16. Lee Y-M, Kaplan MN. Primary sclerosing cholangitis. N Engl J Med 1995;332:924–933.

SUGGESTED READING

1. Kaplan NM. Primary biliary cirrhosis. N Engl J Med 1987;316:521–528.

16 Extrahepatic Cholestasis

Stones and Malignancies

Matthew Estill and Salam F. Zakko

CONTENTS

1. INTRODUCTION

The right and left hepatic ducts unite to form the common hepatic duct in the porta hepatis. The common hepatic duct is joined by the cystic duct to form the common bile duct, which enters the second portion of the duodenum through the ampulla of Vater. The common bile duct runs within the wall of the duodenum for 1–2 cm, and its termination is marked by a contractile smooth muscle band called the sphincter of Oddi. The main pancreatic duct enters the common bile duct in its distal segment, and the head of the pancreas lies adjacent to the distal common bile duct. Extrahepatic cholestasis is defined as a mechanical obstruction to the flow of bile from the liver into the duodenum that occurs at any point from the hepatic ducts to the ampulla of Vater (Fig. 1).

2. ETIOLOGY

Gallstones and malignancies are the most common causes of extrahepatic cholestasis, whereas strictures, sclerosing cholangitis, sphincter of Oddi dysfunction, and chronic inflammation are much rarer. This chapter will focus on the more common causes, namely gallstones and malignancies.

Choledocholithiasis is the term given to the presence of common bile duct stones. These are associated with cholelithiasis (gallstones in the gallbladder) in 95% of cases.

From: *Diseases of the Liver and Bile Ducts: Diagnosis and Treatment*
Edited by: G. Y. Wu and J. Israel © Humana Press Inc., Totowa, NJ

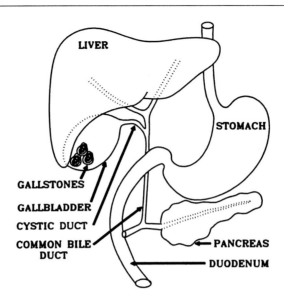

Fig. 1. Anatomy of the biliary system.

Most bile duct stones originally form in the gallbladder, migrate through the cystic duct, and lodge in the distal common bile duct where they may lead to obstruction. Many pass spontaneously into the duodenum, whereas some become impacted at the ampulla of Vater because that is the narrowest portion of the extrahepatic biliary tract. Passage of gallstones from the gallbladder into the common bile duct occurs in approx 10–15% of patients with cholelithiasis. The incidence increases with age, and up to 25% of elderly patients (60–80 yr old) have gallstones in the common bile duct at the time of cholecystectomy *(1)*. There is a 5% incidence of "retained stones" that manifest within 12 mo after cholecystectomy *(2)*. These are stones that present with extrahepatic obstruction after cholecystectomy, but that were not previously suspected or detected. Patients with choledocholithiasis may remain asymptomatic for many years, and be detected incidentally or may present with cholestasis, biliary colic, or a complication such as pancreatitis or cholangitis. Primary bile duct stones are a rare cause of extrahepatic cholestasis in the Western world. In Asia, however, they account for more than 50% of cases *(3)*. They occur in association with chronic hemolytic states (i.e., hereditary spherocytosis), hepatobiliary parasitic infestations (*Clonorchis sinensis*, the Oriental liver fluke), congenital anomalies of the biliary system, and scarred or strictured biliary ducts with chronic bacterial colonization *(4)*. These gallstones are usually black/brown in color and are referred to as pigment stones because they are composed primarily of calcium bilirubinate. Choledocholithiasis that presents more than 12 mo after cholecystectomy is usually due to primary bile duct stones.

Pancreatic head tumors are the most common malignant etiology of extrahepatic cholestasis, and adenocarcinoma is the most common of these. It is twice as common in the head compared to the body or tail of the gland, and is of ductal cell origin in 75–95% of cases *(5)*. Pancreatic adenocarcinoma can obstruct the common bile duct, pancreatic duct, or both. Tumor growth in the pancreatic head, which lies immediately adjacent to the distal common bile duct, causes extrinsic compression leading to partial or complete bile duct obstruction. Occasionally tumor growth into the bile duct can also occur.

Other tumors can cause extrahepatic cholestasis. Cholangiocarcinoma, carcinoma of the ampulla of Vater, and metastatic tumors are less common than pancreatic adenocarcinoma. Benign tumors of the biliary tract are exceedingly rare and include papillomas, adenomas, and cystadenomas. Cholangiocarcinoma has a slight male predominance, occurs in the fifth to sixth decade, and may be associated with sclerosing cholangitis that accompanies ulcerative colitis, and congenital biliary anomalies. Cholelithiasis and choledocholithiasis are not risk factors for cholangiocarcinoma. Cholangiocarcinomas that occur at the convergence of the right and left hepatic ducts are referred to as Klatskin tumors. The ampulla of Vater may be involved in locally spreading duodenal tumors or may be the primary site of sarcomas, adenocarcinomas, or carcinoid tumors. Unlike cholangiocarcinoma and pancreatic carcinoma, these tumors are slower growing, and have a slightly better prognosis. Metastatic lymphomas and carcinomas of colorectal, gastric, and breast origin can spread to lymph nodes in the porta hepatis and produce extrahepatic cholestasis.

3. CARDINAL SYMPTOMS AND SIGNS

3.1. Symptoms

The clinical presentation of extrahepatic cholestasis is variable, ranging from incidental alkaline phosphatase elevation to intermittent biliary colic to severe acute cholangitis or pancreatitis. The clinical presentation is largely dependent on the etiology of obstruction. Choledocholithiasis commonly presents with recurrent episodes of right upper quadrant pain somewhat similar to biliary colic in character (*see* Chapter 17), but with abnormal liver function tests or frank jaundice. With gallstones, the common bile duct obstruction is often intermittent, leading to fluctuations in liver function tests and in the level of pain *(3)*. The symptoms may resolve spontaneously as the obstructing stone passes into the duodenum or may progress to complications such as acute pancreatitis or cholangitis. These complications must be suspected if the patient develops fever, leukocytosis, nonremitting pain, or more generalized pain. Choledocholithiasis may be asymptomatic, especially in the elderly. Rarely, pruritus, diarrhea, intolerance to fatty foods, and/or acholic stools may be the presenting symptoms.

Although the presence of pain may be an important clue to the diagnosis of choledocholithiasis, its absence does not reliably rule out gallstone disease. Nevertheless, painless extrahepatic cholestasis with or without jaundice is most commonly seen in malignancy. Compared to gallstone-related acute biliary colic, a dull, steady abdominal pain with radiation to the thoracolumbar spine may indicate malignant bile duct obstruction. The symptoms of malignant obstruction are often relentless, slowly progressive, and associated with significant weight loss and fatigue.

Finally, it is important to differentiate extrahepatic from intrahepatic cholestasis, a task that is difficult using symptoms and signs alone. A history of drugs, alcohol, or exposure to viruses or environmental toxins raises the suspicion for intrahepatic cholestasis (*see* Chapters 13 and 14). Nausea, vomiting, and pruritus occur with both hepatocellular and biliary tract disease. Dark urine and pale stools confirm a conjugated hyperbilirubinemia, but do not differentiate between hepatocellular or extrahepatic obstructive disease *(6)*. A history of gallstones, prior biliary tract surgery, or high fever suggests extrahepatic cholestasis, whereas a history of alcoholism, hepatitis, or flu-like symptoms suggests intrahepatic or hepatocellular disease.

3.2. Physical Examination

Physical examination may help in differentiating intrahepatic from extrahepatic cholestasis. Ascites, a prominent abdominal venous pattern, asterixis, spider angiomata, palmar erythema, and gynecomastia are seen in patients with chronic hepatocellular disease. Tender hepatomegaly suggests intrahepatic cholestasis due to viral, toxin- or drug-induced hepatitis, arterial vascular insults, and hepatic vein thrombosis. The finding of a palpable gallbladder in the setting of jaundice is thought to suggest a malignant etiology for extrahepatic obstruction rather than gallstones. This is known as the Courvoisier's sign. However, it is rarely encountered in clinical practice. In the absence of pancreatitis, extrahepatic cholestasis produces minimal abdominal tenderness and minimal findings on physical exam. Fever, hypotension, and mental status changes are associated with severe suppurative cholangitis, whereas severe epigastric or periumbilical pain with vomiting suggests pancreatitis. Hemoccult positive stools may suggest hemobilia that can be associated with malignant biliary tract disease or ampullary tumors.

4. DIAGNOSIS

After history, physical examination, and blood testing, 25% of patients in which extrahepatic cholestasis is suspected, are found to have an alternative etiology of the pain or jaundice. Whereas history, physical examination, and laboratory tests alone are 90–95% sensitive, they are only 70–80% specific for the diagnosis of extrahepatic cholestasis in patients with jaundice (6). Therefore, when extrahepatic cholestasis is suspected it must be confirmed by imaging studies. Figure 2 shows a logical diagnostic scheme for the management of patients with suspected cholestasis.

Blood testing in patients with cholestasis invariably shows elevated alkaline phosphatase, which can be confirmed to be of hepatic origin by detecting elevations in other more specific hepatic markers such as 5'-nucleotidase or gamma glutamyl transpeptidase (GGT) (see Chapters 2 and 3). In very early common bile duct obstruction, alkaline phosphatase may be normal. Because acute common bile duct obstruction causes an increase in levels of alkaline phosphatase 1–3 d before total bilirubin, early extrahepatic cholestasis may occur with normal total bilirubin. Bilirubin levels in excess of 10–15 mg/dL are highly indicative of malignant obstruction (7). If blood testing is done in the early phase of the obstruction, the aminotransferases (ALT and AST) may also be elevated. This can confuse the picture with that of acute hepatitic (necroinflammatory) disease. However, the levels of these enzymes decline if cholangitis is not present.

Abdominal ultrasonography is the initial imaging study of choice to investigate suspected extrahepatic cholestasis (see Chapter 5). Key findings include a dilated common bile duct (adjusted for age and body mass index to provide more specificity), dilated intrahepatic ducts, gallstones in the gallbladder or common bile duct, or pancreatic head mass. Its diagnostic accuracy is high for bile duct size. However, due to overlying duodenal loop gas, it usually fails to visualize the distal common bile duct, which is where stones most frequently impact. Hence, the presence of dilated ducts on ultrasound is used as an indirect sign of distal bile duct obstruction. In 20–30% of those patients with choledocholithiasis, the common bile duct is not dilated on ultrasound, especially in early or intermittent obstruction (8). The disadvantages of ultrasonography include its subjectiveness, user dependency, and its low yield in patients who have excessive bowel gas or obesity.

Although computed tomography (CT) scan has a similar yield to ultrasound in cases of extrahepatic cholestasis, CT scan is more costly and exposes the patient to iv contrast and radiation (see Chapter 5). However, it provides better anatomic detail of the pancreas, liver, peritoneum, and retroperitoneal structures. Therefore, if malignancy is strongly suspected, CT scan may be a more useful initial test. It can detect small pancreatic masses, and it is valuable in cancer staging. CT is not as user dependent and is not affected by obesity or bowel gas. Like ultrasound, it has low sensitivity for the detection of common bile duct stones and often cannot pinpoint the level of obstruction. Dynamic CT with continuous bolus iv contrast and helical CT have higher detection rates for pancreatic lesions smaller than 2 cm.

If the diagnosis is still in doubt, a subspecialist may be consulted to perform one of two procedures. These include an endoscopic retrograde cholangio-pancreatography (ERCP), which is normally done by a gastroenterologist, or percutaneous transhepatic cholangiography (PTC), which is done by a radiologist. PTC is technically simple with a success rate of approx 90% in patients with dilated intrahepatic ducts, but only about a 50% success rate when the ducts are not dilated. It carries a 1–10% complication rate, primarily bleeding, sepsis, bile leak,

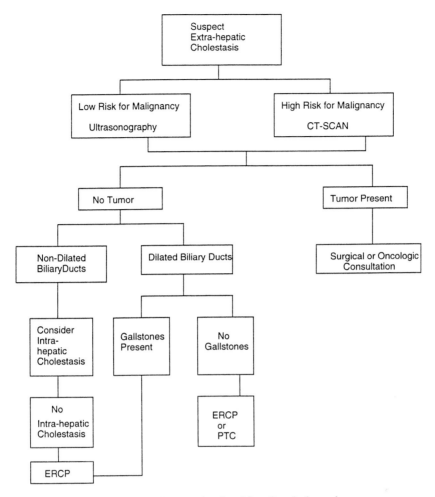

Fig. 2. A diagnostic algorithm for cholestasis.

peritonitis, hematoma, and abscess formation *(6)*. Ascites and severe coagulopathy (prothrombin time greater than 16 s) are relative contraindications. In the absence of common bile duct dilation, PTC should be reserved for those in whom ERCP has been unsuccessful. Theoretically, an ERCP is less invasive because no transhepatic puncture is performed. However, it is still associated with a 1–5% risk of serious complications such as pancreatitis and cholangitis *(9)*. ERCP provides visualization of the pancreatic duct, whereas PTC does not. ERCP is successful in approx 90–95% of cases. It is technically difficult in patients who have duodenal diverticula or who have undergone prior Roux-en-Y intestinal surgery. Selection of ERCP or PTC for any particular patient might depend on any anticipated therapeutic interventions that might be offered by one technique rather than the other, in addition to demonstrating the etiology of ductal dilation. The decision may also be based on local expertise and availability, and should always be made in consultation with a gastroenterologist and/or a surgeon with biliary expertise.

In the event that a tumor is suspected from results of any of the above modalities, a tissue diagnosis can be helpful in cases of extrahepatic cholestasis. Brushings and biopsies taken during ERCP have a sensitivity of 40–60% for cholangiocarcinoma and pancreatic adenocarcinoma, whereas ultrasound-guided percutaneous biopsy has an 80–90% sensitivity and specificity for masses greater than 2 cm *(5)*. Several studies have suggested the possibility of tumor spread, and shorter survival as a result of needle biopsies of pancreatic tumors. Therefore, many reserve this technique to only nonoperative patients or those with unresectable lesions *(10)*. A nondiagnostic or negative tissue biopsy does not rule out malignancy. Hence, for patients with suspected tumors who are operative candidates, a biopsy may be deferred and an experienced pancreatic surgeon should be consulted.

5. TREATMENT

The initial management of extrahepatic cholestasis begins with supportive measures such as hydration, electrolytes, pain control, and aggressive evaluation for cholangitis or pancreatitis. In patients with a high degree of cholestasis (high serum alkaline phosphatase and bilirubin levels), subcutaneous vitamin K (10 mg daily for 3 d) should be supplemented. Pruritus can be treated with bile acid-binding resins such as cholestyramine (4 g q.i.d.). Whereas most patients may be managed on an outpatient basis, prompt evaluation and hospital admission are usually necessary for patients with acute obstruction to monitor for complications. Immediate invasive therapy is rarely necessary in the uncomplicated patient. Analgesia with meperidine 50–100 mg IM every 3–4 h is superior to morphine or codeine derivatives which can provoke sphincter of Oddi spasm, adding to the obstruction. Antiemetics such as prochlorperazine (Compazine) (5–10 mg), or metoclopramide (Reglan) (10 mg) can be used as needed. Figures 3 and 4 show treatment algorithms that may be used for extrahepatic cholestasis.

For uncomplicated cholestasis due to choledocholithiasis, emergent treatment is not necessary unless complications such as cholangitis or worsening pancreatitis were present. Endoscopic sphincterotomy with gallstone extraction provides the lowest procedural morbidity and mortality (6–8% and 1–1.4%, respectively) and has a 90% success rate in the hands of an experienced endoscopist *(9)*. Oral bile acid therapy (ursodeoxycholic acid) for common bile duct stones has a 2-yr success rate of only 10–44% *(11)*. Therefore, although it might be useful in asymptomatic patients with choledocholithiasis who are likely to have cholesterol stones, it has no place in the treatment of cholestasis due to gallstones. The management of uncomplicated choledocholithiasis has undergone rapid evolution in the era of therapeutic endoscopy and laparoscopic surgery. For concurrent cholelithiasis and choledocholithiasis, the timing of cholecystectomy and ERCP or PTC is controversial and continues to evolve. In general, the therapeutic approach is determined by the availability of local expertise in therapeutic ERCP and/or laparoscopic surgery. Laparoscopic cholecystectomy with common duct exploration and stone extraction is slowly becoming available, reducing the need for preoperative ERCP in patients with suspected common duct stones *(12)*. However, laparoscopic common duct exploration adds to the time and morbidity of the operation. In the elderly and high-risk patients (*see* Chapter 17), an ERCP with sphincterotomy and common duct stone extraction without cholecystectomy is acceptable as definitive therapy *(13–16)*. The sphincter of Oddi is the narrowest portion of the common duct, and stones that pass from the gallbladder through the cystic duct usually become lodged there leading to cholestasis and/or pancreatitis. When the sphincter is incised, it is protected against further cholestasis or pancreatitis if more stones were to pass. Follow-up studies have shown that only a minority of patients will need further intervention because of acute cholecystitis developing as a result of the gallbladder stones *(14–16)*.

Treatment of cholestasis due to obstructing pancreatic tumors is directed at either cure or palliation. Because pancreatic tumors respond poorly to chemotherapy or radiation, early surgery is the only hope for cure. The surgical procedure necessary is pancreatoduodenectomy (Whipple resection), which carries a 50% morbidity, and in-hospital mortality of 3–20%. Those figures are very dependent on the expertise at any particular center *(10)*. All patients should be referred to an experienced oncologist after curative resection, because postoperative adjuvant chemotherapy and radiation improve survival.

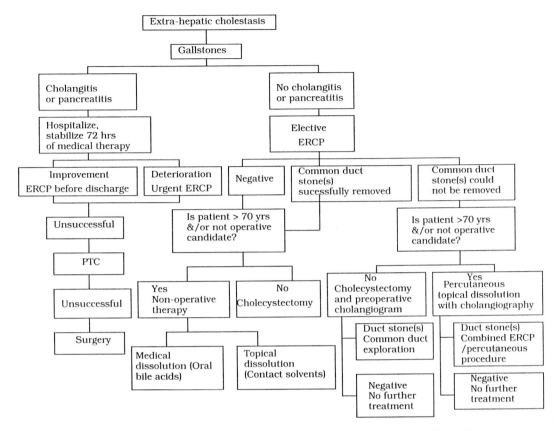

Fig. 3. An algorithm for the treatment of extrahepatic cholestasis caused by gallstones.

The majority of patients with extrahepatic cholestasis due to pancreatic cancer will have nonresectable tumors, and will need palliation with medications and/or with a drainage procedure either surgically, endoscopically, or percutaneously. Palliative surgery can relieve pain, prevent complications such as cholangitis or gastric outlet obstruction, and can alleviate symptomatic jaundice. Choledochojejunostomy and cholecystojejunostomy relieve symptomatic jaundice, whereas gastrojejunostomy relieves gastric outlet obstruction. Many surgeons perform a tumor debulking procedure at the same time. Jaundice along with its accompanying symptoms, such as pruritus, can also be relieved by endoscopic placement of an endoprosthesis or stent. The stent is either a metal mesh or plastic conduit that is placed in the bile duct bridging the obstructing tumor. Endoscopic stenting is successful approx 85% of the time with possibly fewer complications than percutaneous transhepatic stenting. However, this is largely dependent on the expertise available at any particular center *(5)*. Both modalities obviate the need for surgery. However, stents have a limited life span because they tend to obstruct over time due to bacterial colonization. As a result, they need to be replaced every few months. Metallic mesh stents have a significantly longer life span, but they cannot be replaced. The choice of surgical vs nonoperative palliation for patients with pancreatic cancer is largely dependent on patient preference, and is determined after consideration of such factors as the patient's expected length of survival, availability of local expertise, existence of comorbid conditions in the patient, and the time needed for recuperation from surgery. It is not reasonable to subject a patient whose life expectancy is only a few months to a surgical operation that requires a 1–2 mo recuperation period.

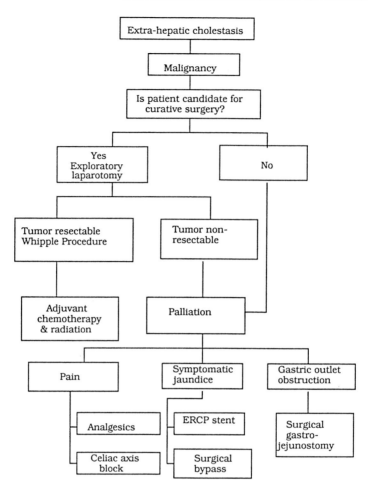

Fig. 4. An algorithm for the treatment of extrahepatic cholestasis caused by malignancy.

Cholangiocarcinoma is a slow growing and almost invariably metastatic tumor by the time of diagnosis. Occasionally, however, early-stage tumors can be treated with surgical resection plus adjuvant radiation and chemotherapy. As with cholestasis due to pancreatic tumors, palliation for cholangiocarcinoma includes endoscopic, percutaneous, or surgical drainage of the biliary tree. Pain relief and occasionally radiotherapy to shrink the obstructing tumor are other options. Carcinoma of the ampulla of Vater is initially diagnosed and treated in an identical fashion to pancreatic carcinoma. Postoperative adjuvant radiation and chemotherapy have been shown to decrease the recurrence rate (17). Because of the rarity of cholangiocarcinoma and ampullary carcinoma, patients should be referred to regional referral centers for treatment.

Pain is the most common and disabling symptom in patients with malignant cholestasis. Hence, adequate narcotic and nonnarcotic analgesia with long-acting agents is important. For refractory pain, palliative techniques such as intraoperative or percutaneous celiac plexus block with ethyl alcohol provide significant relief (18).

6. COMPLICATIONS

A number of secondary conditions can complicate the course of extrahepatic cholestasis or may be manifest on initial presentation. Acute cholangitis can occur when prolonged biliary obstruction results in proliferation of bacteria that normally colonize the biliary tract in many patients. The bacteria invade the biliary system leading to the characteristic presentation of increasing right upper quadrant pain and jaundice with abrupt onset of high, spiking fever and chills due to associated bacteremia. The combination of jaundice, right upper quadrant pain, and fever is referred to as Charcot's triad, and is seen in approx 50% of patients with acute cholangitis. However, its absence does not rule out the diagnosis *(19)*. Atypically, jaundice and fever may be intermittent and pain may be vague or absent. The total bilirubin is greater than 2 mg/dL in 80% of patients *(6)*. In the elderly population, the presentation is usually atypical and all three features of Charcot's triad are rarely present. Hypotension or mental status changes may be the presenting signs. If cultured, bile will grow *Klebsiella, E. coli,* or *Enterococcus* in 75% of patients with early-acute cholangitis *(11)*, whereas polymicrobial growth occurs in 30–50% *(2)*. Blood cultures may grow *E. coli, Klebsiella, Pseudomonas, Enterococcus,* and *Proteus* in decreasing order of frequency *(19)*.

Treatment of acute cholangitis is a medical emergency because, if it is delayed, serious complicating consequences such as septic shock can rapidly result. Hence, when cholangitis is suspected, broad spectrum iv antibiotics must be initiated. Definitive treatment cannot be accomplished without bile duct decompression to allow drainage of the infected bile, which is often purulent. Antibiotic therapy should cover Gram-negative aerobes, anaerobes, and enterococcal species. Traditional "triple antibiotic" therapy includes ampicillin or a third-generation cephalosporin, clindamycin or metronidazole, and gentamicin. However, any combination of parenteral antibiotics effective against *E. coli, Klebsiella,* enterococcal species, and enteric anaerobes is sufficient. In severe infections, two agents for Gram-negative synergy are preferable *(19)*. For milder cases, broad spectrum cephalosporins such as cefotetan or cefoxitin may be used. In mild cases of cholangitis, 75% of patients will show clinical improvement within 12–24 h of initiating antibiotics. A fall in temperature and white blood cell count usually occurs within 2–3 d of antibiotic administration *(4)*. If obstruction of the bile duct continues, however, cholangitis will likely recur. Hence, early biliary decompression is always necessary. For those patients who improve within 12–24 h and remain afebrile for 2–3 d, definitive therapy need not be emergent. If improvement is delayed or the patient deteriorates despite antibiotics, then the common bile duct must be decompressed urgently with either a sphincterotomy or stenting for cholangitis not responding to conservative therapy. This procedure is successful in 97% of patients with dramatic improvement in fever, pain, and serum liver tests *(11)*. Hence, endoscopic drainage has become the treatment of choice and several randomized prospective studies have shown that early endoscopic drainage improves short-term mortality as compared to surgery *(11)*. If endoscopic drainage cannot be accomplished immediately, percutaneous transhepatic drainage of the obstructed biliary system must be attempted. For a small group of patients in whom neither endoscopic nor radiographic drainage procedures are successful, surgery to relieve bile duct obstruction may be life saving.

Extrahepatic cholestasis may be complicated by pancreatitis. Gallstones are the most common cause of nonalcoholic acute pancreatitis in the United States. Biochemical evidence of pancreatitis occurs in up to 15% of patients with acute cholecystitis, and 30% of those with choledocholithiasis *(2)*. It is almost always due to accompanying common bile duct outlet obstruction. Symptoms include moderate-to-severe epigastric and periumbilical pain often extending to the left of the abdominal midline or the lower back, vomiting, and anorexia. Generally, amylase is much higher in gallstone than in alcoholic pancreatitis, whereas lipase levels are elevated in both etiologies *(6)*. Elevation of ALT to greater than three times normal in the setting of elevated amylase and lipase is very specific for the diagnosis of gallstone pancreatitis *(11)*. Amylase and lipase may be mildly elevated in malignant extrahepatic cholestasis or during transient passage of gallstones through the ampulla of Vater. Absence of cholelithiasis on ultrasound during an acute attack does not lower the likelihood of gallstone pancreatitis *(20)*. Because pancreatic tumors rarely present with acute pancreatitis, hyperamylasemia in the setting of extrahepatic cholestasis is more likely a result of gallstone pancreatitis or rarely ampullary tumors.

The initial treatment of gallstone pancreatitis is identical to that for other types of pancreatitis, except that broad-spectrum parenteral antibiotics should be utilized to prevent cholangitis unless the obstruction has subsided. Approximately 95% of patients with acute gallstone pancreatitis will improve with iv hydration, fasting, and analgesia; greater than 90% of common bile duct stones pass spontaneously within the first week *(21)*. In the setting of gallstone pancreatitis, emergent surgical or endoscopic extraction of gallstones retained in the common bile duct has been a subject of much controversy. Two small studies have shown a trend toward improved morbidity and mortality using ERCP and sphincterotomy within 24 h of presentation, largely by reducing the incidence of biliary sepsis *(22,23)*. In general, aggressive endoscopic or operative therapy is reserved for the patient whose condition continues to decline after 72 h of medical management or who shows clear signs of biliary sepsis or cholangitis. All patients must be admitted and closely observed *(24)*.

After recovery from gallstone pancreatitis, all patients should undergo ERCP and gallstone extraction otherwise 25% will develop another attack of pancreatitis within 30 d and 50% within 1 yr *(25)*. In general, cholecystectomy and common duct exploration is recommended after gallstone pancreatitis, but for those with high operative risk or limited life expectancy, sphincterotomy without surgery is an acceptable alternative *(13–16)*. Other options for the high risk patient include medical dissolution therapy with ursodiol for small radiolucent stones, percutaneous chemical contact dissolution therapy with solvents such as methyl-tert-butyl-ether (MTBE) or ethyl propionate (EP) *(see* Chapter 16).

Longstanding extrahepatic cholestasis can lead to secondary biliary cirrhosis, which occurs after years of complete or intermittent bile duct obstruction. It is rare in patients with chole-docholithiasis, but more commonly occurs with longstanding biliary stricture or neoplasia. Once secondary biliary cirrhosis is established, it may progress in severity even if the obstruction is relieved. Up to 10% of patients with biliary obstruction of greater than 1 yr develop progressive periportal fibrosis and cirrhosis on liver biopsy *(4)*.

7. PROGNOSIS

Uncomplicated choledocholithiasis has an excellent prognosis. Over the past 20 yr, major advances in the nonsurgical management of common duct stones have been made. The procedure of endoscopic sphincterotomy and stone extraction has been refined, and now has a very low morbidity and mortality. An analysis of 2347 sphincterotomies in 17 centers showed an overall complication rate of 9.8%, a major complication rate (requiring >10 d in hospital) of 0.6%, and a mortality rate of 0.4% *(25)*. A sphincterotomy does not appear to have any long-term adverse effects. However, a 13% rate of sphincter stenosis over a 6–11-yr follow-up period has been reported *(26)*. Whereas the long-term outcome of patients with cholelithiasis and gallbladder *in situ* who have undergone sphincterotomy is not fully known, the incidence of subsequent cholecystitis or cholangitis is only 10% over 2–5 yr *(27)*. These patients respond well to standard therapy with no significant life-threatening complications. Patients who require subsequent cholecystectomy in this setting usually do so within 1 yr. It is not clear whether cholelithiasis, prior cholangitis, or cystic duct obstruction at ERCP increase the risk for recurrent biliary tract complications in these patients *(11)*.

Cholangitis dramatically worsens the prognosis of extrahepatic cholestasis. For acute suppurative cholangitis, a 30-d mortality of 5% with sphincterotomy and 21% with surgery has been reported. Overall, there is a 10–32% rate of hospital mortality *(11)*. If septic shock or metabolic acidosis occurs, a 20–50% mortality is expected despite surgical or endoscopic drainage. Independent clinical predictors of poor outcome after cholangitis include serious concomitant medical disease, hypoalbuminemia, hyperbilirubinemia, metabolic acidosis, thrombocytopenia, and diabetes mellitus *(4)*. In the elderly, mental status changes and hypotension are the strongest predictors of mortality.

Gallstone pancreatitis has a higher morbidity (25%) and mortality (8%) than other forms of pancreatitis *(28)*. In mild cases, the short-term mortality is 2–8% and does not seem to have improved with early sphincterotomy, whereas in severe cases mortality can be decreased from 20–5% with early ERCP *(22,23)*. Pancreatic necrosis or abscess dramatically worsens the prognosis.

Less than 15% of all patients presenting with pancreatic cancer have a curable lesion *(5)*, and only 10–25% are candidates for surgical resection *(10)*. Of those with resectable lesions, 5-yr survival varies between 15–25%, as distinguished from ampullary carcinoma with a 40–50% 5-yr survival rate *(29)*. Ampullary carcinoma is metastatic or locally advanced in only 20% of cases at the time of diagnosis, with 5-yr survival rate varying 10–40% after pancreaticoduodenectomy with adjuvant chemo- and radiation therapy *(29)*. Cholangio-carcinoma has a prognosis that is similar to that of pancreatic cancer.

8. PREVENTION

Prevention of choledocholithiasis primarily centers on the timing of treatment for cholelithiasis, which is outlined in detail in Chapter 17. Prevention of biliary pancreatitis and cholangitis with sphincterotomy has been described above. For pancreatic and biliary tract malignancy, there are no known preventative measures. Although cigaret smoking has repeatedly been associated with pancreatic adenocarcinoma, smoking cessation has not been shown to lower the risk of developing the disease *(5)*.

9. INDICATIONS FOR CONSULTING THE SUBSPECIALIST

A gastroenterologist, interventional radiologist, or surgeon should be consulted to plan ERCP or PTC and to facilitate early intervention for complications or clinical deterioration. Certainly, a subspecialist should be consulted if any complications of extrahepatic cholestasis occur.

SUMMARY

Extrahepatic cholestasis occurs when a gallstone, tumor, or stricture blocks the flow of bile from the liver into the duodenum.

Extrahepatic cholestasis can be asymptomatic, produce jaundice and/or biliary colic, or present with complications such as biliary pancreatitis, obstructive cholangitis, or secondary biliary cirrhosis.

History, physical examination, and laboratory testing have a greater than 90% sensitivity and 75% positive predictive value for extrahepatic cholestasis.

Abdominal ultrasonography is the initial imaging procedure of choice for suspected extrahepatic cholestasis.

Percutaneous transhepatic cholangiography (PTC) can be done when the biliary ducts are dilated, whereas endoscopic retrograde cholangio-pancreatography (ERCP) can be performed with or without dilated ducts.

Prompt relief of the obstruction is necessary to prevent complications of extrahepatic cholestasis.

REFERENCES

1. Lee S, Kuvel R. Gallstones. In: Yamada T, ed. Textbook of gastroenterology, 2nd ed. Lippincott, Philadelphia, PA, 1995, pp. 2201–2212.

2. Somberg K, Way L, Sleisenger M. Complications of gallstone disease. In: Sleisenger M, Fordtran J, eds. Gastrointestinal disease: pathophysiology/diagnosis/management, 5th ed. Saunders, Philadelphia, PA, 1992, pp. 1816–1823.

3. Gholson C, Bacon B. Gallstones and related biliary diseases,In: Gholson C, Bacon B, eds. Essentials of clinical hepatology. Mosby Year Book, St. Louis, MO, 1992, pp. 113–126.

4. Marks J. Natural history, clinical manifestations, and diagnosis of gallstones. In: Gitnick G, ed. Principles and practice of gastroenterology and hepatology, 2nd ed. Appleton and Lange, Norwalk, CT, 1994, pp. 571–585.

5. Aherndt S, Pitt H. Pancreatic and peri-pancreatic neoplasia. In: Bayless T, ed. Current therapy in gastroenterology and liver disease, 4th ed. Mosby Year Book, St. Louis, MO, 1990, pp. 660–664.

6. Woodley M, Peters M. Approach to the patient with jaundice. In: Yamada T, ed. Textbook of gastroenterology. 2nd ed. Lippincott, Philadelphia, PA, 1995, pp. 893–903.

7. Olen R, Pickleman J, Freeark RJ. Less is better. The diagnostic workup of the patient with obstructive jaundice. Arch Surg 1989;124:791–794.

8. Frank BB. Clinical evaluation of jaundice. A guideline of the Patient Care Committee of the American Gastroenterology Association. J Am Med Assoc 1989;262:3031–3034.

9. Cotton P, Lehman G, Vennes J. Endoscopic sphincterotomy complications and their management: an attempt at consensus. Gastrointest Endosc 1991;37:383–393.

10. Cameron JL, Crist DW, Sitzmann JV. Factors influencing survival following pancreaticoduodenectomy for pancreatic cancer. Am J Surg 1991;161:120–125.

11. Hawes R, Sherman S. Choledocholithiasis. In: Habrich W, Schaffner F, Berk J, eds. Bockus gastroenterology, 5th ed. Saunders, Philadelphia, PA, 1994, pp. 2745–2785.

12. Voyles CR, Sanders DL, Hogan R. Common bile duct evaluation in the era of laparoscopic cholecystectomy. 1050 cases later. Ann Surg 1994;219:744–750.

13. Cotton PB, Vallon AG. Duodenoscopic sphincterotomy for removal of bile duct stones in patients with gallbladders. Surgery 1982;91:628–630.

14. Siegel JH, Safrany L, Ben-Zvi JS. Duodenoscopic sphincterotomy in patients with gallbladders in situ: report of a series of 1272 patients. Am J Gastroenterol 1988;83:1255–1258.

15. Davidson BR, Neoptolemos JP, Carr-Locke DL. Endoscopic sphincterotomy for common bile duct calculi in patients with gallbladder in situ considered unfit for surgery. Gut 1988;29:114–120.

16. Cotton PB. Two to nine year follow up after sphincterotomy in patients with gallbladders. Gastrointest Endosc 1986;32:157–158.

17. Tomkins RK, Saunders K, Roslyn JJ, Longmire WP Jr. Changing patterns in diagnosis and management of bile duct cancer. Ann Surg 1990;211:614–621.

18. Lillemoe KD, Cameron JL, Kaufman HS, Yeo CJ, Pitt HA, Sauter PK. Chemical splanchnicectomy in patients with unresectable pancreatic cancer: a prospective randomized trial. Ann Surg 1993;217:447–457.

19. Lu S, Kaplowitz N. Diseases of the biliary tree. In: Yamada T, ed. Textbook of gastroenterology, 2nd ed. Lippincott, Philadelphia, PA, 1995, pp. 2212–2253.

20. Malini S, Sabel J. Ultrasonography in obstructive jaundice. Radiology 1977;123:429–433.

21. Rattner D. Pancreatitis: surgical considerations. In: Bayless T, ed. Current therapy in gastroenterology and liver disease, 4th ed. Mosby Year Book, St Louis, MO, 1990, pp. 638–642.

22. Neoptolemos JP, Carr-Locke DL, London NJ, Bailey IA, James D, Fossard DP. Controlled trial of urgent endoscopic retrograde cholangiopancreatography and endoscopic sphincterotomy versus conservative treatment for acute pancreatitis due to gallstones. Lancet 1988;2:979–983.

23. Fan ST, Lai EC, Mok FP, Lo CM, Zheng SS, Wong J. Early treatment of acute biliary pancreatitis by endoscopic papillotomy. N Engl J Med 1993;328:228–232.

24. Escourrou J, Cordova JA, Lazorthes F, Frexinos J, Ribet A. Early and late complications after endoscopic sphincterotomy for biliary lithiasis with and without gallbladder in situ. Gut 1984;25:598–602.

25. Freeman ML, Nelson DB, Sherman S. Complications of endoscopic biliary sphincterotomy. N Engl J Med 1993;328:228–232.

26. MacMathuna P, White P, Clarke E, Merriman R, Lennon JR, Crowe J. Endoscopic balloon sphincteroplasty (papillary dilation) for bile duct stones: efficacy, safety, and follow-up in 100 patients. Gastrointest Endosc 1995;42:468–474.

27. Zimmon DS. Alternatives to cholecystectomy and common duct exploration. Am J Gastroenterol 1988;83:1272–1273.

28. Medical Research Council. Multicentre trial of glucagon and aprotinin: death from acute pancreatitis. Lancet 1977;2:632–635.

29. Rosley J, Ferdinand F. Biliary strictures and neoplasms. In: Bayless T, ed. Current therapy in gastroenterology and liver disease, 4th ed. Mosby Year Book, St. Louis, MO, 1990, 613–618.

17   Cholecystitis

Douglas Robertson and Salam F. Zakko

1. INTRODUCTION

Acute cholecystitis is the term used to describe acute gallbladder inflammation. It presents most commonly as a complication of gallstone disease. However, approx 10% of the time it occurs in patients without cholelithiasis and is then referred to as acalculous cholecystitis *(1)*.

The greatest initial challenge for the clinician is to distinguish acute cholecystitis from the more benign condition of biliary colic. Biliary colic is usually caused by the gallbladder contracting in response to a fatty meal and pressing a stone against the gallbladder outlet or cystic duct opening, leading to increased intragallbladder pressure and pain. Alternatively, gallbladder outlet obstruction may be caused by lesions other than stones or spasm. As in acute cholecystitis, biliary colic causes pain in the right upper quadrant. However, unlike acute cholecystitis, the pain is entirely visceral in origin without true gallbladder wall inflammation. As the gallbladder relaxes, the stones often fall back from the cystic duct. Therefore, the attack simply crescendos over a number of hours and then resolves completely. Recurrent cystic duct blockages can progress to total obstruction, causing acute cholecystitis. An episode of prolonged right upper quadrant pain (greater than 4–6 h) should arouse suspicion of an episode of acute cholecystitis, as opposed to an attack of simple biliary colic.

Another term that practitioners may frequently encounter is chronic cholecystitis. Recurrent episodes of colic can lead to fibrotic changes in the gallbladder wall with chronic inflammatory cell infiltration. However, it has been shown that patients with minimal colic can have quite extensive histologic change of their gallbladders *(2)*. Moreover, there is no evidence that

From: *Diseases of the Liver and Bile Ducts: Diagnosis and Treatment*
Edited by: G. Y. Wu and J. Israel © Humana Press Inc., Totowa, NJ

Table 1

American Society of Anesthesiologists (ASA) Physical Status Scale *(13)*

Class 1: A normal, healthy individual.
Class 2: A patient with mild systemic disease.
Class 3: A patient with severe systemic disease that is not incapacitating.
Class 4: A patient with incapacitating systemic disease that is a constant threat to life.
Class 5: A moribund patient who is not expected to survive 24 h with or without operation.

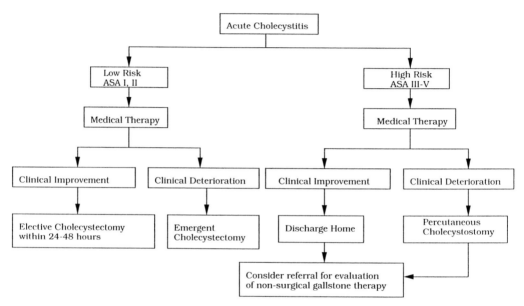

Fig. 3. An algorithm for the treatment of acute cholecystitis.

titis has resolved, the percutaneous catheter could then be utilized to apply one of the newer nonsurgical alternatives for gallstone elimination in these patients *(16)*.

6. COMPLICATIONS

The most common complication of cholecystitis, particularly in patients who delay seeking therapy, is the development of gallbladder gangrene with subsequent perforation. In a recent series of 260 patients with acute cholecystitis, over 20% of patients developed gangrene with 2% experiencing frank perforation *(17)*. Perforation may take a number of forms. Often the fluid from the perforated gallbladder leaks only locally. The result is an abscess which is best diagnosed by CT scan. Less commonly, perforation is not contained in the area of the gallbladder. Such "free" gallbladder perforation into the peritoneum is associated with a very high mortality. Finally, the gallbladder may perforate directly into a local hollow viscus forming a cholecystoenteric fistula. This fistula formation is more commonly the result of long-standing pressure necrosis from stones, rather than a result of acute cholecystitis *(18)*. Gallstones may pass through this fistula into the intestinal lumen. Occasionally, a stone larger than approx 2.5 cm may lodge at the site of the Meckel's diverticulum, which is the narrowest portion of the small intestine, resulting in "gallstone ileus." The mortality from this uncommon complication is approx 20% *(19)*.

Emphysematous cholecystitis is a less frequent complication of cholecystitis that increases by fivefold the risk of gangrene and perforation *(20)*. This particular entity occurs predominately in males, and has a strong association with both diabetes mellitus and acalculous disease. It is often diagnosed on plain film or ultrasound as the presence of air in or directly about the gallbladder. *Clostridium welchii* is the organism most commonly isolated in these cases *(21)*.

Treatment of the above complications includes both aggressive antibiotic therapy and early surgical invention.

7. PROGNOSIS

The overall mortality from an episode of acute cholecystitis is estimated to be approx 3% *(17)*. In young and otherwise healthy patients, however, the overall mortality is probably less than 1%, whereas it can climb to higher than 10% in high risk patients. The development of complications from acute cholecystitis also increases mortality. Another risk factor for severe disease is the presence or absence of stones. Acalculous cholecystitis is associated with a markedly higher overall mortality of approx 30% *(1)*. Although uncommon, the prevalence of acalculous disease appears to be increasing.

8. PREVENTION

Gallstones are exceedingly common. In the United States alone, more than 25 million adults are affected *(22)*. Most will not suffer consequences from their stones and continue to have 'asymptomatic stones,' but some will. The vast majority of patients with cholelithiasis are asymptomatic. In these patients, cholelithiasis may be an incidental finding on an abdominal ultrasound. The likelihood of developing problems from such stone disease is exceedingly small. One study showed that in patients with mild or nonspecific symptoms, the rate of developing complications was approx 1% per yr *(23)*. Furthermore, the initial presenting symptom was not severe. Therefore, treatment of asymptomatic gallstones is not advised *(24)*. When patients present with the initial symptoms from their stones, the likelihood of subsequent symptoms or complications is much higher. Hence, treatment is advised. The National Cooperative Gallstone Study showed that the risk of further symptoms was approx 70% over the next 2 yr after initial presentation *(25)*.

There are a number of treatment options available for patients with symptomatic gallstones. Surgery is the most commonly prescribed modality. The gallbladder, along with its contained stones, is removed under general anesthesia. Recently, the procedure of cholecystectomy is being performed laparoscopically, eliminating the need to cut the rectus abdominis muscle, leading to a significantly shortened hospital stay and convalescence period. However, the laparoscopic procedure carries a higher rate of morbidity in the form of a several-fold increase in the incidence of common bile duct injury *(26,27)*. Ultimately, the choice of technique is based on the experience and preference of the surgeon performing the procedure and the medical condition of the patient.

A number of nonsurgical techniques are now available or are being evaluated. These include medical dissolution with oral bile acids, topical chemical dissolution using solvents to lavage the gallbladder, and extracorporeal lithotripsy. Dissolution with oral bile acids may be appropriate therapy in a patient with small stones (less than 0.2 cm) that "float" during oral cholecystography *(28)*. This form of therapy may take up to 2 yr to complete. Therefore, it is not useful in patients who are acutely symptomatic or those who are having frequent symptoms. However, usually patients become asymptomatic in approx 2–3 mo while on oral bile acids, even though their stones have not yet totally dissolved. In addition, stone recurrence is to be expected in approx 50% of patients, but those may be re-treated with oral bile acids.

Topical dissolution with solvents such as methyl-tert-butyl-ether or, more recently, ethyl propionate is available in a few centers only and on an investigational basis *(16)*. For this procedure, a miniature percutaneous or nasobiliary catheter is placed into the gallbladder and the solvent is infused into and out of the gallbladder to lavage and dissolve the gallstones *in situ*. At the authors' center, a comprehensive standardized automated procedure for topical dissolution is being evaluated with excellent preliminary results *(29)*. It is generally an outpatient procedure that requires no general anesthesia, leaves no surgical scar, and requires no recuperation. Hence, it is clearly a desirable method of treatment for the high-risk patient. Its main disadvantages are that the solvents currently available are only effective against cholesterol stones that are only present in approx 80% of patients with gallstones. In addition, as with medical dissolution, gallstone recurrence is to be expected.

Extracorporeal shock wave lithotripsy, which has gained popularity for the treatment of kidney stones, is still investigational in the United States for gallstone treatment. Only a small number of centers continue to evaluate it. Shock waves are generated outside the patient either using a spark gap electrical discharge, vibrating piezoelectric crystals or an electromagnetically vibrating loudspeaker cone. When focused on the gallstones, the impact of the shock waves disintegrates the stones, regardless of chemical composition, into "sand" or small particles with a large effective surface area that enhances their dissolution with oral bile acids and/or allows gallbladder contractions to expel such particles into the small intestine. Preliminary studies show that it is only effective for patients with solitary stones smaller than 3 cm in diameter. Eighty percent of these patients became stone-free 12 mo after treatment *(30)*.

Whether to proceed with observation, stone removal (nonsurgical therapy), or gallbladder removal in the setting of symptomatic stones is often difficult to determine. A frank discussion of options, risks, and benefits needs to be completed with each patient so that the patient may make a well-informed decision.

9. INDICATIONS FOR REFERRAL TO A SUBSPECIALIST

Any signs of infection or inflammation, including a Murphy's sign or leukocytosis, should prompt the involvement of a surgeon. A consistent history without evidence of peritoneal irritation warrants an evaluation as shown in Fig. 1. The primary care physician may wish to involve a gastroenterologist or surgeon to assist with the decision making process.

SUMMARY

Acute cholecystitis is an acute inflammation of the gallbladder that commonly complicates gallstone disease.

It can present in patients without cholelithiasis (acalculous cholecystitis).

Acute cholecystitis presents with constitutional symptoms and pain of longer duration than simple biliary colic.

Ultrasound of the gallbladder, liver, and abdomen is useful in establishing the diagnosis. When there is doubt, cholescintigraphy may be helpful.

Low risk patients may undergo a cholecystectomy, whereas high risk patients may benefit from the newer nonsurgical modalities.

REFERENCES

1. Barie PS, Fischer E. Acute acalculous cholecystitis. J Am Coll Surg 1995;180:232–242.
2. Nahrwold DL, Rose RC, Ward SP. Abnormalities in gallbladder morphology and function in patients with cholelithiasis. Ann Surg 1976;184:415–421.
3. Morris CR, Hohf RP, Ivy AC. An experimental study of the role of stasis in the etiology of cholecystitis. Surgery 1952;32:673–675.

4. Jivegard L, Thornell E, Svanvik J. Pathophysiology of acute obstructive cholecystitis: implications for non-operative management. Br J Surg 1987;74:1084–1086.

5. Thornell E, Jansson R, Svanvik J. Indomethacin reduces raised intraluminal gallbladder pressure in acute cholecystitis. Acta Chir Scan 1985;151:261–265.

6. Thornell E, Jansson R, Svanvik J. Indomethacin intravenously, a new way for effective relief of biliary pain; a double blind study in man. Surgery 1981;90:468–472.

7. Barbara L, Sama C, Labate AM, et al. A population study on the prevalence of gallstone disease: the Sirmione study. Hepatology 1987;7:913–917.

8. Marton KI, Doubilet P. How to image the gallbladder in suspected cholecystitis. Ann Int Med 1988;109:722–729.

9. Ralls PW, Coletti PM, Lapin SA, et al. Real-time sonography in suspected acute cholecystitis. Radiology 1985;155:767–771.

10. Kim EE, Moon T, Delpassand ES, Podoloff DA, Haynie TP. Nuclear hepatobiliary imaging. Radiol Clin North Am 1993;31:923–933.

11. Fink-Bennett D, Freitas JE, Ripley SD, Bree RL. The sensitivity of hepatobiliary imaging and real time ultrasonography in the detection of acute cholecystitis. Arch Surg 1985;120:904–906.

12. Dayton MT, Doty JE, Sachdeva AK, Peoples JB. The biliary tract. In: Lawrence PF, ed. Essentials of general surgery. Williams & Wilkins, 1988, pp. 231–244.

13. Feigal DW, Blaisdell FW. The estimation of surgical risk. Med Clin North Am 1979;63:1131–1143.

14. Norrby S, Herlin P, Holmin T, Sjodahl R, Tagesson C. Early or delayed cholecystectomy for acute cholecystitis? A clinical trial. Br J Surg 1983;70:163–165.

15. Melin MM, Sarr MG, Bender CE, van Heerden JA. Percutaneous cholecystostomy: a valuable technique in high-risk patients with presumed acute cholecystitis. Br J Surg 1995;82:1274–1277.

16. Zakko SF, Srb S. Chemical contact dissolution of cholesterol gallbladder stones: 100 years later. Recenti Progressi in Medicina 1992;83:416–423.

17. Reiss R, Nudelman I, Gutman C, Deutsch AA. Changing trends in surgery for acute cholecystitis. World J Surg 1990;14:567–570.

18. Roslyn JJ, Thompson JE, Darvin H, DenBesten L. Risk factors for gallbladder perforation. Am J Gastroenterol 1987;82:636–640.

19. Clavien PA, Richon J, Burgan S, Rohner A. Gallstone ileus. Br J Surg 1990;77:737–742.

20. Mentzer RM, Golden GT, Chandler JG, Horsley JS. A comparative appraisal of emphysematous cholecystitis. Am J Surg 1975;129:10–14.

21. Lorenz RW, Steffen HM. Emphysematous cholecystitis: diagnostic problems and differential diagnosis of gallbladder gas accumulations. Hepatogastroenterology 1990;37:103–106.

22. Strom BL, West SL. The epidemiology of gallstone disease. In: Cohen S, Soloway RD, eds. Gallstones. Churchill Livingstone, New York, 1985, pp. 1–26.

23. Friedman GD, Raviola CA, Fireman B. Prognosis of gallstones with mild or no symptoms: 25 years of follow-up in a health maintenance organization. J Clin Epidemiol 1989;42:127–136.

24. Ransohoff DF, Gracie WA. Treatment of gallstones. Ann Intern Med 1993;119:606–619.

25. Thistle JL, Cleary PA, Lachin JM, Tyor MP, Hersh T. The natural history of cholelithiasis: the national cooperative gallstone study. Ann Int Med 1984;101:171–175.

26. Bernard HR, Hartman TW. Complications after laparoscopic cholecystectomy. Am J Surg 1993;165:533–535.

27. National Institutes of Health consensus development conference statement on gallstones and laparoscopic cholecystectomy. Am J Surg 1993;4:390–398.

28. Abranowicz M. Ursodiol for dissolving cholesterol gallstones. Med Lett Drugs Ther 1988;30:81–83.

29. Zakko SZ, Ramsby GR, Chen H, Srb S, Guttermuth C. A comprehensive procedure for contact dissolution of gallbladder (GB) stones. Proceedings of the World Congresses of Gastroenterology, Los Angeles, CA, October 7, 1994.

30. Sackmann M, Delius M, Sauerbrauch T, Paumgartner G, et al. Shock-wave lithotripsy of gallbladder stones: the first 175 patients. N Engl J Med 1988;318:393–397.

VI   Adult Genetic Liver Diseases

18 Genetic Hemochromatosis

Michael L. Schilsky and Irmin Sternlieb

CONTENTS

1. INTRODUCTION

Genetic hemochromatosis is an autosomal recessive disorder in which an inappropriate increase in the absorption of dietary iron is associated with accumulation of this metal within liver cells and in other sites of the body *(1)*. The gene for hemochromatosis has been localized by genetic linkage to the histocompatibility leukocyte antigen (HLA) locus *(2–4)* on chromosome 6. The genetic mutation that gave rise to hemochromatosis seems to originate in a Celtic individual *(5)*. Genetic and population screening studies indicate that the disease occurs in about 1 in 300 of the Caucasian population *(5)*. A candidate gene for hemochromatosis has only recently been identified with the predicted gene product, MHC-H, being a protein that bears resemblance to other major histocompatability (MHC) proteins *(6)*.

2. PATHOGENESIS

The mechanism by which mutations in MHC-H result in the increased iron absorption characteristic of genetic hemochromatosis is unknown. Alterations in the function of the transferrin receptor or of the cellular iron storage protein, ferritin, have been previously excluded. However, abnormal regulation of transferrin receptors and ferritin gene expression in duodenal mucosa may contribute to increased iron absorption *(7–11)*. Data from patients with genetic hemochromatosis who underwent orthotopic liver transplantation (OLT) and instances in which hemochromatotic livers were implanted into recipients without hemochromatosis suggest that the liver and all other affected organs may contain a common defect *(12)*. Without treatment, patients with hemochromatosis continue to accumulate increasing levels

From: *Diseases of the Liver and Bile Ducts: Diagnosis and Treatment*
Edited by: G. Y. Wu and J. Israel © Humana Press Inc., Totowa, NJ

of tissue iron with resultant cellular damage, organ failure, and death *(13)*. The rates of accumulation of tissue iron vary between individuals, being influenced by dietary and genetic factors, as well as by the presence of underlying liver disease *(1)*. Tissue iron levels that are below the threshold for tissue damage may be slightly increased in heterozygotes.

3. CARDINAL SIGNS AND SYMPTOMS

3.1. Symptoms

Homozygotes with genetic hemochromatosis may not manifest symptoms of this disorder until the fourth or fifth decade. However, biochemical signs of iron overload may be recognized much earlier. Expression of the disease varies considerably among patients. Many of the symptoms are nonspecific and can easily be overlooked. Among the most common are decreased libido, impotence, and diminished body hair in males, and weakness, arthritis, abdominal pain, liver disease, and dyspnea in both males and females *(14)*. Diabetes and increased skin pigmentation, once considered as essential features of hemochromatosis, are present infrequently in patients who are recognized at an early stage of the disease.

3.2. Physical Examination

The continual accumulation of hepatic iron in untreated patients results in progressive liver cell damage, collagen deposition, and ultimately cirrhosis and hepatic failure *(13,15)*. Extrahepatic iron accumulation results in cardiac disease with congestive heart failure and arrhythmias, testicular atrophy with associated impotence, diabetes, increased skin pigmentation (so called 'bronze' skin), and infrequently, hypothyroidism. Hepatocellular carcinoma is another serious complication that may arise in patients with genetic hemochromatosis *(16–18)*.

4. DIAGNOSIS

The approach to disease diagnosis is outlined in Fig. 1. The recent discovery that approximately 85% of patients with genetic hemochromatosis are homozygous for a single mutation of MHC-H *(6)*, will permit molecular screening for this disorder for most patients. The utility of molecular genetic testing for this disorder awaits further studies to determine expressivity of the disease in patients homozygous for these mutations. At present, standard biochemical screening should be performed on all suspected patients.

Parameters that indicate abnormal iron accumulation consistent with genetic hemochromatosis include increases in serum iron, transferrin saturation, and ferritin (*see* Table 1). The serologic diagnosis of genetic hemochromatosis may be made utilizing a combination of serum ferritin and transferrin saturation, yielding a sensitivity and specificity of 94% and 86%, respectively, with a predictive accuracy of 0.97 (maximum = 1.0) *(19)*. Magnetic resonance imaging (MRI) can provide evidence for hepatic iron overload in patients with advanced hemochromatosis and may help in its distinction from secondary iron loading *(20–26)*, but is of little or no diagnostic value in most asymptomatic patients.

Liver biopsy should be performed in all patients suspected of having hemochromatosis in order to determine the amount of tissue iron, its cellular distribution, and the stage and severity of tissue injury.

The deposition of excess iron in hepatocytes is characteristic of genetic hemochromatosis, whereas in most other forms of hepatic iron overload, excess iron is localized primarily in Kupffer cells and macrophages, most commonly visualized with Prussian blue staining. Hemosiderin deposits are graded from 0, when no hemosiderin is present, to 4 with severe hemosiderosis. Patients with genetic hemochromatosis most often have grade 3 or 4 siderosis.

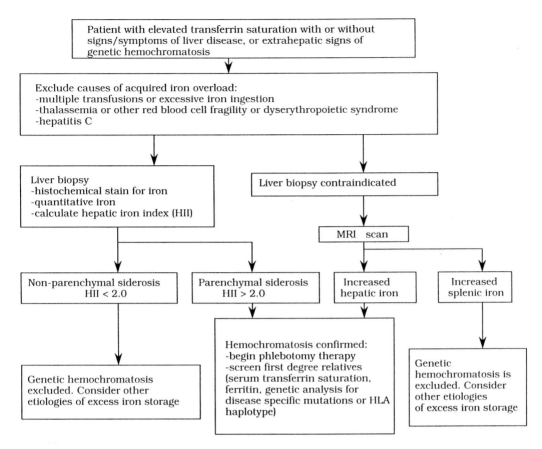

Fig. 1. A scheme for the evaluation of patients with possible genetic hemochromatosis.

Table 1

Tests for Detection of Hemochromatosis

Test	Normal range	Genetic hemochromatosis
Serum iron	50–100 µg/dL	>150 µg/dL
Transferrin saturation	10–40%	>50%
Serum ferritin (males)	20–100 µg/L	>200 µg/L
(females)	20–100 µg/L	>150 µg/L
Liver iron by histochemistry	Absent (grade 0)	Grade 3–4 in parenchymal cells
Hepatic iron content	70–1000 µg/g	>10,000 µg/g[a]
Hepatic iron index[b]	<1.5	>2.0
CT or MRI of liver	No increase in iron	Increased parenchymal iron, lack of iron in spleen

[a]In adult patients with hemochromatosis.
[b]µmoles Fe/g dry weight liver/age (yr).

With advanced siderosis, it may not be possible to identify the primary target cell since excess iron may spill into nonparenchymal cells. Early in the course of iron accumulation, excess iron is present only in periportal hepatocytes at the peripheries of lobules. With progression of the disease, excess iron deposition extends to the centrilobular region *(27)*.

A sample of the liver biopsy should be saved for direct quantitation of hepatic iron content. For liver samples, a whole core of a needle biopsy specimen should be obtained. The specimen should be transferred to a small plastic tube and either frozen or dehydrated for shipment to diagnostic laboratories. Most patients with genetic hemochromatosis have hepatic iron contents in excess of 10,000 µg/g dry liver *(28)*. Since the content of iron may not be as pronounced in asymptomatic patients discovered at an earlier age, and in patients with chronic liver disorders with acquired or secondary iron overload (most commonly viral hepatitis C and alcoholic liver disease), histochemical evaluation for detectable iron often fails to differentiate between these groups (for review, *see* ref. *[29]*). The hepatic iron index, which requires quantitative iron determination (µmoles iron/g dry liver/age in yr) was developed to distinguish between these groups of patients *(30)*. A hepatic iron index of >2 is diagnostic of genetic hemochromatosis *(22,28,30,31)*.

The diagnosis of genetic hemochromatosis is based on the characteristic abnormalities of iron metabolism in the serum, the exclusion of causes of secondary iron overload, liver histology demonstrating excess hepatocellular iron and quantitation of hepatic iron content in order to calculate the hepatic iron index (Table 1). Acquired disorders with iron overload (secondary hemochromatosis) may be the consequence of repeated blood transfusions or excessive iron administration to patients with thalassemia, hereditary spherocytosis, sideroblastic anemia, or porphyria cutanea tarda. Specific features of the hematologic disorders readily distinguish them from genetic hemochromatosis, but alcoholic liver disease and viral hepatitis C often may present difficulties in their differentiation from genetic hemochromatosis. In these disorders, serum iron, transferrin saturation, and ferritin each may be significantly elevated. However, the age-adjusted tissue iron level (hepatic iron index) is below the range seen in genetic hemochromatosis *(29)*.

Once the diagnosis is established, screening of first-degree relatives is mandatory. Screening should be performed by direct mutation analysis or HLA typing, if possible. HLA linkage studies are useful for screening first-degree relatives of individuals in whom the diagnosis cannot be established by direct mutation analysis.

5. TREATMENT

The mainstay of therapy for hemochromatosis is phlebotomy. The removal of 500 mL of blood results in the loss of approx 250 mg of iron. The serum level of ferritin provides only a rough gage of the degree of iron overload, and the amount of iron to be removed. Phlebotomy should be initiated in all patients in whom the diagnosis is established at an interval of 1–2 U weekly, depending on magnitude of iron load (as measured by quantitative hepatic iron determination or degree of siderosis detected histochemically) and the patient's tolerance, or until the hemoglobin falls below 10 g/dL. Phlebotomy, once every 2–4 mo thereafter, may be sufficient to maintain normal iron balance for most patients. Removal of excess tissue iron stores prior to the development of tissue damage improves the life expectancy of patients and prevents the development of cirrhosis *(16,32)*.

In exceptional patients in whom phlebotomy is limited by anemia, treatment may require the use of the chelating agent desferrioxamine, which must be administered by continuous iv or subcutaneous infusion. Dosages of 1–6 mg/m^2 result in the removal of tissue iron and its excretion in the urine *(33)*. The administration of ascorbate with desferrioxamine may accelerate iron removal. However, its use has been associated with cardiac failure and arrhythmias. Therefore, it should not be utilized in the initial phase of treatment.

The development of hepatic failure in hemochromatotics is effectively treated by orthotopic liver transplantation *(12)*, though concurrent heart disease due to iron overload has reduced the survival for these patients, and may even necessitate further phlebotomy treatment post-OLT in some *(34,35)*.

If glucose intolerance has developed, treatment with insulin prevents complications of hyperglycemia. Patients with symptoms of arthritis may benefit from treatment with anti-inflammatory agents.

6. POTENTIAL COMPLICATIONS

In cirrhotic patients with hemochromatosis, the risk of hepatocellular carcinoma is significantly increased *(16,32,36)*. Whether the risk of development of hepatocellular carcinoma is decreased by iron depletion therapy if cirrhosis has already developed has not been established. Diabetes is seen in 30–60% of patients with advanced disease, but is rarely encountered in patients recognized and treated at earlier phases of iron overload *(14)*. Cardiac disease, most commonly congestive heart failure and arrhythmias, remains a significant cause of morbidity and mortality in advanced hemochromatosis *(14,16,32,34–36)*. An increased incidence of infections with *Yersinia enterocolitica* has been reported in patients with iron overload *(37)*. Complications that may arise with desferrioxamine therapy include inflammation at the injection site, anaphylaxis and visual and auditory neurotoxicity *(38)*.

7. PROGNOSIS

Untreated patients with genetic hemochromatosis will develop cirrhosis and ultimately liver failure and extrahepatic symptoms associated with iron overload *(36)*. With early recognition of the disorder and judicious therapy, the prognosis for survival of patients with genetic hemochromatosis improves greatly *(9,16,32,36)*. Treatment prior to the development of cirrhosis results in essentially normal life expectancy *(39)*. Once cirrhosis is present, survival is significantly reduced. Treatment of the iron overload does not affect the diabetes or the course of arthritis.

8. INDICATIONS FOR CONSULTING THE SUBSPECIALIST

The differentiation of hemochromatosis from secondary causes of iron overload often requires liver biopsy, which is performed by the gastroenterologist and hepatologist. When liver biopsy is contraindicated, radiologic consultation for interpretation of an MRI may be necessary. Other problems for which a liver specialist may be consulted include the evaluation of the severity of portal hypertension, screening for hepatocellular carcinoma, and treatment of patients who develop complications of portal hypertension, hepatic insufficiency and encephalopathy, or hepatic failure.

9. REFERENCE LABORATORIES FOR HEPATIC IRON DETERMINATIONS

1. Mayo Medical Laboratory
   Mayo Clinic
   200 1st S. W.
   Rochester, MN 55905
   Telephone 800-533-1710
   Cost: $92
2. Department of Laboratory Medicine
   University of Washington
   1959 N.E. Pacific
   Room NW120, Box 357110
   Seattle, WA 98195
   Telephone 206-548-6066
   Cost: $46

   Department of Laboratory Medicine
   Harbor View Medical Center
   325 9th Avenue, Box 359743
   Seattle, WA 98104
   Telephone 206-731-5853
   Cost: $45
3. University of Massachusetts Medical Center
   Division of Digestive Disease and Nutrition

55 Lake Avenue North
Worcester, MA 01655
Telephone 508-856-3068
Cost: $137

4. Division of Gastroenterology and Hepatology
St. Louis University Health Science Center
3635 Vista Avenue at Grand
St. Louis, MO 63110-0250
Telephone 314-577-8764
Cost: $100

10. REFERENCE LABORATORIES FOR GENETIC STUDIES

Scripps Reference Library
11107 Roselle Street
San Diego, CA 92121
Telephone 619-784-7810/800-788-9709
Fax 619-784-7866

Specimens are submitted to Smith Kline Beecham Laboratories, test number 31354. Requires one lavender top tube, room temperature.

ItxM Diagnostics
3636 Boulevard of the Allies
Pittsburgh, PA 15213
Telephone 412-655-7321/800-967-9672
Fax 412-621-5730

Specimens are submitted in one yellow top tube (ACD), room temperature.

REFERENCES

1. Powell LW, Jazwinska E, Halliday JW. Primary iron overload. In: Brook JH, Halliday JW, Pippard MJ, Powell LW, eds. Iron metabolism in health and disease. Saunders, London, 1994, pp. 227–270.
2. Simon M, Bourel M, Fauchet R, Genetet BG. Association of HLA-A3 and HLA-B1 antigens with idiopathic hemochromatosis. Gut 1976;17:332–334.
3. Simon M, Bourel M, Genetet B, Fauchet R. Idiopathic hemochromatosis: demonstration of recessive transmission and early detection by family HLA typing. N Engl J Med 1977;297:1017–1021.
4. Edwards CQ, Caroll M, Bray P, Cartwright GE. Hereditary hemochromatosis. N Engl J Med 1977;297:7–13.
5. Simon M, LeMignon L, Fauchet R, et al. A study of 609 HLA haplotypes marking for the hemochromatosis gene (1) mapping of the gene near the HLA-A locus and characters required to define a heterozygous population and (2) hypothesis concerning the underlying cause of hemochromatosis HLA association. Am J Hum Genet 1987;41:89–105.
6. Feder JN, Gnirke A, Thomas W, et al. A novel MHC class 1-like gene is mutated in patients with hereditary haemochromatosis. Nat Gen 1996;13:399–408.
7. Whittaker P, Skikne BS, Covell AM, et al. Duodenal iron proteins in idiopathic hemochromatosis. J Clin Invest 1989;83:261–268.
8. Fracanzani AL, Fargion S, Romano R, Piperno A, Arosio P, Ruggeri G, Ronchi G, Fiorelli G. Immunohistochemical evidence for a lack of ferritin in duodenal absorptive epithelial cells in idiopathic hemochromatosis. Gastroenterology 1989;96:1071–1078.
9. Lombard M, Bomford AB, Polson RJ, Bellingham AJ, Williams R. Differential expression of transferrin receptor in duodenal mucosa in iron overload; evidence for a site-specific defect in genetic hemochromatosis. Gastroenterology 1990;98:976–984.
10. McLaren GD, Nathanson MH, Jacobs A, Trevett D, Thomson W. Regulation of intestinal iron absorption and mucosal iron kinetics in hereditary hemochromatosis. J Lab Clin Med 1991;117:390–401.
11. Pietrangelo A, Rocchi E, Casalgrandi G, Rigo G, Ferrari A, Perini M, Ezio V, Cairo G. Regulation of transferrin, transferrin receptor, and ferritin genes in human duodenum. Gastroenterology 1992;102:802–809.

12. Powell LW. Does transplantation of the liver cure genetic hemochromatosis? J Hepatol 1992;16:259–261.

13. Bacon BR, Britton RS. The pathology of hepatic iron overload: a free radical-mediated process? Hepatology 1990;11:127–137.

14. Adams PC, Valberg LS. Evolving expression of hereditary hemochromatosis. Sem Liver Dis 1996;16:47–54.

15. Pietrangelo A. Metals, oxidative stress, and hepatic fibrogenesis. Sem Liver Dis 1996;16:13–30.

16. Niederau C, Fischer R, Sonnenberg A, Stremmel W, Trampesch HJ, Strohmayer G. Survival and causes of death in cirrhotic and noncirrhotic patients with primary hemochromatosis. N Engl J Med 1985;313:1256–1262.

17. Adams PC, Speechley M, Kertesz AE. Long-term survival analysis in hereditary hemochromatosis. Gastroenterology 1991; 01:368–372.

18. Adams PC. Hepatocellular carcinoma in hereditary hemochromatosis. Can J Gastroenterol 1993;7:37–41.

19. Basset ML, Halliday JW, Ferris RA, Powell LW. Diagnosis of hemochromatosis in young subjects: predictive accuracy of biochemical screening tests. Gastroenterology 1984;87:628–633.

20. Brittenham GM, Farrell DE, Harris JW et al. Magnetic susceptibility measurement of human iron stores. N Engl J Med 1982;307:1671–1675.

21. Chezmar JL, Nelson RC, Malko JA, Bernardino ME. Hepatic iron overload: diagnosis and quantification by non-invasive imaging. Gastroenterol Radiol 1990;15:27–31.

22. Bonkovsky HL, Slaker DP, Bills EB, Wolf DC. Usefulness and limitations of laboratory and hepatic imaging studies in iron storage disease. Gastroenterology 1990;99:1079–1091.

23. Gomori JM, Harev G, Tamary H, et al. Hepatic iron overload: quantitative MR imaging. Radiology 1991;179:367–369.

24. Stark DD. Hepatic iron overload: paramagnetic pathology. Radiology 1991;179:333–335.

25. Mitchell DG. Hepatic imaging: techniques and unique applications of magnetic resonance imaging. Mag Res Q 1993;9:103–112.

26. Gandon Y, Guyader D, Heautot JF, et al. Hemochromatosis: diagnosis and quantification of liver iron with gradient-echo MR imaging. Radiology 1994;193:533–538.

27. Alt E, Sternlieb I, Goldfischer S. The cytopathology of metal overload [review]. Int Rev Exp Pathol 1990;31:165–188.

28. Basset ML, Halliday JW, Powell LW. Value of hepatic iron measurements in early hemochromatosis and determination of the critical iron level associated with fibrosis. Hepatology 1986;6:24–29.

29. Bonkovsky HL, Banner BF, Lambrecht RL, Rubin RB. Iron in liver diseases other than hemochromatosis. Sem Liv Dis 1996;16:65–82.

30. Summers KM, Halliday JW, Powell LW. Identification of homozygous hemochromatosis subjects by measurement of hepatic iron index. Hepatology 1990;12:20–25.

31. Sallie RW, Reed WD, Shilkin KB. Confirmation of the efficacy of hepatic tissue iron index in differentiating genetic hemochromatosis from alcoholic liver disease complicated by alcoholic haemosiderosis. Gut 1991;32:207–210.

32. Adams PC, Speechley M, Kertesz AE. Long-term survival analysis in hereditary hemochromatosis. Gastroenterology 1991;101:368–372.

33. Propper RD, Shwin SB, Nathan DG. Reassessment of the use of desferioxamine B in iron overload. N Engl J Med 1977;297:418.

34. Farrell FJ, Nguyen M, Woodley S, et al. Outcome of liver transplantation in patients with hemochromatosis. Hepatology 1994;20:404–410.

35. Westra WH, Hruban RH, Baughman KL, et al. Progressive hemochromatotic cardiomyopathy despite reversal of iron deposition after liver transplantation. Am J Clin Pathol 1993;99:39–44.

36. Bomford A, Williams R. Long-term results of venesection therapy in idiopathic haemochromatosis. Q J Med 1976;45:611–623.

37. Vadillo M, Corbella X, Pac V, et al. Multiple liver abscesses due to Yersinia enterocolitica discloses primary hemochromatosis: Three case reports and review. Clin Infect Dis 1995;21:223,224.

38. Oliveri NV, Buncic JR, Chew E, et al. Visual and auditory neurotoxicity in patients receiving subcutaneous desferrioxamine infusions. N Engl J Med 1986;314:869–873.

39. Fargion S, Mandelli C, Piperno A, et al. Survival and prognostic factors in 212 Italian patients with genetic hemochromatosis. Hepatology 1992;15:655–659.

19 Disorders of Porphyrin Metabolism

Martin Hahn and Herbert L. Bonkovsky

CONTENTS

1. INTRODUCTION

The porphyrias are metabolic disorders, primarily inherited, in which the principal features are disturbances of normal heme and porphyrin metabolism. Deficiency in the activity of one of the enzymes of heme biosynthesis characterizes the various forms of porphyria. Many patients remain asymptomatic carriers of the (genetic) defect, lacking both clinical features and overproduction of heme precursors. Others have so-called latent disease with no clinical symptoms of porphyria, but have elevated porphyrins and/or precursors of heme in the urine or feces. To develop manifest disease, other factors, in addition to the deficient enzyme, are necessary *(1)*. Carriers can be detected only by measuring enzyme activities (e.g., in RBCs, fibroblasts, or lymphocytes); whereas those with chemically active, but clinically latent, disease can be detected also by measurement of porphyrins and/or porphyrin precursors in blood, feces, or urine.

2. PATHOGENESIS

2.1. The Heme Biosynthetic Pathway

The regulation of the heme-biosynthetic pathway provides important clues to the pathogenesis and diagnosis of the various forms of porphyrias (Fig. 1). The sequence of metabolites and

From: *Diseases of the Liver and Bile Ducts: Diagnosis and Treatment*
Edited by: G. Y. Wu and J. Israel © Humana Press Inc., Totowa, NJ

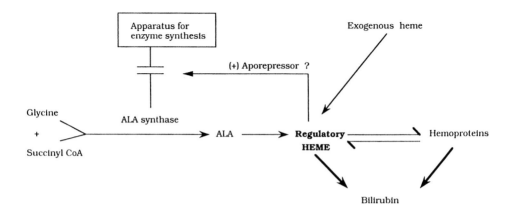

Fig. 1. An overview of hepatic heme metabolism and its regulation by a regulatory heme pool. Source: Bonkovsky HL. Porphyrin and heme metabolism and the porphyrias. In: Zakim D, Boyer TD, eds. Hepatology: a textbook of liver disease, 2nd ed. Saunders, Philadelphia, 1990, p. 386. Used with permission.

enzymes in the heme-synthetic pathway is known and patterns of metabolite excretion are relatively typical for each type of porphyria.

Heme, the end-product of the pathway, is synthesized from succinyl-CoA, glycine, and iron in a series of reactions carried out by eight different enzymes *(1)*. The first step, the formation of delta-aminolevulinic acid (ALA) by condensation of succinyl CoA and glycine, is carried out by the mitochondrial enzyme ALA synthase. ALA is then converted into the monopyrrole porphobilinogen (PBG) by ALA dehydratase (or PBG synthase). In a further series of reactions, several porphyrinogens are synthesized, and finally protoporphyrin is formed. The final enzyme of the pathway, ferrochelatase, inserts iron into protoporphyrin to form the complete heme molecule. Heme is an essential prosthetic group for numerous hemoproteins, including those that carry oxygen (hemoglobin, myoglobin), and many enzymes (mitochondrial and microsomal cytochromes, catalase, peroxidase, and so on).

In normal heme synthesis, most of the actual intermediates are porphyrinogens, the reduced forms of porphyrins. These colorless substances spontaneously oxidize, especially in the presence of oxygen and light, to form the corresponding porphyrins. The latter are reddish-purple and fluoresce bright red when excited by light of 395–410 nm (near UV). The oxidation to porphyrins occurs also within the body, e.g., in liver and skin. The various porphyrins and porphyrinogens differ in the number of carboxylic side chains that are chiefly responsible for their solubility in water. Porphyrins with more carboxyl groups (uro- and heptacarboxy-porphyrin) are more water soluble and, therefore, are excreted mainly into the urine, whereas protoporphyrin carries only two carboxyl groups and is excreted exclusively via bile. Coproporphyrin, which has four carboxyl groups, is excreted into both urine and bile. The initial building blocks of porphyrins, ALA and PBG, are excreted primarily by the kidney. These differences in water solubility partly explain the different porphyrin patterns found in the various porphyrias and are important for diagnostic testing.

2.2. The Regulation of Heme Synthesis

Defective activity of any of the enzymes along the pathway of heme biosynthesis may lead to accumulation of heme precursors proximal to the defective enzyme. In the case of the acute hepatic porphyrias, the so-called regulatory heme pool in the hepatocytes is compromised by this biochemical defect *(2)*, and can only be maintained through compensatory mechanisms, such as decreased repression of ALA synthase (Fig. 1). Induction of clinically manifest disease with symptoms frequently results when these compensatory mechanisms are overcome. For example, after exposure to drugs or chemicals that induce cytochrome P450 enzyme synthesis, exacerbations of acute hepatic porphyrias are triggered. The induction of P450 increases the demand for heme prosthetic groups and depletes the regulatory heme pool, leading to further derepression of porphyrin synthesis and excessive accumulation of porphyrin precursors proximal to the partial enzyme block. The enzymatic defect alone usually is not sufficient to cause disease expression. Thus, the most severe deficiency of regulatory heme and induction of ALA synthase occurs with both increased demand for and decreased heme synthesis, as is the situation in clinically manifest acute hepatic porphyrias.

Hepatic heme metabolism differs in its regulation from heme synthesis in nonhepatic tissues, where ALA synthase is not the rate-controlling enzyme *(1)*. For example, in erythropoietic tissue, heme seems to regulate the transport of iron into normal reticulocytes, thereby regulating the supply of iron for the enzyme ferrochelatase. The latter enzyme may be the rate-limiting step for heme synthesis in some nonhepatic tissues, such as the functioning bone marrow.

In true acute porphyrias in relapse, excretions of ALA and PBG, (as well as of porphyrins), are increased at least fivefold above normal levels. Minor degrees of increased urinary porphyrin excretion (up to 2–3 times normal) without elevation of ALA or PBG occur in a variety of disorders and are termed "secondary porphyrinurias." Because these are unrelated to true porphyrias, modest increases in porphyrin excretion have to be interpreted with caution.

Other factors, notably nutritional state, adrenal and gonadal hormones, as well as tissue iron overload, can affect the activity of the hepatic ALA synthase. For example, starvation can worsen acute porphyric syndromes, but high glucose intake can improve symptoms. These effects are due to carbohydrate repression of hepatic ALA synthase (the so-called "glucose effect") *(2)*. Exogenously administered heme repletes the regulatory heme pool and also leads to repression of ALA synthase, which decreases hepatic overproduction of ALA and PBG. These mechanisms are utilized in the therapeutic strategy of acute attacks (Figs. 1 and 2).

3. CLASSIFICATION AND OVERVIEW OF THE PORPHYRIAS

For the most part, porphyrias are inherited as autosomal dominant diseases, with the exception of congenital erythropoietic porphyria, the porphyria due to deficiency of ALA dehydratase, and some cases of protoporphyria, which follow an autosomal recessive pattern *(3)*.

Depending on the type of porphyria, excessive production of porphyrins occurs chiefly within the liver or the bone marrow, but usually not both *(4)*. Nevertheless, in the inherited forms of porphyria, all cells carry the genetic defect. Only in protoporphyria and hepatoerythropoietic porphyria may overproduction of heme precursors occur both in liver and bone marrow. Most classification schemes take into account the site of porphyrin overproduction (Table 1). These schemes also distinguish acute from chronic porphyrias on the basis of clinical manifestations, the latter representing a more protracted clinical course with dermatological manifestations. These categories are useful for purposes of diagnosis and therapy.

3.1. The Acute Porphyrias

3.1.1. ACUTE INTERMITTENT PORPHYRIA (AIP)

AIP is the most common of the inducible acute hepatic porphyrias encountered in the United States, with an estimated prevalence of the gene of about 1 in 5000 people. It is somewhat more common among people of Scandinavian, British, or Irish descent. Symptoms usually develop

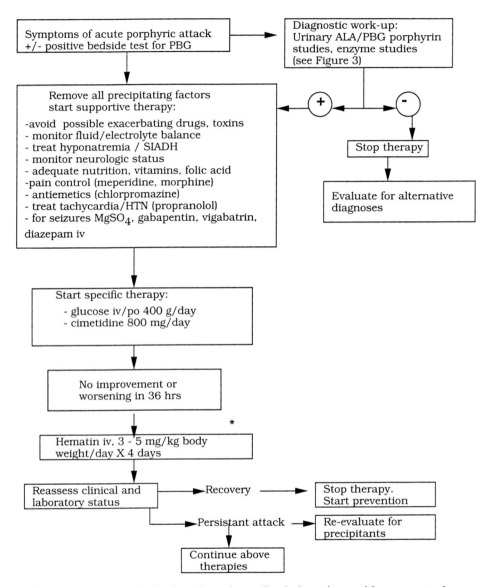

Fig. 2. Therapy of acute porphyria. Start heme immediately in patients with severe attacks, especially with associated paresis, seizures, or psychosis. Abbreviations used: HTN, systemic arterial hypertension MgSO$_4$, magnesium sulfate; SIADH, syndrome of inappropriate secretion of antidiuretic hormone.

in women in their 20s and men in their 30s, although attacks can begin at the extremes of age, as well. The characteristic acute porphyric attacks often occur in response to various precipitating factors (*see* Section 4.3.). Cyclical premenstrual attacks occur in some women, emphasizing the role of hormonal factors in modulating disease activity. The principal biochemical abnormality is elevation of urinary ALA and PBG in patients with latent and, especially, manifest disease. On a milligram basis, the daily excretion of PBG always exceeds that of ALA in AIP patients. Smaller amounts of uro- and coproporphyrin are also excreted in the urine during acute attacks. No cutaneous manifestations are observed. Asymptomatic carriers of AIP, by definition, have no abnormality in the urinary excretion of these precursors and can only be detected by measurement of activity of the defective enzyme PBG deaminase in erythrocytes.

Table 1

Classification of the Porphyrias and Other Disorders of Porphyrin Metabolism

Disorder of Porphyrin Metabolism	Inheritance	Enzyme Defect	Major Site of Abnormality
The Porphyrias			
Acute hepatic porphyrias			
Acute intermittent porphyria	autosomal dominant	porphobilinogen deaminase	liver
Hereditary coproporphyria	autosomal dominant	coproporphyrinogen	liver
Variegate porphyria	autosomal dominant	protoporphyrinogen oxidase	liver
Porphyria due to δ-aminolevulinic acid (ALA) dehydratase deficiency	autosomal recessive	ALA dehydratase	liver
Chronic hepatic porphyrias			
Porphyria cutanea tarda	autosomal dominant or sporadic	uroporphyrinogen decarboxylase (heterozygous)	liver
Mixed hepatic and erythropoietic porphyrias			
Protoporphyria	autosomal dominant	ferrochelatase	bone marrow (liver var.)
Hepatoerythropoietic porphyria	autosomal dominant	uroporphyrinogen decarboxylase (homozygous)	bone marrow and liver
Erythropoietic porphyrias			
Congenital erythropoietic porphyria	autosomal recessive	uroporphyrinogen III cosynthase	bone marrow
Erythropoietic coproporphyria	autosomal dominant	undetermined	bone marrow
Other Disorders of Porphyrin Metabolism			
Intoxications (heavy metals, e.g., <u>lead</u>, (haloaromatic compounds)		variable (e.g., <u>ALA dehydratase</u>)	liver (and others)
Secondary porphyrinurias (diabetes mellitus, anemias, lymphomas, hepatobiliary disease)		mostly normal (rarely mildly decreased)	variable
Hereditary tyrosinemia, Type I	autosomal recessive	fumaryl aceto-acetate-hydrolase (2° inhibition of ALA dehydratase)	liver

3.1.2. HEREDITARY COPROPORPHYRIA (HCP)

The true incidence of this autosomal-dominant inherited disease is not known, because a silent carrier state exists as well. The mean age of onset of symptoms is 28 yr. Women are 2.5 times more frequently affected clinically than are men, although the genetic defect in coproporphyrinogen oxidase occurs with equal frequency in both sexes. The most common mode of presentation is the acute porphyric attack, identical to that occurring with AIP. Attacks are triggered by similar factors as in AIP; usually attacks are less severe and less frequent than in AIP. The other major mode of presentation (29%) is a chronic recurrent vesiculobullous eruption on sun exposed skin (face, dorsa of hands). The principal biochemical abnormality in HCP (even in latent disease) is increased excretion of coproporphyrin III in the feces and (to a lesser extent) in the urine. During an attack, ALA and PBG are elevated in the urine. In contrast to AIP, ALA levels are frequently higher than PBG levels.

3.1.3. VARIEGATE PORPHYRIA (VP)

This autosomal dominant disease is most common (incidence 3 per 1000!) among white South Africans of Dutch descent, in whom it can be traced to a single couple that married in Capetown in 1688. Clinical manifestations are variable—many patients never become symptomatic. Acute attacks are indistinguishable from those of AIP or HCP. Photosensitivity with vesiculobullous lesions similar to HCP or porphyria cutanea tarda occurs alone or in combination with acute attacks. Rare is an isolated acute photoreaction with erythema, pruritus, and urticaria, similar to protoporphyria. Regular chemical findings in VP are increased fecal excretion of proto- and coproporphyrin. Protoporphyrin predominates. Except for prepubertal patients, virtually all patients show this pattern regardless of the symptoms. Urinary findings vary with clinical disease activity—during acute attacks ALA and PBG excretion is increased; in between attacks urinary ALA and PBG levels tend to be normal (unlike in AIP, in which they usually stay somewhat elevated). A characteristic, unique porphyrin accumulates in the plasma of patients with active VP and provides a helpful aid to diagnosis.

3.1.4. PORPHYRIA CAUSED BY SEVERE ALA DEHYDRATASE DEFICIENCY

This autosomal recessive disorder appears to be extremely rare; only a few cases have been described. It is characterized by acute attacks of neurological dysfunction comparable to those with the other acute hepatic porphyrias (AIP, HCP, VP). There are no cutaneous manifestations. Urinary excretions of ALA and coproporphyrin III are consistently elevated, slight increases of PBG and other porphyrins occur. Fecal porphyrin excretion is normal. For unclear reasons, the concentration of zinc protoporphyrin in erythrocytes is increased.

Although the diseases just described are all inherited and the underlying enzymatic defects are present throughout the lives of affected subjects, they are called "acute" porphyrias, because their major clinical manifestation is the acute attack.

In contrast, the so-called chronic phorphyrias, described next, do not cause acute attacks (or, in the case of protoporphyria, do so only rarely and under unusual circumstances).

3.2. The Chronic Porphyrias

3.2.1. PORPHYRIA CUTANEA TARDA (PCT)

In most parts of the world, including the United States, PCT is the most common form of porphyria. It typically presents in middle-aged subjects who are heavy users of alcohol and/ or who take estrogen (e.g., for contraception or therapy of prostatic cancer). The presenting signs are vesicles, bullae, and sores, especially on the dorsal aspects of the face, head, and neck. Hypertrichosis, usually most noticeable on the face, is also common.

The diagnosis is readily established by measurement of urinary porphyrins and by the pattern of these porphyrins, now usually measured by high performance liquid chromatography (HPLC). The typical pattern is a marked increase (>10 times normal) in uro- and heptacarboxyporphyrins. The acute porphyrias that, in relapse, can elevate these porphyrins (Table 2) are excluded by measurements of urinary ALA and PBG, which are normal or near normal in PCT, but markedly increased in the acute porphyrias. Fecal analysis is not usually

Table 2

Usual Chemical Findings In The Porphyrias

	Urine				Feces			Erythrocytes		
	(mg/g creatinine)		(µg/g creatinine)		(µg/g dry weight)			(µg/100 mL packed erythrocytes)		
	ALA	PBG	Uro	Copro	Uro	Copro	Proto	Uro	Copro	Proto
Normal values[a]	<3	<2.5	10–60	50–250	0–5	Tr–50	Tr–120	0–1	0–20	15–60
Acute hepatic porphyrias										
Acute intermittent porphyria										
Latent	↑	↑	N(↑)	N(↑)	N	N	N(↑)	N	N	N
Manifest	↑↑	↑↑	↑	↑	N(↑)	N(↑)	(↑)	N	N	N(↑)
Hereditary coproporphyria										
Latent	N	N	N(↑)	↑↑	N(↑)	↑	N(↑)	N	N	N
Manifest	↑↑	↑↑	↑	↑↑	N(↑)	↑↑	↑	N	N	N
Variegate porphyria										
Latent	N	N	N	↑	N	↑	↑↑	N	N	N(↑)
Manifest	↑↑	↑↑	N(↑)	↑↑	N(↑)	↑	↑↑	N	N	↑↑
ALA dehydrase deficiency	↑↑	N	N(↑)	↑	N	N	N	N	N	N
Porphyria cutanea tarda										
Latent	N	N	↑	N(↑)	↑	N(↑)	N	N	N	↑↑
Manifest	N(↑)	N	↑↑	↑	↑	↑	N	N(↑)	N	↑↑
Protoporphyria										
Latent	N	N	N	N	N	N	↑	N	N	↑↑
Manifest	N	N	N(↑)	N(↑)	N	N(↑)	↑↑	N	N(↑)	↑
Hepatoerythropoietic porphyria	N	N	↑↑	↑	↑↑	↑↑	N	N	N	↑
Erythropoietic porphyrias										
Congenital erythropoietic uroporphyria	N	N	↑↑	↑	–	↑↑	N	↑↑	↑	↑
Erythropoietic coproporphyria	N	N	N	N	N	N(↑)	–	↑	↑↑	↑
Secondary porphyrinurias	N(↑)	N	N(↑)	↑	N	N(↑)	N(↑)	N	N	N(↑)

[a]ALA = δ-aminolevulinic acid; Copro = coproporphyrin; N = normal; PBG = porphobilinogen; Proto = protoporphyrin; Uro = uroporphyrin. (↑) = occasional slight increase; ↑ = increase; ↑↑ = marked increase; – = not tested

From: Bonkovsky, HL. Porphyrin and heme metabolism and the porphyrias. In: Zakim D, Boyer TD, eds. Hepatology a textbook of liver disease.

required for diagnosis, although increased fecal iso-coproporphyrin is a useful marker of PCT. Fecal analysis is also useful for differentiating PCT from HCP or VP.

Coexistent liver disease is the rule in PCT. Formerly, it was ascribed chiefly to alcohol or other toxins, but recent studies have shown that in Italy, Spain, and the United States, most patients with PCT have chronic hepatitis C *(5)*. (This is not true in Germany, Holland, Ireland, New Zealand, or the United Kingdom). The liver disease is usually relatively mild, and most patients do not have cirrhosis. Most PCT patients have moderate hepatic iron overload, and there is growing evidence the hetero- or homozygosity for HLA-linked hemochromatosis is a risk factor for development of overt PCT. Iron in the liver plays an important role in the pathogenesis of overt PCT, and iron removal is the treatment of choice (*see* Section 6.2.).

The enzymatic defect in PCT is a decrease in activity of hepatic uroporphyrinogen decarboxylase (Uro-D), the fifth enzyme of the heme synthetic pathway. In most patients, this is an acquired or sporadic condition, thought somehow due to alcohol, iron, hepatitis C, or other hepatotoxic factors. In about one quarter of patients, there is an inherited defect in Uro-D. Such patients have a 50% reduction in activity of the decarboxylase in erythrocytes, and some of their parents and siblings show similar decreases. However, during active PCT, the decrease in hepatic Uro-D activity is typically greater than 50% (in both acquired and inherited PCT). Also, most subjects with an inherited partial defect in Uro-D activity do not develop overt PCT. Therefore, it is clear that a 50% decrease in activity of this enzyme is not in itself sufficient to cause clinical disease. Other factors, which further decrease Uro-D activity or increase the irreversible oxidation of uroporphyrinogen to uroporphyrin within the liver, are essential in the pathogenesis of PCT.

3.2.2. HEPATOERYTHROPOIETIC PORPHYRIA (HEP)

This is a very severe porphyria which is, fortunately, quite rare. It is manifested in infancy with severe skin changes like those seen in PCT. Later, scarring with acrosclerosis and severe disfigurement usually occurs, although evidence of liver disease usually does not. The abnormalities of porphyrin metabolism resemble those of PCT. The enzymatic defect is a profound decrease in activity of Uro-D (5–10% of normal), usually due to compound heterozygosity, with both alleles coding for defective enzyme molecules.

3.2.3. PROTOPORPHYRIA (PP)

PP is usually a relatively mild form of porphyria with cutaneous clinical features that differ from the other forms of porphyria, as already described. It is the only form of porphyrin in which all urinary porphyrins and porphyrin precursors are normal, because only protoporphyrin is overproduced and over excreted. Its prevalence is estimated to be one per 5000–10,000 people. It is hereditary, although many (perhaps most) patients lack a positive family history, and even detailed evaluations of first degree relatives may fail to reveal other affected persons, suggesting that new mutations account for many instances of the disease. Inheritance of PP is, thus, somewhat uncertain: in some pedigrees it is an autosomal dominant with variable penetrance, whereas, in others, it has been suggested to be an autosomal recessive.

The enzymatic defect in PP is decreased activity of ferrochelatase or heme synthase, the final enzyme of the heme biosynthetic pathway, which carries out the insertion of ferrous iron into protoporphyrin. Because ferrochelatase is a mitochondrial enzyme, it cannot be measured reliably in adult erythrocytes, but rather requires the use of fibroblasts, leukocytes, or liver. Activity of the enzyme in affected persons is typically only approx 20–25% of normal. This is probably due to the fact that the functional enzyme is a homodimer, requiring two normal subunits for activity.

All of the clinical manifestations of PP are due to overproduction of protoporphyrin, which occurs chiefly in the bone marrow. In addition to the cutaneous manifestations, some patients with PP may develop a progressive, fatal hepatopathy, due to accumulation of protoporphyrin in the liver. As described above, the excess of this compound can only be removed from the body by hepatic secretion into the bile. Development of cholestatic liver disease (e.g., due to alcohol, biliary obstruction, etc.) may lead to progressive accumulation of protoporphyrin in hepatocytes and biliary radicles. This, in turn, may worsen cholestasis, setting up a vicious cycle of hepatic dysfunction.

Thus, the potentially serious complications of PP are hepatobiliary. Gallstones, composed chiefly of protoporphyrin, are common, occurring in young patients. Fortunately, development of progressive hepatic fibrosis and pigmentary cirrhosis is rare. All patients with PP should have regular (at least annual) measurement of erythrocytic and plasma porphyrin concentrations and liver chemistries (total bilirubin, ALT, alkaline phosphatase, total protein, and albumin). Those with markedly elevated porphyrins, or any persistent abnormality of liver tests, should be evaluated for gallstone disease and undergo liver biopsy.

3.2.4. Congenital Erythropoietic Porphyria (CEP)

CEP is a very rare form of inherited porphyria which usually is manifest early in life. Infants may pass dark reddish urine, and their wet diapers will fluoresce a bright pink under a Wood's lamp. Their bones and teeth show similar fluorescence. They develop severe skin changes similar to those of PCT or HEP (see above). Increased ineffective erythropoiesis and hemolysis occur, leading to abnormalities of bone structure, splenomegaly, and iron loading.

The main chemical finding is a marked increase in uroporphyrin I in the normoblasts, reticulocytes, and urine. This is due to severe deficiency in activity of the enzyme uroporphyrinogen III (co-) synthase, which normally is present in excess and which efficiently converts hydroxymethylbilane, the final product of the reaction catalyzed by PBG deaminase, to the III isomer of uroporphyrinogen. When activity of the cosynthase is deficient, the bilane spontaneously cyclizes to form the I isomer of uroporphyrinogen. Unlike the III isomer, the I isomer can not be converted to heme. Much of it undergoes irreversible oxidation to uroporphyrin I.

3.3. Other Disorders of Porphyrin Metabolism

3.3.1. Hereditary Tyrosinemia (Type I)

This autosomal recessive disorder is due to a deficiency of the enzyme 4-fumarylacetoacetate hydrolase. This may lead to accumulation of succinylacetone, which is an extremely potent inhibitor of ALA dehydratase. Features of an acute porphyric syndrome, typically with marked elevations of urinary ALA, and normal urinary PBG, may occur in such patients who also develop rapidly progressive liver disease and hepatocellular carcinoma.

3.3.2. Acquired Porphyrinopathies/Secondary Porphyrinurias

Lead poisoning may cause a true toxin-induced porphyria, with neurovisceral symptoms like those of the inherited forms of acute hepatic porphyria and with increased levels of urinary ALA and coproporphyrin during acute manifestations. This is chiefly due to inhibition of ALA dehydratase by lead.

A variety of other chemicals or disorders can lead to mild to moderate increases in urinary porphyrins, generally not more than three times above normal limits. Patients with such conditions are identified, for example, when undergoing a urinary porphyrin screen, as part of a work-up of an unexplained neuropathy or other neuropsychiatric difficulty. Mostly coproporphyrin is found in the urine. In secondary porphyrinurias, fecal porphyrins are normal or only slightly increased, whereas in HCP and VP these are usually markedly elevated, even during clinical remission. Even though some of the patients with secondary porphyrinurias may have abdominal pain, nausea, vomiting, or other symptoms that fit into the broad spectrum of symptoms that have been associated with acute porphyrias, these patients do not have a true porphyria *(6)*. To avoid misdiagnosis, it is important to remember that all acute porphyric syndromes in relapse are associated with large increases in urinary excretion of ALA and/or PBG.

Secondary porphyrinuria also occurs in anemias (particularly aplastic, hemolytic, and pernicious anemia), Hodgkin's disease, leukemias, liver diseases (acute or chronic hepatitis, alcoholic liver disease, and cirrhosis), diabetes mellitus, infections, myocardial infarction, starvation, pregnancy, and after exposure to certain toxins (alcohol, halogenated and haloaromatic compounds, and heavy metals like arsenic, gold, and iron). There are also sporadic reports of increased urinary (copro-) porphyrin excretion in patients that carry the diagnosis of the so-called multiple chemical sensitivity syndrome. In none of these disorders do porphyrin precursors (ALA and PBG) accumulate, and activities of the enzymes of heme biosynthesis are generally within normal limits. The reason for the increase in urinary porphyrins is known for only few of these disorders. For example, in cholestatic liver diseases, the increased urinary porphyrin excretion represents a compensatory increase when bile formation and excretion are impaired. Other proposed explanations for the increased urinary porphyrins include increased synthesis, decreased utilization, and increased oxidation of porphyrinogens to porphyrins (6).

4. CARDINAL SYMPTOMS AND SIGNS

4.1. The Acute Porphyric Attack

The acute attack is the characteristic presentation of the acute hepatic porphyrias (AIP, HCP, VP, and homozygous ALA-D deficiency), lead intoxication, and hereditary tyrosinemia. It is frequently precipitated by ingestion of certain drugs, by infections, fasting, or excessive alcohol ingestion (*see* Table 3). The massive accumulation of porphyrin precursors (ALA and PBG) is associated with, and may to be responsible for, the symptoms and signs of the acute porphyrias. Figure 3 summarizes the clinical signs and symptoms most commonly encountered in attacks of acute intermittent porphyria. Findings in HCP and VP are similar; both also lead to development of cutaneous lesions (discussed below), indistinguishable from those of PCT. Patients with acute porphyric attacks present as acutely ill, usually with severe colicky abdominal pain, characteristically lasting more than 1 d *(6)*. This pain may mimic acute inflammation of a hollow viscus; however, rebound tenderness is distinctly unusual, as the symptoms are usually out of proportion to the physical findings. Severe constipation, nausea, vomiting, as well as purely neurologic symptoms ranging from headaches to psychiatric disturbances, paresthesias, or pareses are common. A progressive neuropathy, with motor fibers affected more than sensory fibers, may supervene. Signs of autonomic instability (tachycardia, postural hypotension, labile hypertension, and urinary incontinence) may accompany the syndrome. Because of cranial, peripheral, or autonomic neuropathy, or because of the associated seizures, patients may be seen primarily by neurologists for evaluation. The neurovisceral features of acute attacks can be divided into five nonexclusive categories of neurologic involvement *(7)*:

1. Autonomic and visceral neuropathy (abdominal pain, constipation, nausea/vomiting, hypotension, and hypertension).
2. Peripheral sensory and/or motor neuropathy (paresthesias, paresis, occasionally respiratory muscle paralysis, and quadriplegia).
3. Bulbar involvement (respiratory, deglutatory, and vagal nuclear damage).
4. Hypothalamic involvement (inappropriate ADH secretion and abnormal release of growth hormone).
5. Cerebral involvement (seizures, coma, psychiatric manifestations such as depression, hysteria, and psychosis).

Table 3

Precipitating Factors of Acute Attacks of Porphyria

Exposure to drugs and chemicals
Barbiturates, hydantoins, sulfonamides, and so on
Alcohol
Luteal phase of the menstrual cycle
Pregnancy
Fasting/starvation
Infection
General anesthesia (rare)
Perioperative period

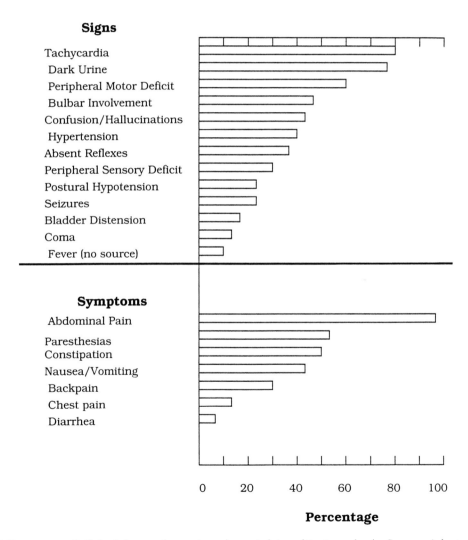

Fig. 3. Frequency of clinical signs and symptoms in acute intermittent porphyria. Source: Adapted from Bonkovsky. In: Zakim and Boyer, eds. loc. Cit. Used with permission.

The combination of intermittent abdominal symptoms and neuropsychiatric manifestations (plus skin lesions in some forms) should lead to a consideration of the diagnosis. The history should focus on previous, similar episodes, precipitating factors, and family history. A thorough history may reveal that patients have passed unusually dark or red urine.

Although the underlying enzymatic defect of acute hepatic porphyrias is expressed in the liver, there are few morphologic abnormalities of the liver. The major abnormalities are found in neural tissue (axonal damage and demyelination, especially after prolonged and repeated attacks). This is consistent with a hypothesis that the neurological/neurovisceral symptoms are caused by heme deficiency within cells of the nervous system in conjunction with a neurotoxic effect of ALA (or another metabolite). The latter is supported by the finding that ALA selectively competes for receptor sites of gamma-aminobutyric acid (GABA), the major inhibitory neurotransmitter in the mammalian nervous system. This partial antagonism to GABA may explain CNS symptoms (e.g., delirium, seizures) in porphyric attacks (8). However, increased levels of ALA do not necessarily correlate well with the severity of attacks. This suggests that pathogenetic factors other than ALA may be involved as well.

4.2. Cutaneous Manifestations

Patients with CEP, HEP, PCT, HCP, or VP (in the case of the latter two with or without associated acute neurovisceral symptoms) may present with vesicles, blisters, and sores on the dorsa of the hands. Less frequently such lesions occur on the forehead, ears, neck, and other sun-exposed areas. They develop at sites of mild trauma and represent injury due to the exposure of excess porphyrins in the skin to light and oxygen. As a result of this so-called photodynamic effect of porphyrins, reactive oxygen radicals are formed that lead to direct tissue damage (lipid peroxidation, lysosomal damage, and complement activation). No acute symptoms occur on exposure to sunlight; the skin damage develops over extended periods of time. Due to a tendency to become infected, these lesions often heal slowly with scarring and leave areas of hypo- or hyperpigmentation and hypertrichosis. In the case of PCT they are often seen in patients with iron overload, alcoholic liver disease, and/or chronic hepatitis C. The history and physical examination, therefore, will reveal symptoms and signs of associated chronic hepatopathy; the family history may be positive for iron storage disease, alcoholism, or porphyria.

In contrast, in PP the cutaneous manifestations are chiefly those of immediate burning, itching, pain, and erythema upon exposure to the sun. This usually is noted shortly after birth and may improve somewhat as patients age (probably mainly due to their avoidance of sunlight). Hives (solar urticaria) and mild blistering may occur. Lichenification of chronically exposed skin, especially over the knuckles, occurs as time goes by (Table 4).

4.3. Precipitating Factors

Certain drugs and other factors are regarded as precipitants for acute attacks (Table 3). This is based on the observation that these factors are frequently associated with subsequent clinical manifestations of acute (hepatic) porphyrias *(8)*. There is also experimental evidence for induction of porphyrin synthesis by many of these factors in animal models and cell culture systems. The classic precipitants, barbiturates (like many other drugs that are implicated in exacerbations), induce cytochrome P450 synthesis in hepatic tissue and lead to increased heme requirement and porphyrin synthesis, as discussed in the section on regulation of the heme biosynthetic pathway.

Aside from the listed drugs (Table 5) and alcohol, exacerbations of acute hepatic porphyrias occur more frequently in women than men. In women, the attacks occur predominantly in the luteal phase of the menstrual cycle, which corresponds to the finding that progesterone and related steroids induce porphyrin synthesis in experimental models. Other precipitating factors are dieting or prolonged fasting, perioperative stress, infection and (rarely) general anesthesia.

Strict avoidance of all precipitating factors is essential, particularly in patients with a history of frequent and severe attacks. The great majority of patients do not develop symptoms, however,

Table 4

Potential Complications of Porphyrias

Systemic changes
Systemic arterial hypertension
Chronic renal failure
Peripheral neuropathy
　　Sensory deficits
　　Motor deficits/muscle atrophy
Seizure disorder
Cholelithiasis (in protoporphyria)
Hemolytic anemia, splenomegaly (in erythropoietic porphyria)
Hepatocellular carcinoma (in acute porphyrias, PCT)
Liver cirrhosis, liver failure (in protoporphyria)
Death (respiratory paralysis, and so on)
Skin changes
　　(in CEP, HCP, HEP, PCT, VP)
　　　　Vesicles, bullae
　　　　Scarring, sclerosis
　　　　Hypo-, hyperpigmentation
　　　　Lichenification
　　　　Hypertrichosis
　　(in protoporphyria)
　　　　Acute photosensitivity reactions: edema, urticaria, erythema
　　　　Chronic: lichenification, mild scarring

following transient exposure to one of these factors during quiescent phases of their illness. Therefore in many patients under physician guidance, oral contraceptive use, pregnancy, hormonal preparations for menopausal symptoms, and moderate alcohol intake are relatively safe and can be permitted.

5. DIAGNOSIS

5.1. Initial Diagnostic Work-Up (Fig. 4)

A good diagnostic strategy will lead to a rapid confirmation or rejection of the suspected diagnosis. Elevated levels of ALA and usually PBG always accompany neurovisceral symptoms during exacerbations of the acute hepatic porphyrias (AIP, HCP, and VP). ALA alone is increased in the porphyria caused by ALA dehydratase deficiency in lead intoxication and in hereditary tyrosinemia. The patterns of porphyrin precursors and porphyrins in urine, feces (or the accumulation of specific porphyrins in erythrocytes) are diagnostic for the different types of porphyrias. Similarly, chronic porphyrias (PCT) and acute hepatic porphyrias in which cutaneous manifestations occur (HCP, VP) are characterized by patterns of elevated levels of porphyrins in urine or feces (Table 2). Complete evaluation of erythrocytic, fecal, plasma, and urinary porphyrins usually suffice for diagnosis; although, by definition, asymptomatic, chemically inactive carriers cannot be diagnosed in this way. They require assays of enzymatic activities and/or molecular studies to detect genetic abnormalities. For some of the enzymes of heme biosynthesis, assays in erythrocytes are available through large commercial laboratories (e.g., for ALA dehydratase or PBG deaminase). However, for the other enzymes, reliable assays are available only in a few specialized centers. Molecular studies are offered only by special labs and generally are indicated only if a defect has been identified in a proband and the rest of the kindred is being evaluated. A high index of suspicion for the diagnosis, prompt recognition of the symptom constellation, and rapid, correct sample collection is crucial for the diagnosis. Between attacks, biochemical abnormalities may resolve and the window for diagnosis may be missed.

Table 5

Drugs And Chemicals in Acute Hepatic Porphyrins

	Unsafe	Safe
Analgesics	Danazol	Acetylsalicylic acid
	Diclofenac	Ibuprofen
	Oxyfenbutazone	Naproxen
	Phenylbutazone	Indomethacin
	Piroxicam	Paracetamol
Opioids	Tramadol	Codeine
	Dextropropoxyphene	Meperidine
	Fentanyl	Methadone
	Pentazocine	Morphine
		Oxycodone
Anesthetics and muscle relaxants	Alcuronium	Bupivacaine
	Barbiturates	Ether
	Fluroxene	Halothane
	Lidocaine	Ketamine(?)
	Mepivacaine	Nitrous oxide
	Methoxyflurane	Procaine
		Propofol(?)
		Succinylcholine
Anticonvulsants	Barbiturates	Bromides
	Carbamazepine	Diazepam(?)
	Clonazepam(?)	Gabapentin
	Felbamate	Magnesium Sulfate
	Hydantoins	Vigabatrin
	Lamotrigine	
	Phenytoin	
	Tiagabine	
	Valproate	
Antibiotics	Cephalosporins(?)	Acyclovir
	Chloramphenicol	Aminoglycosides
	Dapsone	Amphotericin
	Doxycline	Ethambutol
	Erythromycin	Flucytosine
	Griseofulvin	Penicillin
	Metronidazole	Tetracycline(?)
	Sulfonamides	
	Trimethoprim	
Cardiovascular Drugs	Amiodarone	Atropine
	Enalapril	Captopril
	Lidocaine	Digoxin
	Nifedipine	Epinephrine
	Verapamil	Lisinopril
		Losartan
		Nitroglycerin
		Norepinephrine
		Procainamide
		Quinidine
Diuretics and Antihypertensives	α-Methyldopa	Acetazolamide
	Clonidine	Amiloride
	Enalapril	Ethacrynic Acid

	Unsafe	*Safe*
	Furosemide	Lisinopril
	Hydralazine	Losartan
	Spironolactone	Reserpine
	Thiazides	Triamterene
Sedatives and Tranquilizers	Alprazolam	Chloral hydrate
	Chlordiazepoxide	Chlorpromazine
	Flurazepam	Haloperidol
	Meprobamate	Lithium
	Nitrazepam	Midazolam
	Thioridazine	Paraldehyde
	Tricyclic antidepressants	Promazine
		Temazepam
Other	Aminophylline	Allopurinol
	Ergotamine	Chlorpheniramine
	Estrogens[a]	Colchicine
	Metoclopramide	Corticosteroids
	Progestagens[a]	Coumarin
	Sulfonylureas	H2-blockers
		Heparin
		Insulin
		Laxatives
		Loperamide
		Metformin
		Warfarin

Adapted from Bonkovsky HL. Porphyrin and heme metabolism and the porphyrias. In: Zakim D, Boyer TD, eds. Hepatology: A textbook of liver disease, 2nd ed. Saunders, Philadelphia, 1990, p. 399, and recent results in our laboratory.

Those agents marked with (?) are theoretically risky or the reports are controversial.

[a]The female sex steroids are porphyrogenic, but in low doses as oral contraceptives, may help to prevent cyclic monthly attacks of acute porphyria in some women.

Because of the relative rarity of the porphyrias and their complexity, it is recommended that all patients thought to have porphyria be evaluated by, or at least consult with, a physician experienced in dealing with such problems.

Patients with symptoms suggestive of an acute porphyric attack should promptly be evaluated by a bedside qualitative test for PBG (*see* diagnostic algorithm, Fig. 4): The Hoesch test is simpler, less prone to misinterpretation, and better suited as a screening tool than the Watson-Schwartz test (which requires an extraction step). If acute porphyria is suspected, it is not adequate to request a urine porphyrin screen, since this will not detect ALA or PBG. Preparation of the reagent for the Hoesch test requires solution of 2.0 g of p-dimethyl-aminobenzaldehyde in 100 mL of 6M HCl. Add 1–2 drops of fresh urine to 1–2 mL of this modified Ehrlich's reagent. The immediate development of a cherry-red color at the top of the solution, as the urine contacts the reagent, indicates a positive result. Since some medications (e.g., methyldopa, pyridium, laxatives), as well as other factors, may give false-positive results, any positive test should be confirmed by a quantitative determination of ALA and PBG in a 24-h urine collection (protect from light during entire collection period!). The Hoesch and the Watson-Schwartz test usually are not positive if PBG concentrations in the urine are below 10 mg/L (normal upper limit 2.5 mg/L). Therefore, and because some acute porphyric syndromes (ALA dehydratase deficiency, lead intoxication) may not be accompanied by increases in PBG,

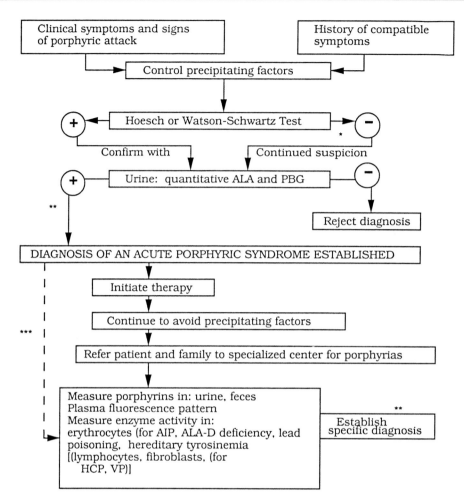

Fig. 4. Diagnostic approach to acute porphyrias. *, Neither Hoesch nor Watson-Schwartz test is positive unless urinary PBG concentration >10 mg/L (normal range >2.5 mg/L). ALA is not detected. **, If ALA/ PBG not distinctly elevated (5–10 times normal), or if only porphyrins in urine are minimally elevated, consider secondary porphyrinurias in the differential diagnosis. ***, Full evaluation of patient and kindred to establish a specific diagnosis is best performed at a special center with expertise in the porphyrias. Some of the tests listed (e.g., the plasma porphyrin fluorescence pattern, erythrocytic ALA-dehydratase, and lymphocytic or fibroblastic enzymatic assays) are not available except in specialized centers.

quantitative determination of ALA and PBG in a 24-h urine should be done in all cases in which there is continued clinical suspicion for the diagnosis of acute porphyria, even if the screening test has been negative or equivocal. Usually, ALA and PBG will be elevated markedly during an attack, provided that the urine sample is handled properly (kept cool and dark). After collection, the urine should be mixed well, the total volume and creatinine concentration measured, and a 30–50-mL portion frozen (<–20°C) in a stout dark plastic bottle until assayed. Quantitation of urinary ALA and PBG is carried out in the United States by several research and by some commercial laboratories. However, many of the latter require the use of different preservatives for the two analytes and, therefore, the collection of two separate urines. We have found that this is unnecessary, provided that the urine is handled as described. Typical costs for quantifying urinary ALA and PBG are $50–100 (Table 6).

Table 6

Typical Costs for Assays of Porphyrins, Porphyrin Precursors,
and Enzymes of the Heme Biosynthetic Pathway

	Analyte	*Typical cost ($U.S.)*
Urine	ALA	20–50
	PBG	20–50
	Total porphyrins	40–80
	Porphyrin fractions	100–200
Feces	Total porphyrins	100–150
	Porphyrin fractions	100–200
Packed Eryhtocytes	Total porphyrins	25–50
	Zinc protoporphyrin	25–50
	ALA dehydratase	100–200
	PBG deaminase	100–200
	Uroporphyrinogen decarboxylase	150–300
PLASMA	Total porphyrins	30–60
	Fluorescent spectrum of porphyrins	50–100

5.2. Diagnosis of Specific Porphyrias

Once the diagnosis of a porphyria is established, further studies can be ordered to establish the precise diagnosis (Table 2). Such evaluations are best carried out at centers with special expertise in evaluation of disorders of porphyrin metabolism. The clinical picture directs the further work-up: If PCT is suspected, a 24-h urine for uroporphyrin quantitation is indicated. Likewise, for diagnosis of AIP, the 24-h urine will show elevations of uro- and coproporphyrin during the attack. For detection of coproporphyrin or protoporphyrin in the diagnosis of variegate porphyria, hereditary coproporphyria, and protoporphyria, fecal porphyrins are preferred (since these porphyrins are primarily or solely excreted via the bile). In the mixed hepatic/erythropoietic porphyrias and the erythropoietic porphyrias, determination of porphyrins in packed erythrocytes can help in the diagnosis, as protoporphyrin frequently accumulates in these cells. Erythrocytes are also used to measure the activity of PBG deaminase (for diagnosis of AIP), ALA dehydratase (for ALA dehydratase-deficiency porphyria), and Uro-D (for familial PCT or HEP). Rarely is it necessary to measure other enzymes of the pathway: Specialized labs may use lymphocytes for determination of coproporphyrinogen oxidase activity (diagnosis of HCP), protoporphyrinogen oxidase (VP), or ferrochelatase (PP). Suspicion of latent disease or screening of asymptomatic family members may warrant such expensive testing.

Secondary porphyrinurias can usually be distinguished from true porphyrias by the only mildly increased urinary excretion of (mostly copro-) porphyrin, and by normal ALA and PBG levels in the urine. Patients usually lack typical symptoms of acute porphyria, and a disorder associated with secondary porphyrinuria may be present *(6)*. Measurements of urinary total porphyrins and porphyrin fractions can be carried out on urines collected and stored as already described for ALA and PBG measurements (vide supra). Stool porphyrins can be carried out on single random stool specimens, although some labs require full 24-h collections. Erythrocytic porphyrin assays and enzymatic activities are carried out on frozen lysates of packed erythrocytes. Plasma porphyrins and the fluorescent spectrum of these porphyrins (particularly useful for diagnosis of variegate porphyria) are also carried out on samples that have been frozen and stored protected from light. Typical costs for these assays are summarized in Table 6.

6. TREATMENT OF PORPHYRIAS

6.1. Treatment of the Acute Attack

Treatment of the acute neurovisceral attack, as may occur in AIP, HCP, VP, homozygous ALA dehydratase deficiency, lead intoxication, or hereditary tyrosinemia, requires immediate removal of all potential precipitating factors (drugs, infections, and so on) along with supportive therapy until the attack resolves. In addition, specific therapies are indicated as outlined below and in the algorithm (Fig. 2). These act directly on the heme biosynthetic pathway and, therefore, lead to a suppression of the porphyrin and precursor production.

Supportive measures include close monitoring of fluid and electrolyte balance. Hyponatremia should be treated with fluid restriction (since it may be due to increased ADH secretion), unless severe vomiting requires fluid replacement. Frequent neurological monitoring to detect signs of progressive paresis (especially of the respiratory muscles) is necessary. Intensive care facilities should be available for patients with such symptoms or with seizures. Pain control can be achieved with acetaminophen, meperidine, or morphine. Addition of chlorpromazine (or prochlorperazine) may not only enhance the analgesic effects of these drugs, but also treat concomitant nausea and vomiting. Tachycardia and hypertension responds well to propranolol, but some patients may develop bradycardia and hypotension, if the dose is not titrated carefully. Some patients may need to be intubated.

Seizure management poses a particular problem, since most of the commonly used anticonvulsants are known inducers of porphyrin synthesis and, therefore, can precipitate attacks (or worsen existing symptoms). Magnesium sulfate ($MgSO_4$), diazepam, clonazepam, and some of the newer anticonvulsants (gabapentin, vigabatrine) seem acceptable for treatment of seizures *(7,9)*. Correcting potential causes for seizures (e.g., electrolyte disturbances) has priority over the use of drugs, however. Lastly, adequate nutrition is of vital importance. Supplementation of the diet with folic acid is recommended, although most authorities do not believe that the very large doses (30 mg/d) recommended by some *(10)* offer a particular benefit. Cimetidine has been reported to blunt experimental porphyrias and to ameliorate some features of acute porphyric attacks *(11)*. It is apparently safe for use in this situation, although the mainstays of therapy are heme and carbohydrates.

In terms of specific measures, carbohydrate administration should be initiated as soon as the presumptive diagnosis is made. A minimum daily intake of 400 g of glucose, either intravenously at 20 g/h or orally (patient may need a naso-enteric tube) should be maintained until all symptoms have subsided. Heme therapy should be started immediately in patients with severe attacks (especially with paresis, seizures, and psychosis) and in patients with mild to moderate attacks who do not improve (or worsen) within the first 36 h of the outlined treatment. As a rule, the earlier heme is given, the more rapid and complete is the recovery *(6,12)*. The usual dose is 3–5 mg/kg body weight per day given once a day. Currently in the United States only one form of heme is FDA-approved—Panhematin® (Abbott). Each vial of Panhematin contains 313 mg of heme as a lyophilized powder. Because of limited stability (rapid formation of toxic by-products), it is important that hematin be dissolved in sterile water immediately before use and that it be infused within 1 h of dissolution (preferably into a large vein to minimize local irritation). To increase stability, hematin can be dissolved in human serum albumin in a molar ratio of 1:1 (prepared by adding 132 mL of 25% human serum albumin to one vial of Panhematin) *(13)*. This leads to formation of methemalbumin, which has been shown to be effective *(14)* and is stable for at least 24 h. The duration of heme therapy needs to be tailored to the individual patient. In most patients 3 d of therapy suffice; therapy for more than 7 d is not usually recommended, although it may, at times, be considered.

Table 7

Management of Cutaneous Manifestations of the Porphyrias

General measures:
   Protect skin from light and trauma; treat secondary skin infections promptly and vigorously.
   Use special clothing that blocks sunlight.
   Opaque sun block preparations (zinc oxide) are somewhat helpful.
   Typical sun block preparations (PABA) are of no benefit, as they do not block out long UV/blue light.
Porphyria cutanea tarda:
   Stop ethanol, estrogen, iron supplements, or other precipitating chemicals.
   Venesection to iron depletion (*see* Table 5).
   Chloroquine or hydroxchloroquine.
   Treat chronic viral hepatitis if present (Interferon, and so on).
   Alkalinize urine.
Protoporphyria:
   Ensure adequate iron.
   Beta-carotene.
   Prevent cholestatic liver diseases: Vaccinate to prevent hepatitis A and B; avoid alcohol excess;
      cholecystectomy for gallstones.
   Splenectomy, if evidence of hemolysis.
   May try oral charcoal or cholestyramine, chenodeoxycholic acid, ursodeoxycholic acid, cysteine.
   Heme infusions.
Liver transplantation.
Hereditary Coproporphyria: Variegate porphyria:
   Avoid precipitating factors (Table 3).
   Prevent cholestatic liver diseases: vaccinate to prevent hepatitis A and B; avoid alcohol excess; avoid
      hepatotoxins; cholecystectomy for gallstones.
   Treat as outlined in Fig. 2.
Congenital erythropoietic porphyria:
   Hypertransfusion.
   Splenectomy (for hemolysis).
   Glucocorticoid trial for anemia.
   Heme infusions.
   Bone marrow transplantation.
Hepatoerythrohepatic porphyria:
   Uncertain, probably for as PCT and CEP.

After the symptoms subside, all treatment can be tapered. It is important to advise patients about their disease, the precipitating factors, and the importance of screening of relatives at-risk.

6.2. Treatment of Cutaneous Manifestations (Table 7)

The cutaneous manifestations of the porphyrias are due to excess porphyrins, made chiefly in the bone marrow or liver, that have been released into the plasma and then been deposited in the skin and subcutaneous tissues. The general principles of therapy are to minimize the overproduction of porphyrins, to maximize their excretion, and to protect the skin from their toxic photodynamic effects.

For cutaneous manifestations of the acute porphyrias (HCP, VP), the methods to diminish porphyrin overproduction have already been described (*see* above). For PCT patients with relatively mild disease, adequate therapy may require only removal of the causative agent (e.g., estrogens, alcohol, haloaromatic chemicals). However, most patients need an additional means to reduce porphyrin overproduction, namely, removal of iron from the liver. This is accom-

Table 8

Recommended Guidelines for Therapeutic Venesection in Therapy of Porphyria Cutanea Tarda

Remove one pint of blood every 7–10 d until iron depletion has been achieved.
Iron depletion is defined as prevenesection hematocrit <34% and one or both of the following:
Serum transferrin saturation (Fe/TIBC) <10%
Serum ferritin <10 ng/mL
Maintaining iron depletion long-term usually is not necessary, but should be done if patient has evidence of homozygous HLA-linked hemochromatosis or if features of PCT recur.
During first 3 yr of remission, check 24 h urinary porphyrin annually in late winter.
Repeat iron depletion if urinary porphyrin >3 times upper limit of normal.

plished most simply and economically by therapeutic venesection, following the guidelines summarized in Table 8. If and when a nontoxic, orally active iron chelator is developed, it may become the treatment of choice, but this development is still some time in the future.

Antimalarials (e.g., [hydroxy-]chloroquine) enhance removal of porphyrins from the liver and perhaps other tissues by forming water-soluble complexes with them. The initial dose should be very low (125 mg 2–3 times a week) to avoid development of an acute liver injury that may occur with rapid, massive mobilization of stored porphyrins. After a month at low dose, these drugs may be increased gradually (over 2–3 wk) to 500 mg/d. Careful retinal examinations should be done prior to and periodically during such therapy, because retinal damage is a potential side effect.

Although not usually necessary, urinary alkalinization will also increase excretion of uroporphyrin. This is accomplished by administration of sodium bicarbonate or sodium citrate/citric acid (Shohls' solution).

For patients with protoporphyria, it is important to ensure that there is no iron deficiency, because such deficiency will worsen protoporphyrin accumulation. High carbohydrate intake and iv infusions of heme, as described for therapy of the acute porphyrias, may also reduce protoporphyrin overproduction. The latter is generally reserved for severely affected persons with evidence of hepatic dysfunction because of the expense and inconvenience of heme therapy. Efforts have been made to enhance biliary secretion of protoporphyrin by administration of bile salts (chenodeoxycholic, ursodeoxycholic acid), and to increase fecal excretion of secreted protoporphyrin by interruption of its enterohepatic cycling (cholestyramine, large doses of activated charcoal). Unfortunately, these treatments rarely seem to be of much clinical benefit.

For protection against cutaneous phototoxicity of protoporphyrin, beta-carotene is a somewhat effective medication. It must be used chronically in doses sufficient to achieve serum levels of 600–800 µg/dL. The usual dose in adults is 120–180 mg/d. Beta-carotene formerly was available in the United States as Solatene®. The same preparation is now available as Lumitene®, from Equivalent Pharmaceutical Industries. Recently, oral cysteine has also been said to be of benefit in PP. However, experience is limited and, on the whole, it seems less effective and less well tolerated than beta-carotene.

Patients with PP also require continuous monitoring of hepatic function, because some develop pigmentary cirrhosis with all the usual complications of decompensated liver disease (ascites, edema, encephalopathy, portal hypertension, hepatocellular carcinoma). Hepatic decompensation may occur rapidly. Those with very high plasma (>100 µg/dL) or RBC (>1,000 µg/dL PRBC) protoporphyrin concentrations or those with abnormal liver chemistries should undergo liver biopsy. Those with advanced fibrosis or cirrhosis should be considered for therapy with heme and liver transplantation.

Pigment gallstones, composed chiefly of protoporphyrin, are common in protoporphyria. Cholecystectomy is indicated, especially if the patient is otherwise in good condition for surgery.

P
inhe
(fre
A
Ir
duri
estal
A
expe
E
Ti
alon
C
term
C
ity w
Pr
essen

We
from N
and do
the Nal

1. Kap
   JL, e
2. Tsch
3. Tsch
   bolic
4. Bonl
5. Bonl
   USA
6. Bonk
   a tex
7. Bonk
8. Bren
   (GAI
9. Krau
   Neur
10. Wide
    to the
11. Horie
    for ac
12. Must
    ders.
13. Bonk
    evide
14. Ande
    tion o
    Libbe

7. POTENTIAL COMPLICATIONS (TABLE 4)

Aside from the chronic skin changes in PCT, HCP, and VP, there are long-term complications of porphyrias that may explain the decreased life expectancy of many patients. Chronic renal failure and hypertension have been found with increased frequency in patients with AIP (and VP). Patients with frequent and severe attacks may have a persistent motor neuropathy, with pareses or muscle atrophy (6,7,15). Sensory neuropathy occurs as well. A seizure disorder has been described in porphyric patients. Many patients with such seizures have been made worse by therapy, because most anticonvulsants are porphyrogenic (Table 5). Recently, an increased risk of development of hepatocellular carcinoma has been found in patients with AIP in Europe (16). This has not yet been confirmed among AIP patients in the United States. Hepatobiliary accumulation of protoporphyrin in protoporphyria can lead to cholelithiasis, as well as to liver failure, with progressive cholestasis. Hemolytic anemias and associated splenomegaly occur in protoporphyria and the erythropoietic porphyrias. PCT is associated with liver disease ranging from fatty liver to cirrhosis. Causative factors include alcohol, chronic hepatitis C, and iron overload. The accumulation of uroporphyrin itself is also potentially hepatoxic. Very important is the fact that the risk of hepatocellular carcinoma is increased in patients with PCT, particularly if hepatic fibrosis or cirrhosis is present (17). It is unclear whether this is due to the PCT per se (porphyrins in the liver leading to critical metabolic disturbances) or to the factors that led to the development of PCT (hepatotoxic chemicals, alcoholic liver disease, iron overload, chronic hepatitis C). It is often recommended that patients with PCT, particularly those with fibrosis or cirrhosis, undergo periodic screening for hepatocellular carcinoma with serum alpha-fetoprotein measurements and hepatic ultrasound. Similar recommendations have, in fact, been made for all patients with cirrhosis (see Chapter 12). Although these recommendations seem reasonable, studies done to date have failed to show improvement in duration of survival among those screened (18).

8. PROGNOSIS

With avoidance of precipitating factors, the severity and frequency of exacerbations of the acute hepatic porphyrias is markedly decreased. Residual neurologic deficits are frequent with more severe disease. As mentioned, hepatocellular carcinoma is more frequent in patients with long-standing PCT, which impacts significantly on the prognosis. Mortality rates from attacks of acute hepatic porphyrias have decreased dramatically to under 10% since the advent of hematin therapy. Life expectancy of patients with latent or mild disease is nearly normal.

For patients with PCT, the most important factor in improving symptoms and prognosis is judicious therapy with periodic iron removal by phlebotomy. Alcohol and estrogen avoidance further prolongs the length of the remission. Efforts should be made to eradicate HCV, when present. The extent of liver disease is a major factor influencing the risk of relapse and development of hepatocellular carcinoma.

9. PREVENTION

The strict avoidance of factors that precipitate acute attacks of hepatic porphyrias or cutaneous symptoms in PCT has been emphasized already. Patients should be well informed about the mechanism of their disease and should understand the importance of adequate nutrition, avoidance of sun exposure, and so on. A list of drugs that are likely to be harmful or safe, respectively, should be provided (Table 5). However, since many drugs have not been

Strategies for molecular therapy of this disorder are under active investigation. Some authors have recommended the use of vitamin E in infants diagnosed with α1AT deficiency. This antioxidant acts as a free-radical scavenger, theoretically decreasing the oxidative injury that stimulates fibrogenesis (28). Because the binding domain of the α1AT is recognized prior to intracellular retention, the manufacture of a peptide that could saturate this site might allow the release of mutant α1AT into the serum. Such a release would not only decrease the amount of damaging intracellular protein, but should provide higher serum levels of active α1AT to requisite tissues. Another strategy aims to manipulate the intracellular degradation system that is able to eliminate some of the mutant protein in those deficient patients who manifest liver injury (29). In addition, efforts are underway to introduce the gene for normal α1AT into affected hosts by way of viral vectors and liposome technology (30–33). Although this strategy will not effectively treat the liver disease, it may be effective for the therapy of emphysema associated with α1AT deficiency.

The understanding of the mutations that cause the disease make this genetic syndrome an excellent model for gene therapy. We have initiated experiments to develop a gene therapy approach for the treatment of the liver disease of α1AT deficiency (34). We have successfully employed α1AT hammerhead ribozymes in both retroviral vectors and in a novel SV40 vector system to selectively inhibit the production of α1AT mRNA and protein in tissue culture. This represents an early stage in the daunting task of developing a gene therapy approach that can be applied successfully in man.

5. PROGNOSIS

5.1. Prognosis in the Pediatric Population

The prevalence of neonatal cholestasis is estimated to be 1 in 2000 live births, with 30–40% of such cases being the result of α1AT deficiency. Retrospective data on the prognosis of α1AT deficiency in the pediatric population has been discouraging. For example, a 1990 review of 98 children with α1AT deficiency noted 50–60% of patients either received a transplant or required one (35). However, prospective analysis of kindreds has yielded more encouraging data regarding the morbidity and mortality of this disorder. Much of the epidemiologic work on α1AT deficiency is from Norway where the prevalence of the Pi*Z allele is relatively high. A 1976 prospective study by Sveger screened 200,000 newborns, identifying 125 children with homozygous α1AT deficiency. Of these 125 patients, 11% presented with neonatal cholestasis and 6% had various other indications of liver disease, but the remaining 83% were apparently healthy (19). An 8-yr follow-up study found that two of the affected individuals died of complications of cirrhosis, whereas the rest remained healthy (20). Further evidence that homozygosity for α1AT deficiency can carry a relatively favorable prognosis is provided by the observation that the frequency of PiZZ in newborns and in adults is approximately identical.

5.2. Prognosis in Adults

α1AT deficiency often presents in adults with end-stage liver disease and portal hypertension. In these individuals the prognosis of their disease can be estimated using the Child-Pugh score, as in other causes of cirrhosis. The risk of hepatocellular carcinoma and cholangiocarcinoma appears to be increased, especially in males (36). This conclusion has been based on retrospective data generated by analysis of 17 autopsied patients from Sweden. Although phenotypic PiZZ heterozygotes are at the highest risk for developing cirrhosis, the incidence of end-stage liver disease in partial deficiency states has been reported. Phenotypes described to have developed cirrhosis include PiMZ, PiSZ, and PiFZ (37).

6. PREVENTION

6.1. Screening

α1AT deficiency has been suggested as an appropriate disease for screening of the general population in which at-risk phenotypes are prevalent *(38)*. In fact, α1AT deficiency does meet many of the key requirements of a screening test: affected patients are asymptomatic in the early stages, the incidence of the PiZ phenotype is relatively common in certain populations, many patients will manifest clinical symptoms later in life (pulmonary or hepatic), and both primary and secondary prevention measures are available for the pulmonary manifestations of the disease. Simple α1AT levels are unacceptable as screening measurements, as the occurrence of false positives and negatives is too high; the best test would be phenotyping. Although the diagnosis of α1AT deficiency can be made prenatally by chorionic villus sampling, it is expensive and technically difficult. In practice, the diagnosis is often made in infancy in cases in which a high level of suspicion exists.

6.2. Prevention of Hepatic Complications

Once the diagnosis is confirmed by Pi typing and/or liver biopsy, preventive measures can be recommended. Breast feeding for the first year of life has been suggested to reduce hepatic manifestations of the disorder *(39)*. Care should be taken to supplement breast-fed infants with intramuscular or oral vitamin K. There is no role for α1AT supplementation in the prevention of hepatic complications of α1AT deficiency, because the damage appears to be related to the deposition of abnormal α1AT as opposed to its deficiency *(40)*. Although there are no prospectively tested prediction models for the timing of liver transplantation in patients with α1AT deficiency as in primary biliary cirrhosis and primary sclerosing cholangitis, the progress of this disorder appears to be slow. Management of cirrhosis, as in control of gastrointestinal hemorrhage, ascites, encephalopathy, and screening for hepatocellular carcinoma, should proceed as with other causes of end-stage liver disease. The survival in those patients undergoing liver transplantation appears to be similar to those patients having the procedure for other indications *(41)*. An additional advantage of transplantation is that the recipient will convert to the Pi type of the donor, thereby providing a cure to the disorder.

6.3. Prevention of Pulmonary Complications

Because cigaret smoking and exposure to second-hand smoke has been implicated in the pathogenesis of the pulmonary complications of α1AT deficiency, smoking cessation is essential in those diagnosed with α1AT deficiency *(42)*. Education in high-risk communities may have an effect on smoke exposure to those at risk. The use of genetically engineered replacement α1AT is being actively investigated (27).

7. INDICATIONS FOR CONSULTING THE SUBSPECIALIST

Because the majority of adults who carry the genetic material coding for α1AT deficiency, even homozygotes for Pi*Z, do not suffer from liver disease, recognition of this abnormality does not necessarily imply the need for hepatologic evaluation. Therefore, those adults or children who are found to have an at-risk phenotype during the evaluation of a family member should be screened for evidence of hepatitis or liver dysfunction prior to referral. Elevated aminotransferases, liver synthetic dysfunction, or a lesion suggestive of primary hepatic malignancy should be further investigated. Since liver biopsy is usually an integral part of this evaluation, referral to the gastroenterologist/hepatologist should be made at this time. Patients who present with manifestations of chronic or decompensated liver disease should be referred directly. The subset with decompensated liver disease or hepatocellular carcinoma should be sent to a center that offers liver transplantation, because this may be the only means to alter the natural history of such patients.

8. CONCLUSIONS

α1AT deficiency is a relatively common genetic disorder that can be related to the development of chronic liver disease. Screening of family members, avoidance of hepatotoxins, and a thorough investigation for other forms of liver insult (especially viral hepatitis) should be instituted. Although there is no specific therapy available to prevent the hepatic manifestations of the disorder, disease progression is often slow. Careful screening for hepatocellular carcinoma seems indicated. Management of the manifestations of chronic liver disease can forestall the eventual need for liver transplantation. Discovery of a suspicious lesion or clinical evidence of decompensation should prompt referral to a center offering orthotopic liver transplantation. As the molecular defect becomes more thoroughly understood and the tools of gene therapy are developed, our understanding and management of this disorder may change dramatically.

SUMMARY

Alpha-1-Antitrypsin (α1AT) deficiency is the most common inborn error of metabolism, causing cholestasis and cirrhosis and the eventual need for liver transplantation.

Hepatotoxicity is thought to result from intracellular accumulation of abnormal human α1AT gene product.

Less than 20% of homozygous PiZZ individuals develop liver disease.

α1AT presents in a variety of ways including neonatal jaundice, progressive hepatitis, cirrhosis with portal hypertension or synthetic dysfunction, and hepatocellular carcinoma.

Heterozygosity for α1AT may be a predisposing factor for liver disease.

Liver transplantation offers survival rates similar to those in other indications; recurrence of α1AT in transplanted patients has not been reported.

REFERENCES

1. Eriksson S. Studies in alpha-1-antitrypsin deficiency. Acta Med Scand Suppl 1965;432:1–85.
2. Gans H, Sharp HL, Tan BH. Antiprotease deficiency and familial infantile liver cirrhosis. Surg Gynec Obstet 1969;129:289–299.
3. Aagenaes O, Matlary A, Elgjo K, Munthe E, Fagerhol M. Neonatal cholestasis in alpha-1-antitrypsin deficient children: clinical, genetic, histological and immunohistochemical findings. Acta Paediat Scand 1992;61:632–642.
4. Stevens PM, Hnilica V, Johnson PC, Bell RL. Pathophysiology of hereditary emphysema. Ann Intern Med 1971;74:672–680.
5. Kennedy M, Brett W. Monozygotic twins with alpha-1-antitrypsin deficiency (Letter). Lancet 1985;1(8427):527–528.
6. Nukiwa T, Satoh K, Brantly M L, et al. Identification of a second mutation in the protein-coding sequence of the Z type alpha-1-antitrypsin gene. J Biol Chem 1986;261:15,989–15,994.
7. Cox DW, Woo SLC, Mansfield T. DNA restriction fragments associated with alpha-1-antitrypsin indicate a single origin for deficiency allele PI Z. Nature 1985;316:79–88.
8. Roychoudhury AK, Nei M. Human polymorphic genes: world distribution. Oxford Univ Press, New York, 1988, pp. 132–135.
9. Cox DW. Alpha-1-antitrypsin deficiency. In: Scriver CR, Beaudet AL, Sly WS, Valle D, eds. The metabolic basis of inherited disease, 6th ed. McGraw-Hill, New York, 1989, pp. 2409–2437.
10. Crystal RG. The alpha-1-antitrypsin gene and its deficiency states. Trends Genet 1989;5:411–417.
11. Cox DW, Smyth S. Risk for liver disease in adults with alpha 1-antitrypsin deficiency. Am J Med 1983;74:221–227.
12. Wu Y, Whitman I, Molmenti E, Moore K, Hippenmeyer P, Perlmutter DH. A lag in intracellular degradation of mutant alpha-1-antitrypsin correlates with the liver disease phenotype in homozygous PiZZ alpha-1-antitrypsin deficiency. Proc Natl Acad Sci USA 1994;91:9014–9018.
13. DeCroo, S, Kamboh MI, Ferrell RE. Population genetics of alpha-1-antitrypsin polymorphism in US whites, US blacks and African blacks. Hum Hered 1991;41:215–221.

14. Nukiwa T, Brantly ML, Ogushi F, Fells GA, Crystal RG. Characterization of the gene and protein of the common alpha-1-antitrypsin normal M2 allele. Am J Hum Genet 1988;43:322–330.
15. Kidd VJ, Wallace RB, Itakura K, Woo SLC. Alpha-1-antitrypsin deficiency detection by direct analysis of the mutation in the gene. Nature 1983;304:230–234.
16. Lomas DA, Evans DL, Finch JT, Carrell RW. The mechanism of Z alpha-1-antitrypsin accumulation in the liver. Nature 1992;357:605–607.
17. Sifers RN, Rogers BB, Hawkins HK, Finegold MJ, Woo SLC. Elevated synthesis of human alpha1-antitrypsin hinders secretion of murine alpha-1-antitrypsin from hepatocytes of transgenic mice. J Biol Chem 1989;264:15,696–15,700.
18. Loebermann H, Tokuoka R, Deisenhofer J, Huber R. Human α1-proteinase inhibitor: crystal structure analysis of two crystal modifications, molecular model and preliminary analysis of the implications for function. J Mol Biol 1984;177:531–536.
19. Sveger T. Liver disease in alpha-1-antitrypsin deficiency detected by screening in 200,000 infants. N Engl J Med 1976;294:1316–1321.
20. Sveger T. Prospective study of children with alpha-1-antitrypsin deficiency: eight year old follow-up. J Pediatr 1989;104:91–94.
21. Moroz SP, Cutz E, Cox DW, Sass-Kortsak A. Liver disease associated with alpha-1-antitrypsin deficiency in childhood. J Pediatr 1976;88:19–25.
22. Clark P, Breit SN, Dawkins RL, Penny R. Genetic study of a family with two members with Weber-Christian disease (panniculitis) and alpha-1-antitrypsin deficiency. Am J Med Genet 1982;13:57–62.
23. Fortin PR, Fraser RS, Watts CS, Esdaile JM. Alpha-1 antitrypsin deficiency and systemic necrotizing vasculitis. J Rheum 1991;18:1613–1616.
24. Lewis JH, Iammarino RM, Spero JA, Hasiba U. Pittsburgh: an alpha-1-antitrypsin variant causing hemorrhagic disease. Blood 1978;51:129–137.
25. Owen MC, Brennan SO, Lewis JH, Carrell RW. Mutation of antitrypsin to antithrombin: alpha-1-antitrypsin Pittsburgh (358 met-to-arg), a fatal bleeding disorder. New Engl J Med 1983;309:694–698.
26. Moroz SP, et al. Membranoproliferative glomerulonephritis in childhood cirrhosis associated with alpha-1-antitrypsin deficiency. Pediatrics 1976;88:19–25.
27. Wewers MD, Casolaro A, Sellers S, et al. Replacement therapy for alpha-1-antitrypsin deficiency associated with emphysema. N Engl J Med 1987;316:1055–1062.
28. Pittschieler K. Heterozygotes and liver involvement. Acta Paediatr 1994;393:21S–23S.
29. Perlmutter DH. Clinical manifestations of alpha-1-antitrypsin deficiency. Gastroenterology Clin N Am 1995;24:27–43.
30. Garver RI Jr, Chytil A, Courtney M, Crystal RG. Clonal gene therapy: transplanted mouse fibroblast clones express human alpha-1-antitrypsin gene in vivo. Science 1987;237:762–764.
31. Kay MA, Baley P, Rothenberg S, et al. Expression of human alpha-1-antitrypsin in dogs after autologous transplantation of retroviral transduced hepatocytes. Proc Natl Acad Sci USA 1992;89:89–93.
32. Lemarchand P, Jaffe HA, Danel C, et al. Adenovirus-mediated transfer of a recombinant human alpha-1-antitrypsin cDNA to human endothelial cells. Proc Natl Acad Sci USA 1992;89:6482–6486.
33. Brantly M, Courtney M, Crystal RG. Repair of the secretion defect in the Z form of alpha-1-antitrypsin by addition of a second mutation. Science 1988;242:1700–1702.
34. Ozaki I, Duan L, Liu SL, Pomerantz RJ, Zern MA. Application of ribozymes for gene therapy of liver disease in a1-antitrypsin deficiency. Molecular diagnosis and gene therapy. Kluwar Academic Publishers, Dordrecht, Netherlands, 1996, pp. 106–115.
35. Ibarguen E, Gross CR, Savik SK, Sharp HL. Liver disease in alpha-1-antitrypsin deficiency: prognostic indicators. J Pediatr 1990;117:864–870.
36. Eriksson S, Carlson J, Velez R. Risk of cirrhosis and primary liver cancer in alpha-1-antitrypsin deficiency. N Engl J Med 1986;314:736–739.
37. Campra JL, Craig JP, Peters RL, Reynolds TB. Cirrhosis associated with partial deficiency of alpha-1-antitrypsin in adults. Ann Intern Med 1973;78:233–238.
38. Sveger T. Screening for alpha-1-antitrypsin deficiency. Acta Paediatr 1994;393:18S–20S.
39. Udall JN Jr, Dixon M, Newman AP, Wright JA, James B, Bloch KJ. Liver disease in alpha 1-antitrypsin deficiency. A retrospective analysis of the influence of early breast- vs bottle-feeding. JAMA 1985;253:2679–2682.
40. Psacharopoulos HT, Mowat AP, Cook PJ, Carlile PA, Portmann B, Rodeck CH. Outcome of liver disease associated with alpha-1-antitrypsin deficiency (PiZ). Implications for genetic counseling and antenatal diagnosis. Arch Dis Child 1983;58:882–887.
41. Esquivel CO, Marino IR, Fioravanti V, Van Thiel DH. Liver transplantation for metabolic disease of the liver. Gastroenterol Clin North Am 1988;17:167–175.
42. Burdelski M. Diagnostic, preventive, medical and surgical management of alpha-1-antitrypsin deficiency in childhood. Acta Paediatr 1994;393:33S–36S.

SUGGESTED READING

1. Alagille D. Alpha-1-Antitrypsin deficiency. Hepatology 1984;4:11S–14S.
2. Deutsch J, Becker H, Aubock L. Histopathological features of liver disease in alpha-1-antitrypsin deficiency. Acta Paediatr 1994;393:8S–12S.
3. Eriksson SG. Liver disease in alpha 1-antitrypsin deficiency. Aspects of incidence and prognosis. Scand J Gastroenterol 1985;20:907–911.
4. Massi G, Chiarelli C. Alpha-1-antitrypsin: molecular system and the Pi system. Acta Paediatr 1994;393:1S–4S.
5. Poley JR. Malignant liver disease in alpha-1-antitrypsin deficiency. Acta Paediatr 1994;393:27S–32S.

VII   Pediatric Liver Diseases

21 Wilson's Disease

Michael L. Schilsky and Irmin Sternlieb

1. INTRODUCTION

Wilson's disease is an autosomal recessive disorder due to inheritance of two mutant alleles of a putative copper transporter (ATP7B) encoded by a gene on chromosome 13 *(1–5)*. Biliary copper excretion is reduced resulting in the accumulation of copper, first in the liver and later in other organs of homozygotes *(6,7)*. The abnormal accumulation of copper results initially in liver injury, followed by accumulation of copper in the brain, kidneys, and in other organs. The condition of the liver to the injury is determined by a balance between cell death, inflammation and regeneration. When cell death is overwhelming, fulminant hepatitis results. Most often, cell injury and inflammatory changes are chronic, leading to fibrosis and cirrhosis. Unless treated, liver disease progresses to hepatic insufficiency and death. Individuals who are heterozygous for the Wilson's disease mutation may manifest minor abnormalities in copper metabolism, but do not develop the disease and do not require treatment *(8)*.

2. CARDINAL SIGNS AND SYMPTOMS

The signs and symptoms of Wilson's disease vary widely. Hepatic manifestations generally occur during childhood and adolescence, whereas neurologic or psychiatric symptoms tend to occur later.

From: *Diseases of the Liver and Bile Ducts: Diagnosis and Treatment*
Edited by: G. Y. Wu and J. Israel © Humana Press Inc., Totowa, NJ

2.1. Hepatic

Early on, patients are asymptomatic. Histologic sections of liver biopsy specimens obtained during this early stage, when the diagnosis may be suspected because of a family history of Wilson's disease or the fortuitous discovery of a reduced serum ceruloplasmin concentration, often reveal only microvesicular or macrovesicular fatty changes, with glycogen deposits in nuclei or nuclear cytoplasmic invaginations (9). At this stage, histochemical staining for copper or copper-binding protein is more often than not nonrevealing. However, electron microscopy may demonstrate specific ultrastructural abnormalities of mitochondria (10,11). With time, fibrosis and cirrhosis appear and, along with these changes, signs and symptoms related to portal hypertension. With progression of liver disease, hepatic insufficiency with associated coagulopathy and encephalopathy may be evident.

A minority of patients develop a picture of fulminant hepatitis, most often during the second decade of life. The presence of an associated nonimmune hemolytic anemia and fulminant hepatic failure suggests the diagnosis of Wilson's disease. Unlike other presentations in which there is no gender preference, Wilsonian fulminant hepatitis occurs three times more frequently in females (12). A peculiarity of this form of fulminant hepatitis is its association with inappropriately low serum aminotransferases and alkaline phosphatase values (12–17).

Some patients may display a histologic picture of chronic active hepatitis with inflammatory infiltrates, interface necrosis, and bridging fibrosis (18). Though these represent only approx 5% of patients with Wilson's disease, the inability to distinguish them on the basis of histology alone often confounds and delays diagnosis.

2.2. Neurologic and Psychiatric Disease

Though often manifesting later than hepatic disease, there is a wide range (8–50 yr) for the onset of neurologic or psychiatric symptoms (8). Most neurologic signs and symptoms are related to motor abnormalities. They may be classified as Parkinsonian with dystonia and rigidity, or as choreic or pseudosclerotic with tremors or dysarthria (19). Symptoms range widely in severity; however, unless treated, progressive deterioration with dysphagia, dysarthria, drooling, tremors, severe hypertonia with contractures and subsequent motor deficits occur along with progression of the liver disease. With rare exceptions, Kayser-Fleischer rings are present in all patients with neurologic or psychiatric Wilson's disease. However, Kayser-Fleischer rings have also been found in the corneas of patients with long-standing cholestatic syndromes. Magnetic resonance imaging (MRI) and computerized tomography (CT) may reveal basal ganglia lesions, which should suggest a diagnosis of Wilson's disease (20,21).

Psychiatric symptoms are wide ranging, from mild behavioral changes and deterioration of school work to severe psychosis and depression (8). Untreated, these patients go on to manifest neurologic symptoms as well as hepatic disease.

3. DIAGNOSIS

The diagnosis of Wilson's disease may be established by a combination of clinical and laboratory examinations (Table 1). The appropriate collection of specimens to avoid contamination is important. For accurate determination of serum ceruloplasmin and copper, subjects should ideally be fasted for 8 h prior to blood collection. The blood should be properly centrifuged and the serum separated and shipped to diagnostic laboratories the same day, or stored at 4°C until delivery. For copper quantitation in liver samples, a whole core of a needle biopsy specimen should be obtained with a copper-free needle, such as a Jamshidi needle. The specimen should be transferred to a small plastic tube and either frozen or dehydrated for shipment to diagnostic laboratories. Copper content may

Table 1

Diagnostic Testing for Wilson's Disease

Test	Normal range or findings	Wilson's disease	Comment
Serum ceruloplasmin	20–40 mg/dL	<20 mg/dL	in 95% patients and 20% of heterozygotes
Corneal slit-lamp exam	Normal	Kayser-Fleischer rings	absent early on in disease
Serum copper	60-120 μg/dL	<60 μg/dL	often above normal range in fulminant hepatitis
24-H urinary copper	<100 μg/24 h	>100 μg/24 h	may be within normal range in asymptomatic patients; in fulminant hepatitis or following chelating agent may exceed 1000 μg/24 h
Hepatic copper	<50 μg/g dry wt	>250 μg/g dry wt	may be elevated in chronic cholestatic syndromes, in syndromes with idiopathic copper toxicosis
Hepatic histology	Normal	Abnormal	most often hepatocellular steatosis with glycogen nuclei, fibrosis, and cirrhosis; chronic active hepatitis in 5%
Rhodanine histochemistry	Negative	Positive	can be negative early on in disease, positive in cirrhotic livers but not in all nodules
Electron microscopy	Normal	Abnormal	mitochondrial alterations when steatosis present, dense lysosomes in later stages
Brain MRI or CT	Normal	Abnormal	alterations in basal ganglia and other less specific changes

also be determined on paraffin-embedded specimens. However, this is less desirable than measurements made on fresh specimens.

The approach to diagnosis for asymptomatic patients, and for patients with hepatic, neurologic, or psychiatric disease are outlined in Figs. 1–3. Once a diagnosis of Wilson's disease is established, screening of siblings by clinical and biochemical evaluation is mandatory. Family screening may also include genetic studies that search for common patterns of polymorphism surrounding the Wilson's disease gene (22). This haplotype analysis is most practical since the large number of mutations of the ATP7B gene (currently over 60 have been identified) are present among patients, but requires the identification of a propositus. At this time, these studies are available only from a few research laboratories. Genetic studies should be used to complement and not supplant a full clinical and biochemical screening for Wilson's disease.

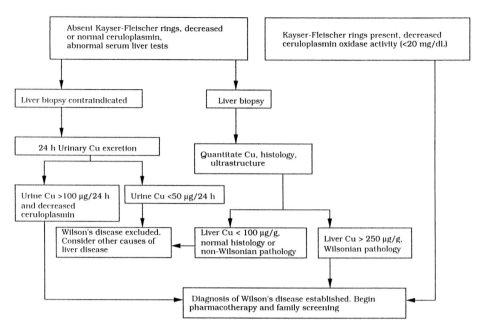

Fig. 1. A scheme for establishing the diagnosis of asymptomatic or hepatic Wilson's disease.

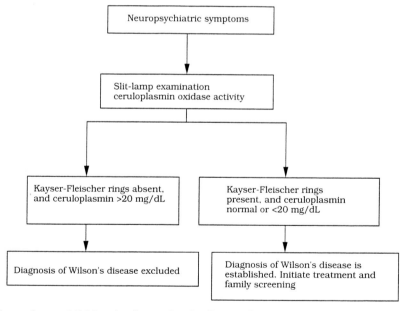

Fig. 2. A scheme for establishing the diagnosis of Wilson's disease with neuropsychiatric presentation.

4. TREATMENT

4.1. Symptomatic Patients

Symptomatic patients should be treated with chelating agents. The agents of choice are penicillamine (with supplemental pyridoxine, 25 mg/d) and trientine, which cause marked increases in urinary copper excretion, in divided dosages of up to 1.5–2.0 g/d *(8,23,24)*. Trientine may be effective in patients who react adversely to penicillamine *(24)*. Improvement of clinical and biochemical parameters may occur over months to a year. In patients with severe

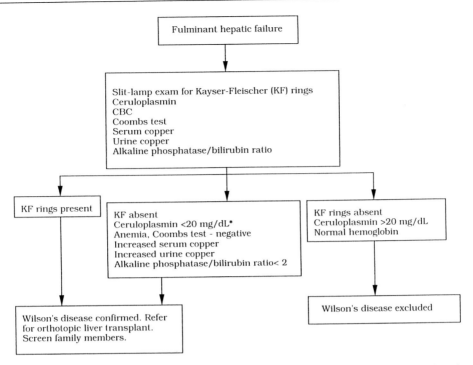

Fig. 3. A scheme for establishing the diagnosis of Wilsonian fulminant hepatitis. Ceruloplasmin can be decreased because of hepatic biosynthetic failure independent of Wilson's disease.

hepatic insufficiency not responding to therapy within 90 d, or patients with fulminant hepatitis, orthotopic liver transplantation (OLT) should be considered *(12)*. Patients with intractable neurologic symptoms may benefit from the addition of the parenteral chelating agent dimercaptopropanol (British Anti-Lewisite or BAL), which may augment copper excretion above levels achieved by oral agents alone *(25)*. Most patients with neurologic or psychiatric symptoms who underwent OLT did so for hepatic insufficiency. However, some showed improvement of neurologic abnormalities and loss of Kayser-Fleischer rings (if present before) *(12)*. OLT is not indicated for the treatment of neurologic Wilson's disease in the absence of hepatic indications for transplantation.

4.2. Asymptomatic Patients

Treatment of asymptomatic patients or maintenance therapy for patients who were previously symptomatic, and who responded favorably to treatment, includes the same agents, penicillamine (with supplemental pyridoxine, 25 mg/d), at maintenance dosages (750–1000 mg/d), or trientine, at maintenance dosages (750–1000 mg/d), or zinc salts (150 mg elemental zinc in divided doses) *(26)*. Zinc appears to act by preventing dietary copper absorption *(27)*. Treatment of newly diagnosed patients may begin as early as 3 yr of age *(8,28)*. For children less than 40 kg, a dosage of 0.02 g penicillamine or trientine per kg body weight, rounded to the nearest 125 mg, may be administered. No studies are available regarding an appropriate pediatric dosage of zinc. However, there are reports in which the adult dosages (150 mg in three divided doses) were tolerated without any ill effect *(29)*.

4.3. Treatment During Pregnancy

Therapy for Wilson's disease should be continued throughout pregnancy with dose modification for penicillamine and trientine during the last trimester to 500 mg/d, and to 250 mg/d for the last six wk, if caesarian section is anticipated or until wound healing has occurred *(8,30,31)*, and continuation of maintenance dosages for zinc *(32)*. No teratogenic effects of penicillamine, trientine, or zinc in humans have been noted.

4.4. Monitoring of Pharmacotherapy

The major goals of monitoring include determinations of the adequacy of the chosen therapy, appropriate screening for potential drug reactions or intolerance, and determining compliance with therapy.

The most important gauge of adequacy of therapy is the patient's clinical response. Regression of symptoms is the major early goal in symptomatic patients. Improvement or normalization of abnormal laboratory parameters represent positive responses that may require months to a year to become evident. Improvement in prothrombin time may be delayed or may persist indefinitely in some patients. Leukopenia and thrombocytopenia due to hypersplenism may not be influenced by any form of treatment, but may be well tolerated by the patients.

The estimation of the nonceruloplasmin copper (total serum copper minus copper content of ceruloplasmin) is a valuable gauge of therapeutic efficacy, with a value of <10 µg/dL as a goal. Along with reductions of serum nonceruloplasmin copper, urinary copper excretion for patients on chelating agents should decline over time from values exceeding 1000–500 µg/24 h. Doctors should alert patients to be vigilant for fever, rash, or lymphadenopathy during the first few weeks of therapy. Complete blood counts and urine screening for cellular elements and protein should be performed at intervals.

In effectively treated patients, values of non-ceruloplasmin copper of >10 mg/dL and a urinary copper excretion of <500 µg/d should suggest noncompliance. For patients on zinc therapy, compliance may be gauged by determination of urinary zinc content. Other effective measures for monitoring compliance include pill counts, periodic corneal slit-lamp exams to exclude a recurrence of Kayser-Fleischer rings, and biochemical screening to exclude changes in hepatic function or increases in non-ceruloplasmin serum copper.

5. POTENTIAL COMPLICATIONS

Complications in patients with neurologic symptoms include progression of symptoms and failure to respond to therapy in patients in whom the delayed diagnosis has resulted in irreversible neurologic damage. Progression or recurrence of neurologic or hepatic disease may occur due to non-compliance with therapy.

Other complications include reactions to pharmacotherapy, progression of disease despite therapy, or non-compliance.

Sensitivity reactions to penicillamine occur in approx 10% of patients, including fever, rashes, neutropenia, or thrombocytopenia. Lupus-like syndromes, nephropathy with proteinuria, progyric changes in the skin, and elastosis perforans serpingosa and, very rarely, Goodpasture's syndrome. Trientine therapy has rarely been associated with a lupus-like syndrome and a sideroblastic anemia that is reversible upon discontinuation of chelational therapy *(24)*.

6. PROGNOSIS

Untreated patients with Wilson's disease suffer progressive hepatic injury leading to hepatic insufficiency, irreversible central nervous system changes, and death. The prognosis for patients with appropriate pharmacotherapy is excellent. Even in patients with chronic active hepatitis and cirrhosis caused by Wilson's disease, pharmacotherapy resulted in 100% 5-yr survivals for compliant patients *(18)*. Discontinuation of pharmacotherapy may result in symptom recurrence and eventual liver failure. One year survival of patients with Wilson's disease who underwent hepatic transplantation was approx 80%, and these patients did not require further treatment for Wilson's disease *(12)*. The development of hepatocellular carcinoma in patients with Wilson's disease is rare, despite the presence of cirrhosis.

7. INDICATIONS FOR CONSULTING THE SUBSPECIALIST

A specialist should be consulted to assist in the diagnosis of Wilson's disease in patients with conflicting or borderline laboratory values. Other indications include inexperience with Wilson's disease and its treatment, failure of patients to respond to initial pharmacotherapy, or problems relating to monitoring for compliance. Patients with Wilsonian fulminant hepatitis should be referred without delay to a center which performs OLT.

8. CONCLUSIONS

Given the ability to effectively treat, prevent and even reverse the manifestations of this disorder, it is essential to consider the diagnosis of Wilson's disease in a young person with unexplained hepatic or neurologic findings or symptoms. Several pharmacologic agents are available, and lifelong compliance with therapy is associated with excellent prognosis.

OLT is lifesaving for patients with fulminant Wilsonian hepatitis, and should be utilized for individuals in whom hepatic insufficiency is progressive despite pharmacotherapy.

9. REFERENCE LABORATORIES FOR COPPER AND CERULOPLASMIN OXIDASE DETERMINATIONS

1. National Center for The Study of Wilson's Disease
   St. Luke's/Roosevelt Hospital
   432 West 58th Street, Suite 614
   New York, NY 10019
   Cost: $75
2. Mayo Medical Laboratory
   Mayo Clinic
   200 1st S. W.
   Rochester, MN 55905
   Telephone 800-533-1710
   Cost: $35

SUMMARY

Wilson's disease should be considered in patients with unexplained liver disease with or without extrahepatic symptoms.

Early recognition and treatment prevent extrahepatic complications.

REFERENCES

1. Frydman M, Bonne-Tammir B, Farrer LA, Conneally PM, Magazanik A, Ashbel S, Goldwitch Z. Assignment of the gene for Wilson disease to chromosome 13: linkage to the esterase D locus. Proc Natl Acad Sci USA 1985;82:1819–1821.
2. Tanzi RE, Petrukhin K, Chernov I, Pellequer JL, et al. The Wilson disease gene is a copper transporting ATPase with homology to the Menkes disease gene. Nat Genet 1993;5:344–350.
3. Bull PC, Thomas GR, Rommens JM, Forbes JR, Cox DW. The Wilson disease gene is a putative copper transporting P-type ATPase similar to the Menkes gene. Nat Genet 1993;5:327–337.
4. Yamaguchi Y, Heiny ME, Gitlin JD. Isolation and characterization of a human liver cDNA as a candidate gene for Wilson disease. Biochem Biophys Res Commun 1993;197:271–277.
5. Petrukhin K, Lutsenko S, Chernov I, Ross BM, Kaplan JH, Gilliam TC. Characterization of the Wilson disease gene encoding a P-type copper transporting ATPase: genomic organization, alternative splicing, and structure/function predictions. Hum Mol Genet 1994;3:1647–1656.

6. Frommer DJ. Defective biliary excretion of copper in Wilson's disease. Gut 1974;15:125–129.

7. Sternlieb I, van den Hamer CJA, Morell AG, Alpert S, Gregoriadis G, Scheinberg IH. Lysosomal defect of hepatic copper excretion in Wilson's disease (hepatolenticular degeneration). Gastroenterology 1973;64:99–105.

8. Scheinberg IH, Sternlieb I. Wilson's disease. Saunders, Philadelphia, 1984.

9. Alt E, Sternlieb I, Goldfischer S. The cytopathology of metal overload [review]. Int Rev Exp Pathol 1990;31:165–188.

10. Sternlieb I. Mitochondrial and fatty changes in hepatocytes of patients with Wilson's disease. Gastroenterology 1968;55:354–367.

11. Sternlieb I. Fraternal concordance of types of abnormal hepatocellular mitochondria in Wilson's disease. Hepatology 1992;16:728–732.

12. Schilsky ML, Scheinberg IH, Sternlieb I. Liver transplantation for Wilson's disease: indications and outcome. Hepatology 1994;19:583-87.

13. Shaver WA, Bhatt H, Combes B. Low serum alkaline phosphatase activity in Wilson's disease. Hepatology 1986;6:859–863.

14. Wilson RA, Clayson KJ, Leon S. Unmeasurable serum alkaline phosphatase activity in Wilson's disease associated with fulminant hepatic failure and hemolysis. Hepatology 1987;7:613–615.

15. McCullough AJ, Fleming CR, Thistle JL, Baldus WP, Ludwig J, McCall JT, Dickson ER. Diagnosis of Wilson's disease presenting as fulminant hepatic failure. Gastroenterology 1983;84:161–167.

16. Berman DH, Leventhal RI, Gavaler JS, Cadoff EM, Van Thiel DH. Clinical differentiation of fulminant Wilsonian hepatitis from other causes of hepatic failure. Gastroenterology 1991;100:1129–1134.

17. Sallie R, Katsiyiannakis L, Baldwin D, et al. Failure of simple biochemical indexes to reliably differentiate fulminant Wilson's disease from other causes of fulminant liver failure. Hepatology 1992;16:1206–1211.

18. Schilsky ML, Scheinberg IH, Sternlieb I. Prognosis of Wilsonian chronic active hepatitis. Gastroenterology 1991;100:762–767.

19. Walshe JM, Yealland M. Chelational treatment of neurological Wilson's disease. Q J Med 1993;86:197–204.

20. Starosta-Rubinstein S, Young AB, Kluin K, Hill G, Aisen AM, Gabreilsen T, Brewer GJ. Clinical assessment of 31 patients with Wilson's disease: Correlations with structural changes on magnetic resonance imaging. Arch Neurol 1987;44:365–370.

21. van Wassenaer-van Hall HN, van den Heuvel AG, Algra A, et al. Wilson disease: findings at MR imaging and CT of the brain with clinical correlation. Radiology 1996;198:531–536.

22. Petrukhin K, Fischer SG, Pirastu M, et al. Mapping, cloning and genetic characterization of the region containing the Wilson disease gene. Nat Gen 1993;5:338–343.

23. Walshe JM. Copper chelation in Wilson's disease. A comparison of penicillamine and triethylene tetramine dihydrochloride. Q J Med 1973;42:441–452.

24. Scheinberg IH, Jaffe ME, Sternlieb I. The use of trientine in preventing the effects of interrupting penicillamine therapy in Wilson's disease. N Engl J Med 1987;317:209–213.

25. Scheinberg IH, Sternlieb I. Treatment of the neurologic manifestations of Wilson's disease. Arch Neurol 1994;51:545–554.

26. Brewer GJ, Dick RD, Yuzbasiyan-Gurkan V, Johnson V, Wang Y. Treatment of Wilson's disease with zinc XIII. Therapy with zinc in presymptomatic patients from the time of diagnosis. J Lab Clin Med 1994;123:849–858.

27. Cousins RJ. Absorption, transport, and hepatic metabolism of copper and zinc: special reference to metallothionein and ceruloplasmin. Physiol Rev 1985;65:238–309.

28. Collins JC, Scheinberg IH, Sternlieb I. Penicillamine prophylaxis for asymptomatic children with Wilson's disease. Hepatology 1993;18:128A.

29. Hoogenraad TU, Koevoet R, de Ruyter Korver EG. Oral zinc sulfate as long-term treatment in Wilson's disease (hepatolenticular degeneration). Eur Neurol 1979;18:205–211.

30. Walshe JM. Pregnancy in Wilson's disease. Q J Med 1977;181:73–83.

31. Walshe JM. The management of pregnancy in Wilson's disease treated with trientine. Q J Med 1986;58:8–87.

32. Brewer JB, Yuzbasiyan-Gurkan V. Wilson's disease. Medicine 1992;71:139–163.

22

Neonatal Jaundice

When Is it Physiologic?

Christopher J. Justinich and Jeffrey S. Hyams

1. INTRODUCTION

Virtually all infants develop hyperbilirubinemia with serum bilirubin levels of at least 1.4 mg/dL (24 µmol/L) in the first 7 d of life. Clinically apparent jaundice develops in greater than one third of healthy newborns. In most cases, the jaundice is "physiologic" or associated with breast-feeding *(1)*. Physiologic jaundice is generally defined as a benign increase in serum unconjugated bilirubin in newborns. Clinically apparent jaundice does not appear before 36 h of age, total serum bilirubin levels do not generally exceed 12 mg/dL (204 µmol/L), and clinical jaundice resolves within 7–10 d. Conjugated bilirubin does not exceed 2 mg/dL (34 µmol/L). Practitioners caring for newborns must recognize the clinical and laboratory features of jaundice which are "pathologic," leading to appropriate diagnosis and management. The morbidity and mortality associated with neonatal jaundice can be attributed to the underlying disease process, as well as from the neurologic sequelae of kernicterus. These complications are largely preventable with timely diagnosis and treatment.

From: *Diseases of the Liver and Bile Ducts: Diagnosis and Treatment*
Edited by: G. Y. Wu and J. Israel © Humana Press Inc., Totowa, NJ

2. BILIRUBIN METABOLISM AND PATHOPHYSIOLOGY

The following is a brief review of bilirubin formation and its metabolic fate, with particular reference to factors leading to increased serum bilirubin levels in newborn infants. Readers are referred to more comprehensive reviews for greater detail (*see* Chapter 14) *(2,3)*. Bilirubin is formed as a metabolic product of heme, the vast majority arising from the breakdown of hemoglobin from red blood cells. Neonates tend to be polycythemic, possessing a relatively greater red blood cell mass than older children and adults. In addition, neonatal red blood cells have a shorter half life, and these two factors account for a higher daily production of bilirubin in term infants compared with older children and adults. Heme is oxidized to biliverdin by the enzyme heme oxygenase, then rapidly reduced to bilirubin by biliverdin reductase. Bilirubin is poorly soluble in water, so almost all circulating bilirubin is bound to albumin. This becomes crucial when drugs competing for albumin-binding sites displace bilirubin, or when other factors, such as acidosis decrease the affinity of bilirubin for albumin *(4)*. These conditions allow fat-soluble free bilirubin to traverse the blood-brain barrier and enhance central nervous system toxicity.

The hepatic sinusoidal membrane possesses a specific bilirubin carrier that allows the rapid uptake of bilirubin from circulating bilirubin-albumin complexes *(5)*. The bilirubin then binds to intracytoplasmic proteins that help prevent bilirubin from refluxing back into the circulation *(6)*. Conjugation of bilirubin with glucuronic acid takes place in the smooth endoplasmic reticulum, catalyzed by bilirubin glucuronosyltransferase. This enzyme reaches mature levels in the first week of life in term infants, as opposed to a delay in premature infants *(7)*, a factor that promotes hyperbilirubinemia in these babies.

Any factors that increase the production of bilirubin may overwhelm the infant's ability to metabolize and excrete bilirubin, leading to jaundice. These factors include polycythemia, the presence of extravascular blood, for example from a cephalohematoma or hemolysis from drugs, blood group incompatibilities, hemoglobinopathies, and red cell enzyme or membrane abnormalities (Table 1). Delay in passage of meconium and other factors that enhance the enterohepatic circulation of bilirubin may also lead to jaundice *(8,9)*. Miscellaneous factors include hypothyroidism, sepsis or congenital infection leading to hemolysis, and specific inborn errors of bilirubin metabolism such as Crigler-Najjar syndrome (*see* Chapter 23).

3. DIAGNOSIS

The most important aspect of the history is the timing of the onset of clinically apparent jaundice. Physiologic jaundice by definition does not start in the first 36 h of life, so jaundice presenting earlier should be investigated. A family history of blood dyscrasias, previous infants with pathologic hyperbilirubinemia, and prematurity or other complications of pregnancy or delivery will all increase the risk of pathologic jaundice.

The physical examination may be helpful in several regards, but will not replace the need for laboratory investigations if the jaundice is of concern. Clinical assessment of jaundice is best performed in conditions of white or natural lighting. Increasing jaundice in newborns tends to progress in a cephalocaudal manner *(10)*, starting with the head and neck with bilirubin levels 4–8 mg/dL (68–136 μmol/L), upper trunk 5–12 mg/dL (85–204 μmol/L), lower trunk and legs 8–16 mg/dL (136–272 μmol/L), with the whole body including palms and soles invariably seen at levels greater than 15 mg/dL (255 μmol/L). Evidence of bruising or hematomas should be sought, as well as hepatosplenomegaly, which may accompany hemolysis and/ or extramedullary hematopoiesis, and, in extreme cases of hemolysis, hydrops fetalis.

Initial laboratory investigations are aimed at determining if jaundice is due to unconjugated hyperbilirubinemia, whether the level and timing are consistent with physiologic jaundice, and

Table 1

Causes of Neonatal Unconjugated Hyperbilirubinemia

1. Physiologic jaundice.
2. Breast milk jaundice.
3. Enhanced hemolysis.
     Isoimmune hemolytic disease.
     Red cell membrane abnormality.
     Red cell enzyme abnormality.
     Hemolysis from congenital infection/sepsis.
     Polycythemia.
     Extravasated blood.
4. Hereditary.
     Crigler-Najjar Syndrome.
     Gilbert's syndrome.
     Lucey-Driscoll syndrome.
5. Endocrinopathies.
     Hypothyroidism.
     Hypopituitarism.
6. Enhanced enterohepatic circulation.
     Bowel obstruction.
     Breast feeding.

(Adapted from Gourley GR: Jaundice. In: Wyllie R, Hyams JS, eds. Pediatric gastrointestinal disease-pathophysiology, diagnosis, management. Saunders, Philadelphia, 1993, p. 297, with permission.)

to determine if the level of hyperbilirubinemia warrants consideration of specific therapy. Hyperbilirubinemia consistent with breast milk jaundice generally does not require investigation or treatment, but a fall in bilirubin levels after a short trial of formula feeding may help confirm the diagnosis (10). Conjugated hyperbilirubinemia greater than 2 mg/dL (34 μmol/L) should prompt investigation without delay, and generally consultation with a pediatric gastroenterologist/hepatologist (see Chapter 23). Investigation is also indicated for unconjugated hyperbilirubinemia in the first 36 h of life, bilirubin levels of greater than 12 mg/dL (204 μmol/L), and significant jaundice persisting beyond 10 d or increasing at a later age. The first step is to search for hemolytic disease, which is the most common underlying cause (Fig. 1). Maternal and fetal blood types, a direct Coombs test, a complete blood count, blood smear, and a reticulocyte count will distinguish the major causes of unconjugated hyperbilirubinemia. If the Coombs test is positive, then the likely diagnosis is isoimmunization due to feto-maternal blood group incompatibility. This may involve either major or minor blood group determinants. The Coombs-negative infant with a high hematocrit and normal blood smear likely has polycythemia as a cause of jaundice. Infants with a relatively low hematocrit and high reticulocyte count will often have nonimmune hemolysis from abnormalities in red blood cells. A clue to this diagnosis will be abnormal red cell morphology on the blood smear. Abnormalities include hemoglobinopathies, red cell enzyme deficiencies, and red cell membrane abnormalities. If the infant is anemic, but the blood smear is normal, then extravasated blood giving an increased load of bilirubin is likely, for example, from a cephalohematoma.

4. DIFFERENTIAL DIAGNOSIS OF UNCONJUGATED HYPERBILIRUBINEMIA

Below is a brief review of the causes of unconjugated hyperbilirubinemia.

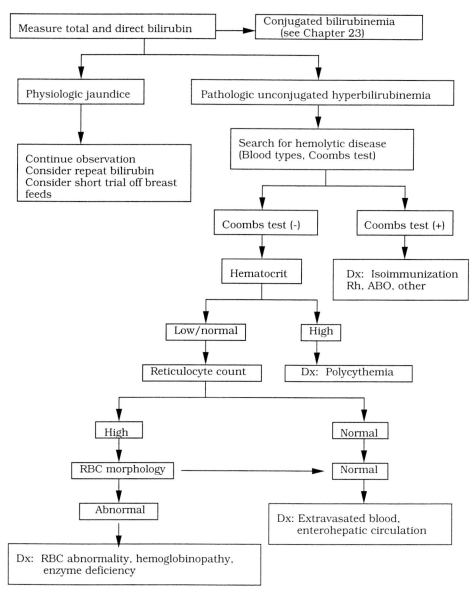

Fig. 1. A schematic diagram for an approach to diagnosis of unconjugated hyperbilirubinemia. Adapted from ref. *(12)*.

4.1. Physiologic Jaundice

"Physiologic jaundice" is unconjugated hyperbilirubinemia that appears in healthy infants over 36 h of age. The peak total bilirubin is generally less than 12 mg/dL (204 μmol/L), and jaundice clinically resolves by 7–10 d *(1)*. Factors promoting jaundice in these normal newborns include increase in bilirubin production from relative polycythemia with decreased RBC survival, and perhaps delay in conjugation due to decreased levels of glucuronosyltransferase. These factors are often accentuated in premature infants.

4.2. Breast Milk Jaundice

It is clear that normal breast-fed infants tend to have higher bilirubin levels than formula-fed infants, both in the first 5 d of life (early phase), and even more accentuated after 5 d (late phase) *(11)*. This is likely part of the spectrum of physiologic jaundice, as levels generally remain below 20 mg/dL (340 μmol/L), and spontaneous resolution is the rule. Appreciable levels of bilirubin usually do not appear until 3–4 d of life, but may persist for weeks or even months. The pathogenic mechanisms thought to be important include the presence of factors that inhibit conjugation (e.g., hormone, free fatty acid), or enhance the enterohepatic circulation of bilirubin, thereby increasing the bilirubin burden *(12)*. Discontinuation of breast-feeding is generally not necessary, although a trial of formula feeding for 48–72 h leading to a decrease in total bilirubin helps confirm the diagnosis if this is in question.

4.3. Hemolytic Disease

Increased hemolysis of any cause will increase the burden of unconjugated bilirubin that the neonate will need to metabolize, and mechanisms to conjugate and excrete bilirubin can become overwhelmed. The commonest abnormality is isoimmunization from ABO blood group incompatibility between the mother and fetus. Rh incompatibility is seen less commonly since the advent of Rho immune globulin to prevent sensitization of Rh-negative mothers for subsequent pregnancies *(13)*, but tends to be more severe than ABO incompatibility. Occasionally, minor blood group incompatibilities (Kell, Duffy) lead to significant isoimmunization. Rare red cell membrane abnormalities, such as hereditary spherocytosis, and red cell enzyme abnormalities, such as glucose-6-phosphate dehydrogenase or pyruvate kinase deficiency, may similarly present in the newborn period with hyperbilirubinemia. Sepsis or congenital infections may also cause hemolysis, but this is rarely an isolated finding, and often conjugated hyperbilirubinemia and liver dysfunction will be present. The presence of significant polycythemia or extravasated blood increases bilirubin burden and may result in jaundice.

4.4. Hereditary Hyperbilirubinemia

Crigler-Najjar syndrome *(14)* results from a metabolic defect in bilirubin conjugation leading to severe unconjugated hyperbilirubinemia (*see* Chapter 23). Lucey-Driscoll syndrome *(15)* is a transient unconjugated hyperbilirubinemia associated with a circulating inhibitor of glucuronosyltransferase. This is found in maternal and infant serum and is thought to be related to gestational hormones. Gilbert's syndrome is a benign mild unconjugated hyperbilirubinemia related to decreased glucuronosyltransferase and is generally not recognized until after puberty. This late onset is thought to be related to hormonal influences, especially from estrogen. It is believed that some infants with transient neonatal hyperbilirubinemia are actually an early manifestation of Gilbert's syndrome, brought out by the effects of maternal estrogen on the fetus *(16)*.

4.5. Endocrinopathies

Both hypothyroidism and hypopituitarism *(17)* can cause unconjugated hyperbilirubinemia that resolves when replacement therapy is given. The exact mechanism for hyperbilirubinemia is unknown. Congenital hypothyroidism should be diagnosed by routine neonatal screening. Hypopituitarism presents with hypoglycemia, features of hypothyroidism or cortisol deficiency, and micropenis.

4.6. Enhanced Enterohepatic Circulation of Bile

Conjugated bilirubin is secreted into the intestinal lumen where, under normal circumstances, enteric bacteria transform it into urobilinogen and it is excreted into the stools. Any factor that delays passage of bilirubin-rich meconium (e.g., bowel obstruction) or interferes with development of normal bacterial flora (e.g., antibiotic therapy) may, therefore, enhance reabsorption of bilirubin and contribute to hyperbilirubinemia *(8,9)*.

5. TREATMENT OF UNCONJUGATED HYPERBILIRUBINEMIA

Treatment is directed at decreasing levels of unconjugated hyperbilirubinemia, thereby reducing the risks of bilirubin toxicity on the central nervous system (*see* Section 6.). The method used depends on the magnitude and anticipated rise in bilirubin, and the presence of other risk factors that may increase susceptibility for kernicterus. One must be mindful of drugs that may displace bilirubin from albumin. Prevention of Rh isoimmunization by the widespread use of Rho immune globulin (RhoGAM) has greatly reduced complications related to Rh incompatibility *(13)*.

Phototherapy is the mainstay of therapy of moderate unconjugated hyperbilirubinemia, to prevent progression to levels requiring exchange transfusion. Controversy exists regarding the timing and absolute level of bilirubin requiring phototherapy in the healthy newborn, and readers are referred to the American Academy of Pediatrics practice parameters on the management of hyperbilirubinemia *(18,19)*. These guidelines recommend phototherapy for normal term infants for total bilirubin exceeding 15 mg/dL (255 μmol/L) at 24–48 h of life, 18 mg/dL (310 μmol/L) at 48–72 h, and 20 mg/dL (340 μmol/L) over 72 h of age. Others have proposed a more conservative approach to treatment in otherwise healthy infants with unconjugated hyperbilirubinemia. Premature infants are at increased risk of toxicity from hyperbilirubinemia; guidelines for treatment are reviewed in the National Institute of Child Health and Human Development Phototherapy Study *(20)*, and are beyond the scope of this review. The apparatus used, as well as the optimal color (white, blue, and green) *(21)*, has been the subject of some debate; the optimal wavelength is approx 460 nm. Phototherapy causes photo-oxidation of bilirubin in the skin to water soluble photoisomers, the most important being lumirubin *(22)*, which is excreted in bile and urine.

Exchange transfusion is employed when rapid reduction in serum bilirubin is desired. Most often this technique is employed in the setting of hemolysis causing early, rapidly progressing severe hyperbilirubinemia. Readers are referred to the specific guidelines for term and preterm infants mentioned above, and to general neonatology references *(23)*.

Recently, interest has evolved in the use of metalloporphyrins as specific inhibitors of heme oxygenase to prevent bilirubin production from heme *(24)*. This treatment is considered experimental at this time, but may have a role in isoimmune hemolytic hyperbilirubinemia and in hereditary hyperbilirubinemia.

6. COMPLICATIONS OF UNCONJUGATED HYPERBILIRUBINEMIA

Untreated severe hyperbilirubinemia results in serious central nervous system sequelae, including bilirubin encephalopathy characterized by seizures and opisthotonos, and kernicterus *(3,25)*. Kernicterus is a condition that is frequently fatal, in which autopsy reveals staining of the basal ganglia and related structures with bilirubin. Survivors of kernicterus often manifest severe neurologic complications, characteristically choreoathetotic cerebral palsy and hearing loss. Kernicterus is clearly related to extremely high levels of unconjugated hyperbilirubinemia (>30 mg/dL, 510 μmol/L). However, lower bilirubin levels have been associated with kernicterus in the presence of complicating factors such as prematurity, anoxia, hypoalbuminemia, and presence of drugs which displace bilirubin from circulating albumin.

7. INDICATIONS FOR CONSULTING THE SUBSPECIALIST

Consultation with a subspecialist should be considered in any infant with conjugated hyperbilirubinemia. In cases of unconjugated hyperbilirubinemia, a referral should be obtained if a cause cannot be found, and the patient does not respond to therapy. When this is occurs, consideration should be given to the presence of possible inborn errors of bilirubin metabolism.

8. CONCLUSIONS

Most cases of jaundice in neonates are benign and self-limited. However, jaundice may be a sign of serious underlying disease with significant morbidity and even mortality. This may be as a result of the underlying disease itself, or due to the devastating neurologic sequelae of kernicterus. Pathologic hyperbilirubinemia must be recognized early by primary care providers, leading to timely diagnosis and treatment.

SUMMARY

Neonatal jaundice is usually benign and self-limited, but may be a feature of serious underlying disease.

Features of pathologic jaundice include onset within 36 h of life, total bilirubin levels exceeding 12 mg/dL, and conjugated bilirubin levels exceeding 2 mg/dL.

Significant hyperbilirubinemia in the neonate signals the need for prompt evaluation of underlying causes and the need for specific therapy.

The goals of therapy are twofold: to treat the underlying pathologic process if possible, and to avoid the development of kernicterus with serious neurologic sequelae.

A referral should be obtained if conjugated bilirubin is increased or if unconjugated hyperbilirubinemia without identifiable cause does not respond to therapy. Consideration should be given to possible diagnosis of inborn errors of bilirubin metabolism.

REFERENCES

1. Maisels MJ, Gifford K. Normal serum bilirubin in the newborn and the effect of breast-feeding. Pediatrics 1986;78:837–843.
2. Gourley GR. Jaundice. In: Wyllie R, Hyams JS, eds. Pediatric gastrointestinal disease, lst ed. Saunders, Philadelphia, 1993, pp. 293–308.
3. Gourley GR. Bilirubin metabolism and neonatal jaundice. In: Suchy FJ, ed. Liver disease in children, lst ed. Mosby, St. Louis, 1994, pp. 105–125.
4. Ebbesen F, Foged N, Brodersen R. Reduced albumin binding of MADDS-a measure of bilirubin binding-in sick children. Acta Paediatr Scand 1986;75:550–554.
5. Berk PD, Stremmel W. Hepatocellular uptake of organic anions. In: Popper H, Schaffner F, eds. Progress in liver diseases, vol. VIII. Grune and Stratton, New York, 1987, pp. 125–144.
6. Levi AJ, Gatmaitan Z, Arias IM. Two hepatic cytoplasmic protein fractions, Y and Z and their possible role in the hepatic uptake of bilirubin, sulfobromophthalein and other anions. J Clin Invest 1969;48:2156–2167.
7. Kawade N, Onishi S. The prenatal and postnatal development of UDP-glucuronyl-transferase activity towards bilirubin and the effect of premature birth on this activity in the human liver. Biochem J 1981;196:257–260.
8. Poland RL, Odell GB. Physiologic jaundice: the enterohepatic circulation of bilirubin. N Engl J Med 1971;284:1–6.
9. Rosta J, Makoi Z, Kertesz A. Delayed meconium passage and hyperbilirubinemia. Lancet 1986;2:1138.
10. Kramer LI. Advancement of dermal icterus in the jaundiced newborn. Am J Dis Child 1969;118:454–458.
11. Gartner LM. On the question of the relationship between breastfeeding and jaundice in the first 5 days. Sem Perinatol 1994;18:502–509.
12. Gourley GR. The pathophysiology of breast milk jaundice. In: Polin RA, Fox WW, eds. Fetal and neonatal physiology. Grune and Stratton, New York, 1992, pp. 1173–1179.
13. Clarke CA. Prevention of Rh-hemolytic disease. Br Med J 1967;4:484–485.
14. Crigler JF, Najjar VA. Congenital familial nonhemolytic jaundice. Pediatrics 1952;10:169–180.
15. Arias IM, Wolfson S, Lucey JF, et al. Transient familial neonatal hyperbilirubinemia. J Clin Invest 1956;44:1442–1150.
16. Odell GB, Gourley GR. Hereditary hyperbilirubinemia. In: Lebenthal E, ed. Textbook of gastroenterology and nutrition in infancy, 2nd ed. Raven Press, New York, 1989, pp. 947–967.
17. Thompson GN, McCrossin RB, Penfold JL, et al. Management and outcome of children with congenital hypothyroidism detected on neonatal screening in South Australia. Med J Aust 1986;145:18–22.
18. American Academy of Pediatrics Practice Parameter: management of hyperbilirubinemia in the healthy term newborn. Pediatrics 1994; 94:558-65.

are evidenced by normal plasma disappearance of BSP, and indocyanine green, and radiologic visualization of the biliary tree by cholecystographic agents (2).

Crigler-Najjar syndrome Types I and II can be differentiated by bile pigment analysis. In type I, the bile contains only small amounts of unconjugated bilirubin and in some cases, traces of bilirubin glucuronides. In contrast, the bile of patients with Crigler-Najjar syndrome Type II contains significant amounts of bilirubin glucuronides, although less than 50% of estimated daily bilirubin production is excreted into bile. The proportion of bilirubin monoglucuronide in bile exceeds 30% of total conjugated bilirubin, reflecting the reduced hepatic bilirubin-UGT activity in the liver (11).

Liver biopsy is not usually necessary for the diagnosis and reveals no significant abnormality. In several patients with Crigler-Najjar syndrome type I, pigment plugs were observed in bile canaliculi and bile ducts, probably resulting from biliary excretion of unconjugated bilirubin or its photoisomers. Electron microscopy of the liver reveals no specific pathologic change. Hepatic bilirubin-UGT activity is undetectable in Crigler-Najjar syndrome type I, whereas a small amount of activity (4–12% of normal) is usually detectable in the liver biopsy specimens from patients with Crigler-Najjar syndrome type II (2).

1.1.4. Genetic and Prenatal Diagnosis

The availability of modern molecular biological techniques has made it feasible to identify sequence abnormalities of the UGT1 gene from genomic DNA extracted from any nucleated cell, such as blood leukocytes, buccal smear, amniotic cells, or chorionic villus samples (7). Such genetic analysis assists in the diagnosis of Crigler-Najjar syndromes without having to obtain a liver biopsy. It also helps in the identification of heterozygote carriers and genetic counseling. Genomic DNA analysis of chorionic villus biopsy samples or amniotic cells has been used to make prenatal determination of the bilirubin-UGT genotype in cases in which a previous sibling was born with Crigler-Najjar syndrome (12).

1.2. Gilbert's Syndrome

Gilbert's syndrome, one of the most common inherited disorders in humans, is characterized by mild, fluctuating unconjugated hyperbilirubinemia (13). In adults, serum bilirubin levels usually range from 1– 5 mg/dL, but may increase to up to 10 mg/dL in physically or mentally stressful situations. As in Crigler-Najjar syndrome type II, the bilirubin monoglucuronide to diglucuronide ratio in the bile is higher than that in normals, usually exceeding 30% of total (normally 80–90% of pigments excreted in bile is bilirubin diglucuronide) (14). Other than bilirubin concentrations, all serum biochemical tests are within normal limits. Although Gilbert's syndrome is generally considered innocuous, it may be associated with higher levels of serum bilirubin during the neonatal period (see Section 1.2.2.).

1.2.1. Molecular Genetics

Recently, a variant promoter upstream to the first exon of bilirubin-UGT has been found to be associated with Gilbert's syndrome. Normally, the promoter consists of A(TA)6TAA, whereas subjects with Gilbert's syndrome are homozygous for a variant promoter that contains two extra nucleotides: A(TA)7TAA. The variant promoter is thought to reduce the expression of hepatic bilirubin-UGT1 (15). However, this reduction is not sufficient to cause hyperbilirubinemia in all persons, because daily serum bilirubin production is an important variable. In adult females, the daily bilirubin production is lower than in males. As a result, the full clinical manifestation of Gilbert's syndrome is unusual in females.

1.2.2. Relationship of Gilbert's Syndrome with Neonatal Hyperbilirubinemia

As the daily bilirubin production is higher in neonates than it is in adults, the presence of a Gilbert's-type promoter upstream to bilirubin-UGT1 may be expected to result in higher serum bilirubin levels. Indeed, in a study involving a large number of healthy, full-term, newborn Greek babies, without glucose-6-phosphatase deficiency or any other evidence of hemolysis, mean serum bilirubin levels at 72 h after birth were found to be significantly higher in neonates homozygous for the Gilbert genotype. This finding indicates that the Gilbert-type promoter is one of the determinants of the level of hyperbilirubinemia in otherwise healthy newborns *(1,2)*. The precise increase in the risk for the adverse effect of neonatal jaundice in babies homozygous for the Gilbert genotype remains to be determined.

2. BILIRUBIN TOXICITY

Unconjugated bilirubin is potentially toxic. However, in physiological states, binding to plasma albumin, rapid uptake by hepatocytes, and an efficient conjugation mechanism protect the body from the toxic effects of bilirubin *(2)*. Therefore, the manifestation of its toxicity is largely limited to the neonatal life, and in subjects with inherited disorders of bilirubin conjugation. Degeneration of brain tissue, associated with yellow pigmentation was first reported in 1949 *(16)*. The association of kernicterus, or bilirubin-induced encephalopathy with severe unconjugated hyperbilirubinemia was subsequently established. Whereas the cerebral toxicity has received the most attention, other organ systems are also affected *(2)*.

2.1. Cerebral Toxicity: Clinical Features of Bilirubin Encephalopathy

High serum unconjugated bilirubin levels (usually over 20 mg/dL) in the newborn may result in clinical evidence of brain damage, ranging from subtle neurological abnormality to severe encephalopathy or fully developed kernicterus (1). Bilirubin encephalopathy may occur at lower bilirubin concentrations in small premature babies or in the presence of acidosis, hypoxia, sepsis, and the use of drugs that compete with bilirubin for albumin binding. Overt kernicterus most commonly occurs at 3–6 d of life, and is evidenced by the loss of the moro reflex, truncal hypertonicity, and opisthotonus from a startling stimulus. Survivors may develop irreversible hearing loss, muscle spasticity, paralysis of upward gaze, athetosis, and mental retardation in various combinations or may have no residual brain damage *(17)*. Some infants who have more modest hyperbilirubinemia may not have overt signs of kernicterus, but may have a higher incidence of impairment of neurological and intellectual function in later years. In some children with Crigler-Najjar syndrome Type I, bilirubin encephalopathy may present late with cerebellar symptoms *(2)*. The occurrence of kernicterus is usually limited to the neonatal period and the first few months of life. However, in patients with inherited deficiency of bilirubin glucuronidation, kernicterus may occur during adolescence or early adulthood.

The brain, particularly basal ganglia, hippocampus, thalamus, and nuclei of the cerebellum, pons, and medulla are grossly pigmented in infants dying in acute bilirubin encephalopathy *(18)*. Although the term kernicterus refers to this pigmentation, children dying of chronic bilirubin encephalopathy after the neonatal period do not exhibit cerebral bilirubin deposition. The clinical manifestations usually precede histological evidence of brain damage. Within 72 h of onset of kernicterus, no specific cellular pathology is noticed by light microscopy. After 72 h, the pigmented areas show cytoplasmic degeneration, loss of Nissl substance, development of fine vacuoles, and distortion of nuclear chromatin. Focal necrosis of neurons and glial cells occurs later and gliosis of the affected areas is seen in chronic cases. These histologic lesions are not present from the onset of clinical kernicterus, and may not be the initiating pathophysiological events in bilirubin-induced brain damage *(2,18)*.

Nonspecific signs of encephalopathy in the neonate may result from other causes, such as cerebral hemorrhage and, therefore, kernicterus cannot be always diagnosed without pathological documentation. In the absence of specific neuropathological lesions, yellow discoloration of the brain at autopsy is not pathognomonic of bilirubin encephalopathy, because in the presence of hyperbilirubinemia, the brain may acquire yellow pigmentation in the setting of other forms of injury. Such lesions need to be excluded on clinical or pathological basis (1,2,17). Conversely, prolonged storage of brain tissue in formaldehyde may result in the loss of initially present pigmentation. Thus, in the absence of neuronal degeneration, bilirubin-staining alone does not establish the diagnosis of classic kernicterus (17).

The prognostic significance of a moderate degree of hyperbilirubinemia is not entirely clear. Serum bilirubin levels that are not high enough to cause kernicterus have been reported to result in an increased incidence of neurologic abnormalities or decreased intellectual performance later in life.

2.1.1. Blood–Brain Barrier and Cerebral Bilirubin Clearance

A series of interfaces between the plasma and brain, termed the blood-brain barrier, regulates the influx of blood-borne substances into the brain. Capillary endothelial cells and adjoining foot processes of astroglial cells represent the structural component of the blood–brain barrier. Transporter and carrier proteins that mediate the influx of nutrients, ions, and water into the cerebrospinal fluid and brain constitute the functional component of the barrier (17,19). Although the immaturity of the blood–brain barrier has been implicated in the vulnerability of neonates to bilirubin encephalopathy, bilirubin encephalopathy does occur in adults in the presence of severe unconjugated hyperbilirubinemia and transfer of plasma bilirubin into adult brain has been documented. Indeed, studies of transfer of lipophilic substances from blood to brain showed no difference between neonates and adults. Furthermore, an inefficient blood-brain barrier would permit albumin to enter the brain along with bilirubin, thereby mitigating the toxic effect of bilirubin. Therefore, immaturity of blood-brain barrier may not be a major cause of the susceptibility of neonates to bilirubin-encephalopathy (2,17).

The transport of bilirubin between plasma and brain is bidirectional. Bilirubin may bind with greater avidity to neonatal brain cell membranes, thereby reducing the clearance of bilirubin from brain. Cerebral bilirubin clearance may be further reduced in the presence of hypoxia and acidosis. Lower affinity of bilirubin for neonatal albumin and lower plasma albumin concentration in neonates may be other factors that contribute to higher incidence of bilirubin toxicity in neonates (2,17).

Experimentally, the blood–brain barrier can be unilaterally and reversibly opened without causing brain damage by infusion of hypertonic urea or arabinose. The hyperosmolarity-associated shrinkage of the capillary endothelial cells results in temporary opening of the tight junctions. When the blood–brain barrier is opened in newborn rats by this technique, intravenously administered albumin-bound bilirubin rapidly enters the brain. Following the reversal of the blood-brain barrier, bilirubin is rapidly cleared from the brain. The clearance of bilirubin from brain parallels its clearance from serum, suggesting that bilirubin is cleared by diffusion or transport back into the general circulation. However, damaged brain, which may be edematous, may bind bilirubin and be unable to clear bilirubin rapidly and, therefore, be more vulnerable to bilirubin toxicity (20).

2.1.2. Biochemical Mechanisms of Bilirubin Toxicity

Bilirubin has a broad range of toxicity on organs, cells, subcellular organelles, and cellular functions. It is not clear which of these toxic effects are relevant in bilirubin encephalopathy. Bilirubin inhibits DNA, RNA, and protein synthesis in brain cells. Bilirubin uncouples oxidative phosphorolyation and inhibits ATPase activity of brain mitochondria. All toxic effects of bilirubin are inhibited by binding of bilirubin to albumin (2).

2.2. Bilirubin Nephrotoxicity

Deposition of unconjugated bilirubin in the renal medulla results in medullary necrosis and formation of bilirubin crystals on the renal papillae in hyperbilirubinemic infants and in Gunn rats. In adult Gunn rats, an abnormality of the ascending loop of Henle leads to an impairment of urinary concentration, which is ameliorated by reduction of serum bilirubin levels. The urinary concentration defect has not been found in mature neonates with hyperbilirubinemia or in patients with Crigler-Najjar syndrome type I who survive to adult age (2,21).

3. TREATMENT

Conventional treatment aims at reducing serum bilirubin levels. As discussed above, serum bilirubin levels are reduced by induction of bilirubin-UGT activity by phenobarbital treatment in patients with Crigler-Najjar syndrome type II, but not in type I. Phenobarbital also normalizes serum bilirubin concentrations in Gilbert's syndrome. However, this innocuous condition does not need treatment.

3.1. Phototherapy

Because all its polar groups are engaged by internal hydrogen bonding, bilirubin IXα is insoluble in water. Exposure to light promotes the formation of geometric isomers of bilirubin IXα that lack internal hydrogen bonds, are more polar than bilirubin, and are excreted in bile without conjugation (2). Bilirubin photoisomers excreted in bile undergo reconversion to the hydrogen-bonded structure and may form bilirubin "plugs" within bile ducts. Subsequently, stable structural changes occur in the molecule, resulting in the formation of irreversible photoproducts. Phototherapy is the mainstay of medical therapy for severe unconjugated hyperbilirubinemia of the newborn. In patients with Crigler-Najjar syndrome type I, and in severe cases of Crigler-Najjar syndrome type II, phototherapy needs to be continued until the disease is reversed by liver transplantation. Fluorescent lamps with devices for shielding the eyes, or "light blankets" are available and effectively lower serum bilirubin levels. After children reach 3 or 4 yr of age, phototherapy becomes progressively less effective due to thickening of the skin, increased skin pigmentation, and decreased surface area in relation to body mass (1,22).

3.2. Exchange Transfusion and Plasmapheresis

In neurological emergencies, plasmapheresis or exchange transfusion rapidly reduce serum bilirubin concentration. Because bilirubin is tightly bound to plasma albumin, removal of albumin results in the withdrawal of equimolar amounts of bilirubin. This is followed by mobilization of tissue bilirubin stores to the plasma (1).

3.3. Orthotopic Liver Transplantation

Because, at present, there is no other definitive long-term treatment for patients with this condition, orthotopic liver transplantation has become a standard treatment of Crigler-Najjar syndrome type I. Although this procedure is not without risk in these individuals, it has cured several patients, and has dramatically changed the prognosis of Crigler-Najjar syndrome type I. Because a segment of a normal liver is sufficient to reduce serum bilirubin levels, auxiliary grafting of a liver segment has been performed in several cases. Opinions differ as to the optimum time for liver transplantation. Some investigators believe that the transplantation should be performed around the age of 6–8 yr, before the onset of clinical bilirubin encephalopathy (1,23).

3.4. Experimental Methods

3.4.1. INHIBITION OF HEME OXYGENASE

Noniron metalloporphyrins, such as tin-protoporphyrin or tin-mesoporphyrin are "dead-end" inhibitors of microsomal heme oxygenase, which is rate-limiting in the production of bilirubin. Administration of these compounds suppresses neonatal hyperbilirubinemia in animals. Injection of tin-mesoporphyrin temporarily reduces serum bilirubin levels in patients with Crigler-Najjar syndrome type I, and can be used to reverse an encephalopathic crisis. However, the effect does not last for a long time (24).

3.4.2. INDUCTION OF BILIRUBIN-OXIDIZING ENZYMES

The induction of P-450c results in increased oxidative degradation of serum bilirubin in Gunn rat liver, with consequent reduction of serum bilirubin levels. Several naturally occurring indoles extracted from cruciferous vegetables, such as cabbage, cauliflower, and Brussels sprouts induce P-4501A1 and 1A2 in rat liver and intestine. One such inducer, indole-3-carbinol, is being studied for a potential therapeutic effect in Gunn rats and in Crigler-Najjar syndrome type I *(25)*.

3.4.3. REDUCTION OF INTESTINAL REABSORPTION

Oral administration of charcoal, agar, or cholestyramine interferes with the intestinal absorption of unconjugated bilirubin, increasing the efficacy of phototherapy. Calcium salts have a similar effect on patients undergoing phototherapy for Crigler-Najjar syndrome type I, but not in patients with Crigler-Najjar syndrome type II, who are usually not treated by phototherapy *(1,2)*.

3.4.4. EXPERIMENTAL

Transplantation of hepatocytes and gene therapy as new therapeutic approaches are under investigation.

3.4.4.1. Liver Cell Transplantation. This technique is being evaluated as a potential treatment for Crigler-Najjar syndrome type I. Hepatocyte transplantation by portal venous infusion of hepatocytes, intraperitoneal injection of microcarrier-bound hepatocytes, or intraperitoneal implantation of alginate-polylysine-encapsulated hepatocytes resulted in a reduction of serum bilirubin levels in Gunn rats. Transplantation of isolated liver cells into the spleen also results in biliary excretion of conjugated bilirubin and reduction of serum bilirubin levels. After intrasplenic injection, a great majority of the hepatocytes rapidly translocate to the liver, where, in the absence of immune rejection, they survive and function throughout the lifespan of recipient rodents (26).

3.4.4.2. Gene Therapy. Because the metabolic defect in Gunn rats and in Crigler-Najjar syndrome type I results from lesions of a single gene, supplementation with a normal bilirubin-UGT gene is an attractive potential therapeutic modality. Bilirubin disposal is a multistep process mediated by several proteins preferentially expressed in the liver. Therefore, gene therapy for bilirubin-UGT deficiency must be directed at the hepatocyte. Methods for gene introduction into the liver using recombinant viruses or ligands that mediate receptor-directed endocytosis are being evaluated for this purpose. In an *ex vivo* approach, liver cells harvested from a mutant subject by partial hepatectomy are established in primary culture and transduced with normal (therapeutic) genes using recombinant retroviruses. In an in vivo approach, the deficient gene is carried by recombinant adenoviruses. The use of these vectors led to long-term correction of the metabolic defect in Gunn rats *(27,28)*.

4. PREVENTION: GENETIC COUNSELING

4.1. Genotypic Diagnosis and Carrier Identification

Because Crigler-Najjar syndromes are inherited as autosomal recessive characteristics if both parents are heterozygous carriers for the disorder, the probability of the offspring having the disease is 1:4, being an asymptomatic carrier is 1:2, and being homozygous normal is 1:4. In many cases, the parents are known to be blood relatives, which increases the chance of the offspring having this rare disorder. Because the phenotypic manifestation of the disease can be cured by liver transplantation in the future, patients with homozygous genotypic abnormality are expected to have children. If one parent is homozygous for the disease gene and the other is an asymptomatic carrier, the probability of the offspring having the disease is 1:2, the remainder will be asymptomatic carriers. In many cases, there is no known consanguinity, and the chromosomes derived from the father and the mother may contain different mutations (compound heterozygosity). Often, there is no known history of inherited jaundice in any other member of the kindred.

Currently several research laboratories are capable of performing molecular genetic analysis of DNA extracted from blood leukocytes or buccal smears for identifying the mutations that can cause Crigler-Najjar syndromes (8,10,15). The effect of observed mutations can be evaluated by expression of mutagenized bilirubin-UGT mRNAs. This allows the identification of heterozygous carriers, which can be used for prenatal or preconceptional genetic counseling.

4.2. Prenatal Diagnosis

Recently, it has been possible to use molecular genetic techniques to identify sequence abnormalities in the bilirubin-UGT gene from genomic DNA extracted from amniotic cells or chorionic villus samples (12). Such definitive identification of the genotype of the fetus should greatly facilitate the genetic counseling and may aid in the institution of early treatment during the neonatal and even prenatal life.

SUMMARY

The three grades of inherited deficiency of bilirubin-UDP-glucuronosyltransferase (UGT) are: complete deficiency (CN type I), severe partial deficiency (CN type II), and mild reduction in enzyme activity (Gilbert's syndrome).

CN type I is a recessive disorder characterized by severe unconjugated hyperbilirubinemia leading to kernicterus and death. Phototherapy, intermittent plasmapheresis and, finally, liver transplantation are the main treatment modalities.

CN type II (Arias syndrome), is characterized by somewhat lower serum bilirubin levels than CN type I. Bilirubin levels can be reduced by at least 25% by phenobarbital treatment. Kernicterus is rare.

Gilbert's syndrome is characterized by mild fluctuating unconjugated hyperbilirubinemia. It is innocuous and no treatment is required.

High serum unconjugated bilirubin levels in the newborn may result in clinical features of brain damage (kernicterus).

Bilirubin encephalopathy may occur in adolescents and adults in the presence of serum unconjugated hyperbilirubinemias.

ACKNOWLEDGMENTS

This work was supported in part by the following NIH grants: RO1-DK 46057 (to JRC); RO1-DK 39137 (to NRC). Y. I. was supported by an NIH Hepatology Training Grant T32-DK-

07218 and an APF fellowship grant. The authors acknowledge the help of Indrajit Roy Chowdhury in preparing the manuscript.

REFERENCES

1. Roy Chowdhury J, Jansen PLM. Metabolism of bilirubin. In: Zakim D, Boyer TD, eds. Hepatology: a textbook of liver disease, 3rd ed. Saunders, Philadelphia, 1996, pp. 323–347.
2. Roy Chowdhury J, Roy Chowdhury N, Arias IM. Hereditary jaundice and disorders of bilirubin metabolism. In: Sciver, Boudet, Sly, Valle, eds. The metabolic and molecular bases of inherited disease, 7th ed. McGraw Hill, New York, 1995, pp. 2161–2208.
3. Crigler JF, Najjar VA. Congenital familial non-hemolytic jaundice with kernicterus. Pediatrics 1952;10:169.
4. Wolkoff AW, Roy Chowdhury J, et al. Crigler-Najjar syndrome (Type I) in an adult male. Gastroenterology 1979;76:840–848.
5. Arias IM, Gartner LM, Cohen M, Benezzer J, Levi AJ. Chronic nonhemolytic unconjugated hyperbilirubinemia with glucuronyltransferase deficiency: Clinical, biochemical, pharmacologic, and genetic evidence for heterogeneity. Am J Med 1969;47:395.
6. Gollan JL, Huang SM, Billing B, Sherlock S. Prolonged survival in three brothers with severe type II Crigler-Najjar syndrome. Ultrastructural and metabolic studies. Gastroenterology 1975;68:1543.
7. Roy Chowdhury J, Roy Chowdhury N. Unveiling the mysteries of inherited disorders of bilirubin glucuronidation. Gastroenterology 1993;105:288–293.
8. Bosma PJ, Roy Chowdhury N, Goldhoorn BG, et al. Sequence of exons and the flanking regions of human bilirubin-UDPglucuronosyltransferase gene complex and identification of a genetic mutation in a patient with Crigler-Najjar syndrome, Type I. Hepatology 1992;15:941–847.
9. Huang TJ, Lahiri P, Oude Elferink RPJ, et al. Mechanism of inherited deficiencies of multiple UDP-glucuronosyltransferase isoforms in two patients with Crigler-Najjar syndrome, Type I. FASEB J 1992;6:2859.
10. Ritter JK, Yeatman MT, Ferriera P, Owens IS. Identification of a genetic alteration in the code for bilirubin UDP-glucuronosyltransferase in the UGT1 gene complex of a Crigler-Najjar syndrome, Type I. J Clin Invest 1992;90:150.
11. Roy Chowdhury J, Roy Chowdhury N, Wu G, Shouval R, Arias IM. Bilirubin monoglucuronide and diglucuronide formation by human liver in vitro: assay by high pressure liquid chromatography. Hepatology 1981;1:622.
12. Sengupta KS, Gantla VR, Bommineni P, et al. Prenatal identification of Crigler- Najjar syndrome type 1 genotype by analysis of chronic villus sample DNA. Hepatology 1994;13:320A.
13. Gilbert A, Lereboullet P. La cholemie simple familiale. Semin Med 1991;21:241.
14. Powell LW, Hemingway E, Billing BH, Sherlock S. Idiopathic unconjugated hyperbilirubinemia (Gilbert's syndrome): a study of 42 families. N Engl J Med 1967;277:1108.
15. Bosma PJ, Roy Chowdhury J, Bakker C, et al. A sequence abnormality in the promoter region results in reduced expression of bilirubin-UDP-glucuronosyltransferase-1 in Gilbert syndrome. N Engl J Med 1995;333:1171–1179.
16. Mollison PL, Cutbush M. Hemolytic disease of the newborn: criterial of severity. Brit Med J 1949;1:123.
17. Schenker S, Hoyumpa AM, McCandless DW. Bilirubin toxicity to the brain (kernicterus) and other tissues. In: Ostrow JD, ed. Bile pigments and jaundice. Marcel Dekker, New York, 1986, pp. 395–419.
18. Turkel SB, Miller CA, Guttenberg ME, Moynes DR, Hodgman JE. A clinical pathologic reappraisal of kernicterus. Pediatrics 1982;69:267.
19. Cornford EM, Braun LD, Oldendorp WH, Hill CA. Comparison of lipid-mediated blood brain barrier penetrability in neonates and adults. Am J Physiol 1982;243:C161.
20. Laas R, Helmke K. Regional cerebral blood flow following unilateral blood-brain barrier alteration induced by hyperosmolar perfusion in the albino rat. In: Cervos-Navarro J, Fritschka E, eds. erebral circulation and metabolism. Raven, New York, 1981, pp. 317–321.
21. Engle WD, Avant BS Jr. Neonatal hyperbilirubinemia and renal function. J Pediatr 1982;100:113–116.
22. Berk PD, Martin F, Blaschkle TF, Scharschmidt BF, Plotz PH. Unconjugated hyperbilirubinemia: physiological evaluation and experimental approaches to therapy. Ann Intern Med 1975;82:552.
23. Kaufman SS, Wood RP, Shaw BW, et al. Orthotopic liver transplantation for type I Crigler-Najjar syndrome. Hepatology 1986;6:1259.
24. Galbraith RA, Drummond GS, Kappas A. Suppression of bilirubin production in the Crigler-Najjar, Type I syndrome: studies with heme oxygenase inhibitor-tin-mesopor. Pediatrics 1992;89:175.
25. Kapitulnick J. The role of cytochrome P-450 in the alternate pathways of bilirubin metabolism in congenitally jaundiced Gun rats and infants with the Crigler-Najjar syndrome, Type I. Int Bilirubin Workshop, Trieste, 1992, p. 53.
26. Demetriou AA, Levenson SM, Whiting J, et al. Replacement of hepatic functions in rats by transplantation of microcarrier-attached hepatocytes. Science 1986;233:1190.

27. Takahashi M, Ilan Y, Sengupta K, Roy Chowdhury N, Roy Chowdhury J. Induction of tolerance to recombinant adenoviruses by injection into newborn rats: long term amelioration of hyperbilirubinemia in Gunn rats. J Biol Chem 1996;271:26,536.
28. Ilan Y, Attavar P, Takahashi M, et al. Induction of central tolerance by intrathymic inoculation of adenoviral antigens into the host thymus permits long-term gene therapy in Gunn rats. J Clin Invest 1996;98:2640.

SUGGESTED READING

1. Suchy FJ, Shneider BL. Neonatal jaundice and cholestasis in liver and biliary diseases. Williams and Wilkins, Philadelphia, 1996, pp. 495–510.
2. Schenker S, Hoyumpa AM, McCandless DW. Bilirubin toxicity to the brain (kernicterus) and other tissues. In: Ostrow JD, ed. Bile pigments and jaundice. Marcel Dekker, New York, 1986, pp. 395–419.

24 Neonatal Cholestasis

Colston F. McEvoy and Frederick J. Suchy

CONTENTS

1. INTRODUCTION

Cholestasis is a decrease in bile flow caused by impaired secretion by hepatocytes or to obstruction of bile flow through the intra- or extrahepatic bile ducts. It presents clinically with conjugated hyperbilirubinemia, but the consequences of chronic cholestasis are related to the retention of other potentially noxious substances that are normally excreted into bile, including bile acids, copper, and lipids, and to a deficiency of micelle-forming bile acids within the intestinal lumen that are essential for dietary lipid and fat-soluble vitamin absorption. Injury to hepatocytes and the biliary system may be progressive from the underlying disease and from secondary effects of cholestasis, leading to fibrosis and cirrhosis. The numerous conditions manifesting as neonatal cholestasis are shown in Table 1.

Urgent evaluation of the cholestatic infant is critical to the treatment of life-threatening metabolic or infective liver diseases and for the surgical management of biliary anomalies *(1)*.

The approach to the evaluation of the infant with cholestatic liver disease is outlined in Fig. 1. Measurement of serum conjugated bilirubin levels is the most important initial test. Cholestatic jaundice may occur in the neonate along with a severe acute illness, sometimes leading to hepatic failure or can be an isolated finding. Because of otherwise good health and appearance of some infants, cholestasis may be misinterpreted as physiologic hyperbilirubinemia or the jaundice sometimes associated with breast feeding (*see* Chapter 22, this volume). However, cholestatic liver disease should be excluded in any infant who is jaundiced beyond 14 d of age *(2)*. Acholic stools are observed in severe liver dysfunction and with biliary obstruction, but the physician may be misled by stools that are only lightly pigmented or

From: *Diseases of the Liver and Bile Ducts: Diagnosis and Treatment*
Edited by: G. Y. Wu and J. Israel © Humana Press Inc., Totowa, NJ

Table 1

Differential Diagnosis of Neonatal Cholestasis

1. Disorders of the Bile Ducts.
   Extrahepatic biliary atresia
   Paucity of interlobular bile ducts
   Alagille's syndrome
   Choledochal cysts
   Neonatal sclerosing cholangitis
   Spontaneous perforation
   Bile duct stenosis
   Inspissated bile plug
   Cystic fibrosis
   Caroli's disease
   Cholelithiasis
   Tumors/masses
2. Neonatal Hepatitis.
   Idiopathic
   Viral
       Rubella
       Cytomegalovirus
       Herpeviruses
       Reovirus type II
       Human herpesvirus 6
       Adenovirus - Enteroviruses
       Hepatitis B - Hepatitis C
       ? Other non A, B, C, D, E
       HIV
   Bacterial and parasitic
       Bacterial sepsis
       Syphilis
       Listeriosis
       Tuberculosis
       Toxoplasmosis
       Other
3. Toxic.
   Drugs
   Parenteral nutrition
4. Idiopathic Cholestasis.
   Byler's disease
   Hereditary cholestasis with lymphedema
   Benign recurrent cholestasis
   North American Indian cholestasis
5. Metabolic Diseases.
   Amino acids
       Tyrosinemia
   Lipids
       Neimann-Pick type C
       Gaucher's disease
       Wolman's disease
       β-oxidation defects
   Urea cycle
       Arginase deficiency

Table 1 *(continued)*

Carbohydrates
  Galactosemia
  Fructosemia
  Type IV glycogenosis
Bile acid biosynthesis
  Peroxisomal defects
  3β-hydroxy-Δ5C$_{27}$-steroid dehydrohydrogenase deficiency
  Δ^4-3-oxosteroid-5β-reductase deficiency
Defective oxidative phosphorylation
Other
  Alpha-1-antitrypsin deficiency
  Hypopituitarism (septo-optic dysplasia)
  Hypothyroidism
  Neonatal hemochromatosis
6. Miscellaneous Associations.
  Shock/hypoperfusion
  Histiocytosis X
  Intestinal obstruction
  Erythrophagocytic histiocytosis
  Neonatal lupus erythematosus
  Indian childhood cirrhosis
  Extracorporeal membrane oxygenation
  Autosomal trisomies
  Graft vs host disease
  Donahue's syndrome

intermittently pigmented with evolving obstruction. The urine is usually dark, but this is easily missed. Bleeding secondary to vitamin K deficiency can be a presenting feature of neonatal cholestasis.

Variable elevations of serum direct bilirubin, aminotransferase levels, serum alkaline phosphatase, and serum lipids are observed, but are not specific. However, these tests along with the blood glucose, ammonia levels, and coagulation studies may provide insight into the severity of the liver dysfunction. Unfortunately, no single test or group of tests has proven to be of satisfactory discriminatory value in distinguishing infants with intra- and extrahepatic cholestasis, because at least 10% of infants with intrahepatic cholestasis will have sufficient bile secretory failure so as to have diagnostic tests that overlap with biliary atresia *(3–5)*.

Ultrasonography is a useful initial study for assessing the size and composition of the liver and can usually demonstrate the presence and size of the gallbladder, detect stones and sludge in the bile ducts and gallbladder, and demonstrate cystic or obstructive dilatation of the biliary system *(6)*. Unfortunately, dilatation of the intrahepatic bile ducts is not usually seen in extrahepatic biliary atresia. Computed tomography and magnetic resonance imaging provide similar information to that obtained by ultrasonography, but are less suitable for use in infants because of the need for contrast and for heavy sedation or general anesthesia *(6)*.

Hepatobiliary scintigraphic imaging with agents such as technetium 99m iminodiacetic acid derivatives is often used in evaluating the cholestatic infant *(7)*. Pretreatment with phenobarbital for a period of 5 d is required to stimulate bile flow and enhance visualization of the bile tract. Hepatic uptake of isotope occurs rapidly in patients with biliary atresia because liver function is usually preserved early in the disease, but excretion into the intestine is absent even on scanning 24 h later. In contrast, uptake is poor in cases of neonatal hepatitis, but excretion

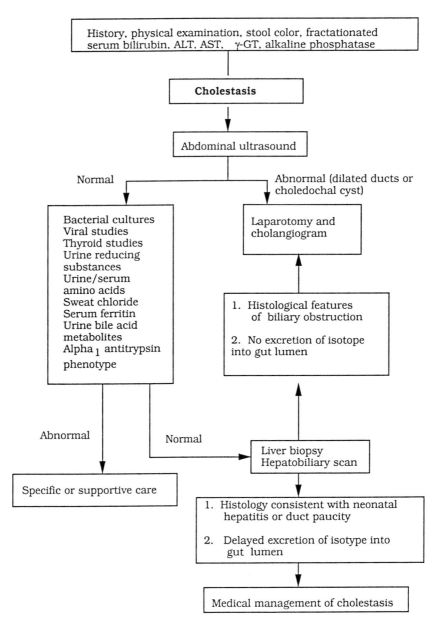

Fig. 1. Schematic diagram for evaluation of neonatal cholestasis.

into bile in the intestine may eventually be detected. In practice, the distinction between severe hepatocellular disease and biliary obstruction may not be reliably made using this technique, and equivocal results may further delay diagnosis and treatment.

Percutaneous transhepatic cholangiography or endoscopic retrograde cholangiography (ERCP) may be of value in visualizing the biliary tract in selected cases, but are technically demanding in infants *(8)*.

Percutaneous liver biopsy is particularly useful in the evaluation of the cholestatic patient *(5,9)*. A diagnosis of extrahepatic biliary atresia can be successfully made on the basis of clinical and histologic criteria in 90–95% of patients. In the small number of cases in which doubt about the diagnosis persists, the patency of the biliary tree can be directly examined at the time of a mini-laparotomy and operative cholangiogram. Liver tissue can also be examined by electron microscopy, used for enzymatic and genetic analysis, and can be cultured for infectious agents.

2. DISORDERS OF THE BILE DUCTS

2.1. Extrahepatic Biliary Atresia

Extrahepatic biliary atresia is a disorder characterized by a complete obstruction of bile flow due to destruction or absence of all or part of the extrahepatic bile ducts (10). The disorder occurs in 1:10,000 to 1:15,000 live births and accounts for approx one third of the cases of neonatal cholestatic jaundice. It is the single most frequent cause of death from liver disease and of referral for liver transplantation (approx 50% of all cases) in children.

The etiology of extrahepatic biliary atresia is unknown. The disease is not inherited. Because of the inflammatory process and progressive injury to the biliary system, a number of viral agents have been implicated, including cytomegalovirus, rubella virus and, possibly, reovirus type III, but these agents do not account for the majority of cases (11). Extrahepatic anomalies occur in 10–25% of patients and include cardiovascular defects, polysplenia, malrotation, situs inversus, and bowel atresias, suggesting that the pathogenetic process may begin prenatally (12). However, most cases can not be attributed to a failure in morphogenesis or recanalization of the bile duct during embryonic development. Injury to and obliteration of the extrahepatic bile ducts usually progresses postnatally.

Complete fibrous obliteration of all or at least a portion of the extrahepatic bile ducts is pathognomonic (13) (see Fig. 2). In the most common form of atresia (approx 90% of cases), the entire extrahepatic biliary tree is affected. Incomplete forms involving the proximal or distal portions of the bile ducts may also occur. The entire perihilar area often consists of a cone of dense fibrous tissue. The gallbladder is absent or involved in the inflammatory process to some extent in approx 80% of patients. Prior to complete destruction, bile ducts may demonstrate lumina with variable degeneration of epithelial cells, inflammation, and fibrosis in the periductular tissues.

2.1.1. CARDINAL SIGNS AND SYMPTOMS

Most infants with biliary atresia are of normal birth weight and appear healthy at birth (2). Females are affected more commonly than males. Infants appear jaundiced after the period of physiologic hyperbilirubinemia. Patients with complete biliary obstruction develop acholic stools; however, early in the course with incomplete or evolving atresia, stools may appear normally pigmented or only intermittently pigmented (10). Bleeding due to vitamin K deficiency may be a presenting feature.

Moderate hepatomegaly with a firm liver edge is a typical finding (10). The spleen is usually not enlarged early in the course, but will become enlarged as cirrhosis develops. Ascites and edema are not initially present.

2.1.2. DIAGNOSIS

On laboratory evaluation, the serum bilirubin level is variably elevated, often between 6 and 12 mg/dL with at least 50% of the total being conjugated (5,10). Serum aminotransferase and alkaline phosphatase levels are moderately elevated. Liver histology from a liver biopsy done in the first weeks of life generally shows good preservation of the hepatic architecture with a variable degree of bile ductular proliferation, canalicular and cellular bile stasis (14). Portal tract fibrosis, inflammation, and edema are often seen. The presence of bile plugs in portal triads is an important feature of large duct obstruction. Variable injury to the biliary epithelium

family members, indicating that spontaneous mutations can occur or that minimally affected family members go undetected *(31)*.

2.4.1. Cardinal Signs and Symptoms

Chronic cholestasis of varying severity affects most patients. Jaundice and clay-colored stools may be observed during the neonatal period or during the first months of life. Other patients may present because of poor growth. Intense pruritus may be present by 6 mo of age. Xanthomas often develop on the extensor surfaces of the fingers and in creases of the palms and popliteal areas during the first years of life. The liver and spleen are usually normal in size or only slightly enlarged.

Dysmorphic facies, recognized during infancy and becoming more characteristic with age, consists of a broad forehead, deeply set and widely spaced eyes, and a somewhat small and pointed mandible which imparts a triangular appearance to the face *(29)*. A flattened malar eminence and prominent ears are also observed. Extrahepatic anomalies have been described with this syndrome, but there is considerable variability in phenotypic expression. Short stature can only be partially attributed to the severity of chronic cholestasis. Mild to moderate mental retardation affects 15–20% of patients. Congenital heart disease occurs in most patients with peripheral pulmonic stenosis observed in approx 90% of cases. Decreased bone age, variable shortening of the distal phalanges, and vertebral arch defects are frequently present. Ophthalmological examination often reveals a posterior embryotoxon (mesodermal dysgenesis of the iris and cornea). Renal abnormalities and hypogonadism may occur.

2.4.2. Diagnosis

Standard liver tests are altered and of value in establishing the presence of liver disease. Serum bilirubin and aminotransferase levels are often elevated. Serum cholesterol levels of 200 mg/dL or higher and serum triglyceride concentrations ranging from 500–1000 mg/dL are typical. Total serum bile acid concentrations are markedly elevated, but the bile acid profiles in serum, urine and bile do not differ qualitatively from other cholestatic patients.

On liver biopsy, the hallmark of the condition is a paucity of interlobular bile ducts. The only clearly established mechanism for duct paucity is duct destruction rather than a failure of ducts to develop. The histologic features during the first months of life include: significant ballooning of hepatocytes, variable cholestasis, portal inflammation, and giant cell transformation. The number of interlobular bile ducts is often not decreased on initial liver biopsy, but bile duct injury and loss is progressive. Cellular infiltration of portal triads contiguous to interlobular bile ducts, lymphocytic infiltration, and pyknosis of biliary epithelium and periductal fibrosis may be found, leading to paucity of interlobular bile ducts usually after 3 mo. Mild periportal fibrosis is seen, but progression to cirrhosis occurs uncommonly. The extrahepatic bile ducts are patent, but are usually small.

The clinical course is marked by varying degrees of cholestasis, which may be unremitting or sometimes worsened during intercurrent illness. Significant morbidity may result from pruritus, cutaneous xanthomata, and neuromuscular symptoms related to vitamin E deficiency. Treatment should focus on the provision of an adequate caloric intake, the prevention or correction of fat-soluble vitamin deficiencies, particularly vitamin E deficiency, and symptomatic measures to relieve pruritus *(32)*.

Long term prognosis is determined by the severity of the liver disease and associated malformations *(33)*. Progression to cirrhosis and liver failure can occur, but more often severe complications such as bone fractures, intractable pruritus, and xanthoma necessitate liver transplantation. Hepatocellular carcinoma may occur. The severity of associated malformations may decrease survival and preclude candidacy for liver transplantation *(34)*.

2.5. Cystic Fibrosis

Patients with cystic fibrosis may develop cholestasis in the neonatal period *(35)* (*see* Chapter 25, this volume, for more details). Meconium ileus may be associated. Clinical features of cholestatic jaundice and acholic stools can mimic extrahepatic biliary atresia. A reliable sweat chloride analysis may be difficult to obtain in the neonate. Genotype analysis is an alternative method of diagnosis, particularly in the absence of a positive family history. There is no significant difference in the allele frequencies of defined and undefined mutations of the cystic fibrosis gene between patients with and without liver disease *(36,37)*. Bile plugging in portal tracts, bile ductular proliferation, and portal fibrosis are found on liver biopsy. These features of biliary obstruction may necessitate exploratory laparotomy to exclude biliary atresia. The extrahepatic bile ducts appear normal or obstructed by thick, tenacious mucous. Removal of the inspissated material by irrigation can be of value, but the cholestatic liver disease may improve spontaneously *(38)*. The severity of the pulmonary disease and complications of meconium ileus often determine the outcome. Neonatal cholestasis does not necessarily predict progression to biliary cirrhosis in later life.

3. INTRAHEPATIC CHOLESTASIS

3.1. Neonatal Hepatitis

Neonatal hepatitis refers to a pattern of injury typical of the neonatal liver rather than a specific diagnosis, and is characterized by swelling and multinucleated giant cell transformation of hepatocytes, as well as variable cholestasis, inflammation, necrosis, and fibrosis *(1,39)*. The relative incidence of the disorder in early reports varied from 1:2500 to 1:8000 live births. In many series at least one third of the patients with neonatal cholestasis fell into the category of so-called idiopathic neonatal hepatitis. A familial form affects 10% of patients, suggesting causation by an underlying inborn error of metabolism. At present, the incidence of idiopathic neonatal hepatitis is much lower, due to advances in diagnostic methods in virology and inborn errors of metabolism. These allow for a more precise diagnosis of inborn errors of metabolism *(40)*. For example, neonatal hepatitis may be caused by perinatal infection with parvovirus B19 or human herpesvirus-6. Other recent associations include neonatal lupus erythematosus, alpha-1-antitrypsin deficiency, and inborn errors of bile acid metabolism.

3.1.1. CARDINAL SIGNS AND SYMPTOMS

The clinical presentation of neonatal hepatitis is highly variable *(4,5,41)*. In contrast with patients with biliary atresia, the infant with neonatal hepatitis is often born prematurely or of low birth weight. Cholestatic liver disease may be noticed during the neonatal period or escape recognition until 1– 2 mo of age. A hemorrhagic diathesis may result from deficiency of coagulation factors and from thrombocytopenia. Microcephaly and chorioretinitis strongly suggest intrauterine infection with rubella or cytomegalovirus. One third of infants may fail to thrive. Hepatosplenomegaly is usually present. A fulminant course, reflecting massive necrosis of hepatocytes, can occur with herpes simplex infection, enteroviral infections, or with inborn errors such as neonatal iron-storage disease or tyrosinemia.

3.1.2. DIAGNOSIS

Total and conjugated serum bilirubin levels are variably elevated *(5)*. Serum aminotransferases are moderately elevated, but markedly abnormal levels may be found with significant necrosis. Alkaline phosphatase, 5'-nucleotidase, and γ-glutamyltransferase levels are raised, but cannot be reliably used to differentiate the condition from biliary obstruction.

On liver biopsy, the lobular architecture may be severely disturbed with variable swelling, degeneration, and necrosis of hepatocytes and extramedullary hematopoiesis *(5)*. Multinucleated giant cells,

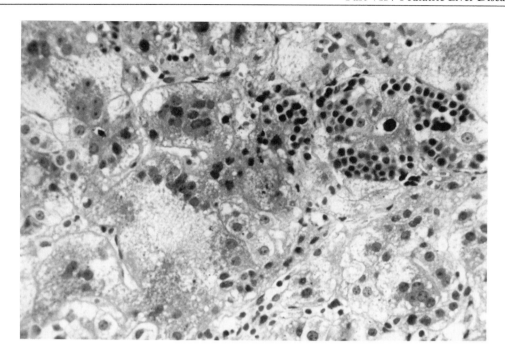

Fig. 3. Liver biopsy from patient with idiopathic neonatal hepatitis showing typical multinucleated giant cells.

thought to form by fusion of hepatocytes, may be prominent throughout the lobule (*see* Fig. 3). Hepatocellular and canalicular bile stasis reflect the severity of cholestasis. Ductular bile plugs and proliferation should be negligible. Periportal and lobular fibrosis may be present. Pseudoacinar arrangement of hepatocyte and steatosis suggest a metabolic basis for the liver disease.

3.1.3. TREATMENT AND PROGNOSIS

There is no specific treatment for neonatal hepatitis. Fat-soluble vitamin deficiencies should be prevented and optimal nutritional support provided with a formula containing medium-chain triglycerides. Approximately 60% of patients with the sporadic form of neonatal hepatitis recover completely, one-third die from rapidly progressive disease, and approx 10% develop chronic liver disease (*41*). In series collected 15–20 yr ago, the outcome was considerably worse in familial cases: 60% of patients died, 30% recovered, and 10% developed chronic liver disease. Many of these patients probably suffered from disorders that can now be readily diagnosed, such as alpha-1-antitrypsin deficiency.

3.2. Alpha-1-Antitrypsin Deficiency

Alpha 1-antitrypsin (α1AT), a 50 kDa glycoprotein synthesized predominantly in liver, is the major serum protease inhibitor and acts to inhibit a broad range of proteolytic enzymes, particularly neutrophil elastase (*42*) (*see* Chapter 20, this volume). The protease inhibitor occurs in over 75 variants, known PI phenotypes, which are each inherited as codominant alleles. The normal phenotype, determined by protein electrophoresis, is designated MM. Patients with a homozygous deficiency state or ZZ phenotype have low serum alpha 1-antitrypsin levels, usually 10–15% of normal values (*43*). The incidence of the PiZZ phenotype is 1:2000 to 1:4000. The deficiency state can be associated with progressive liver disease in infants, children, and adults. Approximately 10–15% of patients with the PiZZ phenotype develop cholestatic jaundice in the neonatal period.

3.2.1. Cardinal Signs and Symptoms in the Neonate

Hepatomegaly and acholic stools are typical in these patients *(42)*. Patients may rarely present with ascites or bleeding. Although asymptomatic, another 40–50% of infants may have abnormal liver biochemical tests in the first months of life. The diagnosis should be made by determination of the α1AT phenotype. Measurement of α1AT levels alone is not reliable, since the protein is an acute phase reactant.

3.2.2. Diagnosis

Liver biopsy in the neonate often shows a giant cell hepatitis. Bile ductular proliferation may be variably observed; paucity of bile ducts may be found later. The presence of periodic acid-Schiff positive, diastase-resistant inclusions within hepatocytes representing the abnormal α1AT is a characteristic feature, but is not usually prominent before 4 mo of age. A variable degree of fibrosis may be present. Cirrhosis has been reported in the neonate.

3.2.3. Prognosis

The course of patients with neonatal liver disease related to α1AT deficiency is variable *(44)*. Rare patients presenting with cirrhosis may deteriorate rapidly within the first months of life. However, in most patients the jaundice clears by 4 mo of age. Nearly equal proportions of patients manifest one of the following outcomes: continued liver dysfunction with progression to cirrhosis and end-stage liver disease by age 10 yr; persistent liver test abnormalities with slow progression to cirrhosis in adolescence or later; mild liver test abnormalities and minimal fibrosis with survival into adulthood; and apparent complete resolution of hepatic disease. Hepatocellular carcinoma may occur in these patients.

3.2.4. Treatment

The treatment of liver disease associated with α1AT deficiency is supportive *(45)*. Liver transplantation, if required, is curative with the patient then assuming the Pi type of the donor organ.

3.3. Progressive Familial Intrahepatic Cholestasis

Progressive familial intrahepatic cholestasis (PFIC), also known as Byler's Disease, is a syndrome in which chronic, unremitting cholestasis develops early in life *(46,47)*. Jaundice, severe pruritus, and growth failure are typical features. Low serum γ-glutamyl transpeptidase and cholesterol levels help to differentiate PFIC from other chronic cholestatic disorders in children. An autosomal recessive pattern of inheritance is likely. The chromosomal locus for progressive familial intrahepatic cholestasis has been recently mapped to 18q21-q22, the same region as benign recurrent intrahepatic cholestasis *(48)*. Progression to cirrhosis and liver failure usually occurs by 3–4 yr of age, but may develop in the neonatal period. Partial external biliary diversion has been used successfully to treat intractable pruritus in these patients; in some cases the cholestasis also improves following the procedure *(49)*. Orthotopic liver transplantation is required in patients with decompensated cirrhosis.

4. INBORN ERRORS OF BILE ACID METABOLISM

The pathways for biosynthesis of bile acids from cholesterol require more than 15 enzymatic steps in the hepatocyte. In multisystem disorders of peroxisomal assembly and function, such as Zellweger syndrome, defective shortening of the cholesterol side chain can result in cholestasis and progressive liver disease. Liver-specific injury occurs in two recently described enzymatic defects affecting modifications of the steroid nucleus: deficiency of 3-hydroxy-5-C27-steroid dehydrogenase/isomerase and 4-3-oxosteroid-5-reductase *(50–52)*. Most patients with these disorders develop progressive jaundice, elevated aminotransferases and conjugated hyperbilirubinemia during the first weeks of life. Giant cell hepatitis is present on liver biopsy. Cases demonstrate an autosomal recessive pattern of inheritance and appear to be fatal if untreated. Cholestatic liver disease results from bile secretory failure and from retention of bile acid precursors that are hepatotoxic. Serum bile acid concentrations are paradoxically normal or low in these patients when measured by routine methods, and seemingly incompatible with a diagnosis of severe cholestasis. The diagnosis is strongly suggested by fast atom bombardment-mass spectrometry (FAB-MS) analysis of urine, which quantitatively indicates an elevated urinary bile acid excretion compatible with cholestasis, but is remarkable for an absence of normal glyco- and tauro-conjugates of primary bile acids. Atypical bile acids, reflecting accumulation biosynthetic precursors, account for up to 90% of total urinary bile acids in these patients.

These inborn errors of metabolism may be effectively treated with bile acid replacement (51). Replacement of exogenous bile acids is necessary for the generation of bile acid-dependent bile flow. Moreover, the feeding of primary bile acids should inhibit bile acid synthesis at the level of 7α-hydroxylase and, thus, significantly decrease the production of toxic bile acid precursors. There is a growing experience with the use of bile acid treatment for disorders involving the steroid nucleus as well as the bile acid side chain. Using the approach of feeding cholic acid or chenodeoxycholic acid often with the addition of ursodeoxycholic acid, most patients have had a remarkable clinical and biochemical improvement, with normalization of serum liver tests and resolution of jaundice. Careful monitoring of urine and plasma samples and titrating therapy according to the disappearance of the unusual bile acid metabolites from urine are required.

5. TOTAL PARENTERAL NUTRITION (TPN)-ASSOCIATED CHOLESTASIS

Infants receiving total parenteral nutrition (TPN) may develop cholestatic liver disease. This risk is highest in premature infants and those who receive minimal enteral feeds and is associated with the duration of therapy. Characteristically, there is a gradual increase in the serum conjugated bilirubin fraction after 2–3 wk of TPN, followed by increases in aminotransferases and alkaline phosphatase. TPN-related liver disease often resolves with the advancement of enteral feedings, but can progress to cirrhosis and hepatic failure. The pathogenesis is unclear and may be multifactorial. Immaturity of the enterohepatic circulation, toxicity of TPN components, systemic infection, deficiencies of specific nutrients, as well as the comorbidities affecting these sick infants, may contribute (53,54). The diagnosis of TPN cholestasis is one of exclusion. Histologic findings include cholestasis in hepatocytes, canaliculi, and Kupffer cells, most predominant in the centrilobular region, as well as portal inflammation with mild bile duct proliferation and, in more severe cases, fibrosis (55). Infants at risk for the development of TPN-related liver disease should have careful monitoring of their biochemical indices and ongoing efforts made to initiate and advance their enteral feedings.

6. MEDICAL MANAGEMENT OF CHRONIC CHOLESTASIS

Efforts should be directed toward promoting growth and development and minimizing discomfort in infants with chronic and sometimes progressive cholestatic liver disease (56).

Failure to thrive is common in children with cholestasis, largely because of impaired fat solubilization and absorption (57). Medium-chain triglycerides (MCT), which do not require bile salt solubilization for absorption, can provide needed calories when given in a commercial formula or as an oil supplement. Some long-chain triglycerides should also be given to prevent the development of essential fatty acid deficiency. Fat malabsorption in cholestatic infants results in deficiencies of fat-soluble vitamins (58). Vitamin A deficiency may manifest as xerophthalmia, night blindness, and thickened skin. Metabolic bone disease with osteoporosis and pathologic fractures can occur from vitamin D deficiency. A degenerative neuromuscular syndrome, characterized by arreflexia, opthalmoplegia, cerebellar ataxia, peripheral neuropathy, and posterior column dysfunction, occurs in children with chronic vitamin E deficiency. Vitamin K malabsorption results in a coagulopathy. Infants with cholestasis should receive supplemental fat-soluble vitamins with doses adjusted according to regularly followed serum vitamin levels and prothrombin time. A water soluble form of vitamin E, d-α-tocopherol polyethylene glycol-1000-succinate (15–25 IU/kg/d), enhances absorption of this vitamin as well as of vitamins A and D, which can be given together as a double dose of standard infant vitamin preparation. Vitamin K may be given orally, 2.5–5 mg twice a week up to daily dose, as needed. Occasionally, infants with advanced liver disease will require intramuscular injection of vitamin K.

Pruritus and xanthomas resulting from chronic liver disease can be sources of significant discomfort for children (59). Pruritus may be observed by 3 mo of age. Efforts to treat these symptoms are aimed at increasing bile flow with medications such as ursodeoxycholic acid (10–20 mg/kg/d) and phenobarbital (3–5 mg/kg/d), or at binding bile acids, cholesterol and other potentially toxic agents in the intestinal lumen with the non-absorbable anion exchange resin, cholestyramine (0.25–0.5 gm/kg/d). These two medications should not be administered simultaneously as cholestyramine will bind ursodeoxycholic acid rendering it ineffective. Rifampicin (10 mg/kg/d) may also be effective in relieving pruritis. Its mechanism of action is unclear.

7. INDICATIONS FOR CONSULTING THE SUBSPECIALIST

Any infant with persistent jaundice beyond 2 wks of age, or an elevated direct bilirubin fraction, should be promptly evaluated. As the evaluation may include a liver biopsy, it is reasonable to refer these infants to a subspecialist.

8. CONCLUSIONS

Cholestasis in the neonate is the clinical and pathological manifestation of a multitude of disorders that affect the bile ducts, hepatocytes, or bile acid metabolic pathways. An expedient workup is necessary in order to identify metabolic diseases responsive to specific medical therapies and assure timely surgical treatment for biliary atresia. Many forms of cholestasis have no specific treatment. They require nutritional support to optimize growth and development. The prognosis of neonatal cholestasis varies greatly depending on the underlying etiology.

SUMMARY

Cholestasis is a decrease in bile flow due to impaired secretion by hepatocytes or obstruction of the intra- or extrahepatic bile ducts.

The causes of cholestasis in the neonate are numerous and include disorders of bile ducts, hepatitis (infectious or idiopathic), familial cholestatic disorders, metabolic disorders, and others.

Infants who have severe or persistent jaundice, or an elevated conjugated bilirubin fraction, should be evaluated. Initial evaluation should include fractionated bilirubin, aminotranferases, alkaline phosphatase levels, and abdominal ultrasound. Further evaluation should be directed by the patient's history, physical exam, and clinical course.

Percutaneous liver biopsy is an important diagnostic tool in the evaluation of neonatal cholestasis. Metabolic diseases amenable to specific medical therapies should be identified and treated promptly.

Biliary atresia should be diagnosed early (by 60 d of age) to optimize the chance for successful surgical treatment.

Medical treatment of cholestasis in infants includes nutritional support with absorbable fats, calories and fat-soluble vitamins. Symptomatic treatment may be required for pruritus and xanthomas.

REFERENCES

1. Watkins JB. Neonatal cholestasis: developmental aspects and current concepts. Semin Liver Dis 1993;13:276–288.
2. Hussein M, Howard E R, Mieli-Vergani G, Mowat A P. Jaundice at 14 days of age: exclude biliary atresia. Arch Dis Child 1991;66:1177–1179.
3. Balistreri WF. Neonatal cholestasis: medical progress. J Pediatr 1985;106:171.
4. Fung KP, Lau SP. Differentiation between extrahepatic and intrahepatic cholestasis by discriminant analysis. J Paediatr Child Health 1990;26:132-35.
5. Lai MW, Chang MH, Hsu SC, Hsu, HC, et al. Differential diagnosis of extrahepatic biliary atresia from neonatal hepatitis: a prospective study [see comments]. J Pediatr Gastroenterol Nutr 1994;18:121.
6. Paltiel HJ. Imaging of neonatal cholestasis. Semin Ultrasound CT MRI 1994;15:290-305.
7. Keller MS. Imaging of the liver and biliary tract. In: FJ Suchy, ed. Liver disease in children. Mosby, Philadelphia, 1994, p. 309.
8. Guelrud M, Jaen D, Mendoza S, Plaz J, Torres P. ERCP in the diagnosis of extrahepatic biliary atresia. Gastrointest Endosc 1991;37:522–526.
9. Hays DM, Woolley MM, Snyder WH Jr, Reed GB, Gwinn JL, Landing BH. Diagnosis of biliary atresia: relative accuracy of percutaneous liver biopsy, open liver biopsy, and operative cholangiography. J Pediatr 1967;71:598.
10. Ohi R, Ibrahim M. Biliary atresia. Sem Pediatr Surg 1992;1:115–124.
11. Brown WR. Lack of conformation of the association of reovirus 3 and biliary atresia: methodological differences. Hepatology 1990;12:1254–1255.
12. Carmi R, Magee C A, Neill CA, Karrer FM. Extrahepatic biliary atresia and associated anomalies: etiologic heterogeneity suggested by distinctive patterns of associations. Am J Med Genet 1993;45:683–693.
13. Tan CE, Driver M, Howard ER, Moscoso GJ. Extrahepatic biliary atresia: a first-trimester event? Clues from light microscopy and immunohistochemistry. J Pediatr Surg 1994;29:808–814.
14. Desmet VJ. Cholangiopathies: past, present, and future. Semin Liver Dis 1987;7:67–76.
15. Karrer FM, Hall RJ, Stewart BA, Lilly JR. Congenital biliary tract disease. Surg Clin North Am 1990;70:1403–1418.
16. Miyano T, Fujimoto T, Ohya T, Shimomura H. Current concept of the treatment of biliary atresia. World J Surg 1993;17: 332–336.
17. Karrer FM, Lilly JR, Stewart BA, Hall RJ. Biliary atresia registry, 1976 to 1989. J Pediatr Surg 1990;10:1076–1081.
18. Laurent J, Gauthier F, Bernard O, et al. Long-term outcome after surgery for biliary atresia. Study of 40 patients surviving for more than 10 years. Gastroenterology 1990;99:1793–1797.
19. Ohi R, Nio M, Chiba T, Endo N, Goto M, Ibrahim M. Long-term follow-up after surgery for patients with biliary atresia. J Pediatr Surg 1990;25:442–445.
20. Karrer FM. Price MR, Bensard DD, et al. Long-term results with the Kasai operation for biliary atresia. Arch Surg 1996;131:493–496.
21. Vacanti JP, Shamberger R C, Eraklis A, Lillehei CW. The therapy of biliary atresia combining the Kasai portoenterostomy with liver transplantation: a single center experience. J Pediatr Surg 1990;25:149–152.
22. Ryckman F, Fisher R, Pedersen S, et al. Improved survival in biliary atresia patients in the present era of liver transplantation. J Pediatr Surg 1993;28:382–385.
23. Ryckman FC, Noseworthy J. Neonatal cholestatic conditions requiring surgical reconstruction. Sem Liver Dis 1987;7:134–154.
24. O'Neill JA Jr. Choledochal cyst. Curr Probl Surg 1992;29:361–410.
25. Savader SJ, Benenati J F, Venbrux AC, et al. Choledochal cysts: classification and cholangiographic appearance. Am J Roentgenol 1991;56:327–331.
26. Todani T, Watanabe Y, Narusue M, Tabuchi K, Okajima K. Congenital bile duct cysts. Classification, operative procedures, and review of thirty seven cases including cancer arising from choledochal cyst. Am J Surg 1977;134:263.
27. Kahn E. Paucity of interlobular bile ducts: arteriohepatic dysplasia and nonsyndromic duct paucity. In: Abramowsky CR, Bernstein J, Rosenberg HS, eds. Transplantation pathology -hepatic morphogenesis. Perspective Pediatric Pathology. Karger, Basel, 1991, p. 168.
28. Hadchouel M. Paucity of interlobular bile ducts. Sem Diagn Pathol 1992;9:24–30.
29. Alagille D, Estrada A, Hadchouel M, Gautier M, Odievre M, Dommergues JP. Syndromic paucity of interlobular bile ducts (Alagille syndrome or arteriohepatic dysplasia): review of 80 cases. J Pediatr 1987;110:195–200.
30. Hol FA, Hamel BC, Geurds MP, et al. Localization of Alagille syndrome to 20p11.2-p12 by linkage analysis of a three-generation family. Hum Genet 1995;95:687–690.
31. Elmslie FV, Vivian AJ, Gardiner H, Hall C, Mowat AP, Winter RM. Alagille syndrome: family studies. J Med Genet 1995;32:264–268.
32. Alagille D. Management of paucity of interlobular bile ducts. J Hepatol 1985;1:561–565.
33. Hoffenberg EJ, Narkewicz MR, Sondheimer JM, Smith DJ, Silverman A, Sokol RJ. Outcome of syndromic paucity of interlobular bile ducts (Alagille syndrome) with onset of cholestasis in infancy. J Pediatr 1995;127:220–224.

34. Tzakis AG, Reyes J, Tepetes K, Tzoracoleftherakis V, Todo S, Starzl TE. Liver transplantation for Alagille's syndrome. Arch Surg 1993;128:337–339.
35. Colombo C, Battezzati PM, Podda M. Hepatobiliary disease in cystic fibrosis. Sem Liver Dis 1994;14:259–269.
36. Colombo C, Apostolo MG, Ferrari M, et al. Analysis of risk factors for the development of liver disease associated with cystic fibrosis. J Pediatr 1994;124:393–399.
37. Mack DR, Traystman MD, Colombo JL, et al. Clinical denouement and mutation analysis of patients with cystic fibrosis undergoing liver transplantation for biliary cirrhosis. J Pediatr 1995;127:881.
38. Festen C, Kuyper F, Holland R, van Haelst U. Neonatal jaundice in cystic fibrosis: a conservative approach is not always justified. Z Kinderchir 1988;43:106,107.
39. Haber BA, Lake AM. Cholestatic jaundice in the newborn. Clin Perinatol 1990;17:483–506.
40. Felber S, Sinatra F. Systemic disorders associated with neonatal cholestasis. Sem Liver Dis 1987;7:108–118.
41. Dick MC, Mowat AP. Hepatitis syndrome in infancy—an epidemiological survey with 10 year follow up. Arch Dis Child 1985;60:512–516.
42. Perlmutter DH. Clinical manifestations of alpha 1-antitrypsin deficiency. Gastroenterol Clin North Am 1995;24:27–43.
43. Povey S. Genetics of alpha 1-antitrypsin deficiency in relation to neonatal liver disease. Mol Biol Med 1990;7:161–172.
44. Sveger T. The natural history of liver disease in alpha 1-antitrypsin deficient children. Acta Paediatr Scand 1988;77:847–851.
45. Perlmutter DH. Metabolic liver disease in childhood. Semin Gastrointest Dis 1994;5:54–64.
46. Whitington PF, Freese DK, Alonso EM, Schwarzenberg SJ, Sharp HL. Clinical and biochemical findings in progressive familial intrahepatic cholestasis. J Pediatr Gastroenterol Nutr 1994;18:134–141.
47. Alonso EM, Snover DC, Montag A, Freese DK, Whitington PF. Histologic pathology of the liver in progressive familial intrahepatic cholestasis. J Pediatr Gastroenterol Nutr 1994;18:128–133.
48. Carlton VE, Knisely AS, Freimer NB. Mapping of a locus for progressive familial intrahepatic cholestasis (Byler disease) to 18q21-q22, the benign recurrent intrahepatic cholestasis region. Hum Mol Genet 1995;4:1049–1053.
49. Whitington PF, Whitington GL. Partial external diversion of bile for the treatment of intractable pruritus associated with intrahepatic cholestasis. Gastroenterology 1988;95:130.
50. Russell DW, Setchell KD. Bile acid biosynthesis. Biochemistry 1992;31:4737–4749.
51. Bjorkhem I. Inborn errors of metabolism with consequences for bile acid biosynthesis. A minireview. Scand J Gastroenterol Suppl 1994;204:68–72.
52. Setchell KD, Suchy FJ, Welsh MB, Zimmer-Nechemias L, Heubi J, Balistreri WF. Delta 4-3-oxosteroid 5 beta-reductase deficiency described in identical twins with neonatal hepatitis. A new inborn error in bile acid synthesis. J Clin Invest 1988;82:2148–2157.
53. Senger HBG, Beyreiss K, Braun W, Raiha N. Evidence for amino acid induced cholestasis in very-low-birth-weight infants with increasing enteral protein intake. Acta Paediatr Scand 1986;75:724–728.
54. Wolf A, Pohlandt F. Bacterial infection: the main cause of acute cholestasis in newborn infants receiving short-term parenteral nutrition. J Pediatr Gastroenterol Nutr 1989;8:297–303.
55. Mullick FG, Moran CA, Ishak KG. Total parenteral nutrition: a histopathologic analysis of the liver changes in 20 children. Mod Pathol 1994;7:190–194.
56. Sokol RJ. Medical management of the infant or child with chronic liver disease. Sem Liver Dis 1987;7:155–167.
57. Kaufman SS, Murray ND, Wood RP, Shaw BW Jr, Vanderhoof JA. Nutritional support for the infant with extrahepatic biliary atresia. J Pediatr 1987;110:679–686.
58. Sokol RJ. Fat-soluble vitamins and their importance in patients with cholestatic liver diseases. Gastroenterol Clin North Am 1994;23:673–705.
59. Ramirez RO, Sokol RJ. Medical management of cholestasis. In: Suchy FJ, ed. Liver disease in children. Mosby, Philadelphia, 1994, p. 356.

SUGGESTED READING

1. McEvoy CA, Suchy FJ. Biliary tract disease in children. Pediatr Clin North Am 1996;43:75–98.
2. Sokol RJ. Fat-soluble vitamins and their importance in patients with cholestatic liver diseases. Gastroenterol Clin North Am 1994;23:673–705.
3. Ryckman FC, Noseworthy J. Neonatal cholestatic conditions requiring surgical reconstruction. Sem Liver Dis 1987;7:134–154.

2.2. Pathogenesis

The abnormally high chloride concentration in sweat (> 60 meq/L) reflects mutations of the CFTR. At present > 85 % of individuals with CF have more than 600 different definable DNA mutations, most commonly the delta F508 phenylalanine deletion. The defect in chloride transport is expressed in the fetus and throughout life, with altered fluidity of secretions. The CFTR is expressed on biliary epithelium, but not on hepatocyte canalicular membranes. As a result, bile is abnormally viscous, promoting sludge and stone formation. A characteristic multinodular biliary fibrosis and biliary cirrhosis (2) evolve slowly during childhood and adolescence although even newborn infants can manifest biliary complications of CF known as the inspissated bile syndrome.

By age 21 approximately 30% of CF individuals have hepatobiliary disease, 5% with cirrhosis (3–5). CF associated liver disease is more prevalent in patients with pancreatic insufficiency and in those who have history of meconium ileus in infancy; no correlation with specific mutations of the CFTR has been found (6).

Cholelithiasis in CF is more common than in the age matched general population, with cholesterol rather than bilirubin the major component of stones (7). Cholelithiasis appears less common in pancreatic sufficient patients and those whose steatorrhea is normalized with enteric coated microsphere enzyme supplements, situations in which excessive fecal bile acid loss does not occur. Asymptomatic atrophy of the gallbladder with microgallbladder is common. Abnormalities of the extrahepatic biliary tree including common bile duct strictures and changes resembling sclerosing cholangitis are reported, presumably a result of inflammatory reaction to viscous bile. However their significance remains controversial (8–10).

2.3. Cardinal Symptoms and Signs

Clinical suspicion of CF is based on the symptoms and signs of multisystemic disease listed in Table 1 and, once considered, should be pursued. At least 15% of adults with CF have glucose intolerance or overt diabetes mellitus, the long-term consequence of pancreatic obstruction (11,12). About five percent of CF patients are diagnosed as adults with nasal polyps, mild chronic lung disease, or chronic pancreatitis, sometimes with normal or inconclusive sweat test.

Infertility in males (approximately 95%) results from in utero destruction of the vas deferens and azospermia. Females have diminished fertility. In neither case is this reproductive failure likely to be a consequence of liver disease.

CF-associated hepatobiliary disease should be considered in the differential diagnosis of abdominal pain in a CF patient and if hepatic or splenic enlargement is noted on physical examination. Diagnosis of CF-associated liver disease (see Fig. 1) requires exclusion of other causes of chronic liver disease and usually does not require liver biopsy. If a biopsy is obtained, there will be evidence of variable sized nodules, bile ductular proliferation, and inspissated mucous secretions within bile ductules without a great deal of intracellular bilirubin stasis. When nutritional status is compromised there may be steatosis as well. Unfortunately the multifocal nature of CF associated liver injury may lead to biopsy sampling errors, including the finding of relatively normal histology in the face of true cirrhosis (13).

Colicky abdominal pain need not reflect hepatobiliary disease. Meconium ileus equivalent or the distal intestinal obstruction syndrome (DIOS) is the most common etiology (14,15). Fibrosing colonic strictures and Crohn's disease should be considered in the differential diagnosis.

Rarely, secondary or reactive amyloidosis complicates CF with deposition in liver, spleen, kidney and elsewhere (16–18). Organomegaly develops and gastrointestinal hemorrhage, not variceal in origin, can be substantial and difficult to localize.

Table 1
Diagnosis of Cystic Fibrosis

Signs and symptoms of multisystemic disease in young individuals, including:

Growth failure
Nasal polyps
Chronic lung disease, *Pseudomonas* colonization
Pancreatic steatorrhea
Acute or chronic relapsing pancreatitis
Unexplained glucose intolerance
Biliary tract disease, unexplained biliary cirrhosis or portal hypertension
Intestinal obstruction, and/or rectal prolapse
Male infertility
Acute hyponatremia

Sweat test:
Pilocarpine-stimulated sweat chloride quantitation

Positive	Equivocal	Normal
> 60 meq/L	40-60 meq/L	< 40 meq/L
↓	↓	↓
Sweat test siblings and offspring	Repeat sweat test	DNA haplotype analysis (blood)
↓	↓	
DNA haplotype	DNA haplotype	

2.4. Treatment and Complications

Therapy of hepatobiliary complications of CF can be considered in two categories, treatments specific to CF and those appropriate to gallstones, biliary cirrhosis and portal hypertension regardless of underlying etiology (Table 2 and Fig. 2).

Fat soluble vitamins A, D, and E are usually supplemented at 200% recommended daily allowance. Oral vitamin K is supplemented as well since patients frequently require broad spectrum antibiotic treatment for chronic pulmonary infection. When discussing long-term vitamin supplementation, the patient should understand that difficulty with night vision is a clinical sign of vitamin A deficiency; that vitamin D, adequate calcium, nutritional supplements, pancreatic enzymes and exercise together can minimize osteoporosis and osteopenia, with bone densitometry used to assess adequacy of calcium, magnesium and vitamin D absorption *(19,20)*; and vitamin E deficiency has long-term consequences of peripheral neuropathy with loss of deep tendon reflexes and gait disturbance. Serum concentrations of these vitamins should be measured and doses adjusted.

Ursodeoxycholic acid (Actigall, CibaGeneva) is a newer therapy that appears effective prophylactically in CF to decrease hepatic inflammation as measured by aminotransferase abnormalities, to improve solubility of bile, thereby decreasing the likelihood of gall bladder sludge and stone formation, and to replete the bile acid pool and improve fat absorption *(21–23)*. The dose is 10–30 mg/kg/d or 300-600 mg daily in divided doses; the lower dose is

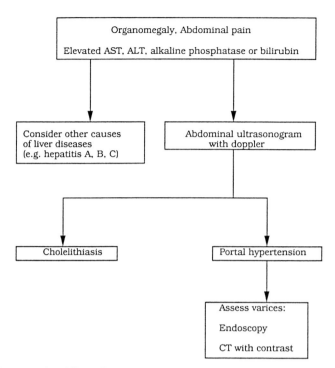

Fig. 1. Diagnosis of CF-associated liver disease signs or symptoms: A scheme for the evaluation of cystic fibrosis-associated liver disease.

recommended for prophylaxis against hepatobiliary inflammation. Pancreatic enzyme supplementation can normalize fat absorption and also seems to decrease the lithogenicity of bile *(24)*.

If gallstones are detected and result in symptoms, the procedure of choice is laparoscopic cholecystectomy; ursodeoxycholic acid does not resolubilize these stones *(24)*. The anesthetic and insufflation agent should be carefully chosen because the patient's pulmonary status is likely compromised. Specifically, regional anesthesia may be preferable to general anesthesia and insufflation with carbon dioxide must be monitored carefully to avoid hypercapnia.

Biliary cirrhosis in CF is often asymptomatic with normal synthesis of albumin and coagulation factors, normal processing of ammonia through the urea cycle and chronic minimal serum aminotransferase, alkaline phosphatase and bilirubin abnormalities. Portal hypertension can be the first and most obvious manifestation of liver disease, characterized by esophageal variceal bleeding or hypersplenism. Ascites, on the other hand, is uncommon probably because the cirrhosis is patchy and multinodular, preserving hepatocellular function until late in the disease process. Spontaneous bacterial peritonitis with abdominal pain and fever has been reported *(25)*. In general, CF-associated hepatobiliary disease responds to the same treatments appropriate for chronic hepatobiliary disease of other etiologies with one exception. Sodium chloride restriction should be modest since CF patients can develop hyponatremia because of loss of salt in sweat and actually require salt tablets in very hot weather *(26)*. Variceal bleeding is treated by emergent resuscitation with ligation or sclerotherapy and standard pharmacotherapies (*see* Chapter 29, this volume). When bleeding becomes refractory, consideration must be given to the options of transjugular intrahepatic portosystemic shunt (TIPS), traditional portosystemic shunts, and orthotopic liver

Table 2
Treatment for Cystic Fibrosis

Nutrition	
	High calorie diet (often 150% RDA, with 30-40% fat content)
	Enteral nutritional supplements containing medium chain triglycerides may be delivered through nasogastric tube or percutaneous gastrostomy
	Supplemental parenteral nutrition
Pancreas	
exocrine	Pancreatic enzyme supplements (enteric coated microspheres)
	Fat soluble vitamin supplements (200% RDA)
	Inhibitors of gastric acid secretion
endocrine	Management of diabetes mellitus
Biliary	
gallstones	Laparoscopic cholecystectomy, when symptomatic
Hepatic	
biliary	Ursodeoxycholic acid may slow progression
cirrhosis	Evaluate for orthotopic liver transplantation when severe or if lung transplantation is under consideration
portal	Variceal bleeding requires band ligation or sclerotherapy and
hypertension	usual pharmacotherapies
	Ascites is controlled with diuretics
	Avoid stringent sodium chloride restriction
	Consider TIPS, shunt surgery and transplantation

transplantation. Shunt surgery and transplantation are also considerations in older CF patients who are candidates for bilateral lung transplantation and have CF-associated hepatobiliary disease (27–29).

Experimental gene therapy in humans to date is directed at respiratory epithelial cells in an effort to improve the pulmonary disease. Development of vectors targeting the biliary epithelium for long term expression may be considerably more difficult (1).

2.5. Prognosis

Hepatobiliary disease is the second most common cause of death in CF. The prognosis for long term survival depends primarily on excellent pulmonary and nutritional management. Approximately 36% of CF patients are adults age 18 and older and, as of 1997, mean survival exceeds 31 years (30,31). In 1991 it was 30.6 years for males and 28.2 years for females, gender differences attributed to abnormal eating patterns common in young women.

With longer survival new complications and associated conditions are described. Among these are Crohn's disease, colonic strictures, amyloidosis, and adenocarcinoma of the bowel and pancreas (32–36). To date there is no report of CF-associated hepatoma.

The primary care physician plays numerous key roles in promptly diagnosing CF and its complications, early referral to a Cystic Fibrosis Center for education and therapy, helping the patient achieve normal growth, providing psychosocial support to patient and family over decades, and arranging genetic diagnosis for the patient, family and at risk pregnancies. These responsibilities can be expected to increase in the future.

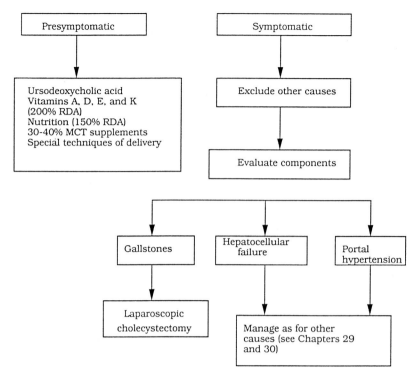

Fig. 2. Treatment of hepatobiliary complications of cystic fibrosis: A scheme for the treatment of hepatobiliary complications of cystic fibrosis.

2.6. Prevention

Cystic fibrosis is a common genetic disease which can be prevented only by identification of carrier parents, fetal genotyping and elective termination of pregnancy. At present newborn screening, although feasible, is used only in pilot programs. Family members of CF patients whose CFTR genotype is known should be offered carrier detection, which identifies approximately 80–90% of heterozygotes.

2.7. Indications for Consulting the Subspecialist

All CF patients should be referred to CF centers for education and multidisciplinary consultations. Management of individualized treatment plans is the responsibility of the patient and practitioner, with assistance as needed from gastroenterology, nutrition, pulmonary, infectious disease and surgical specialists.

Management of acute gastrointestinal hemorrhage and decisions regarding TIPS, other portosystemic shunts and transplantation should involve the hepatologist or gastroenterologist, interventional radiologist, and appropriate surgeons.

3. GALACTOSEMIA

3.1. Introduction

Individuals with classical galactosemia, which is a deficiency of galactose-l-phosphate uridyl transferase (GALT) in liver, erythrocytes and other organs, have lifelong intolerance of dietary lactose and galactose. Consequences include cataracts, intellectual and developmental deficits, and female infertility. This autosomal recessive disorder is variably distributed in different ethnic groups, with incidence as high as 1:18,000 in some northern European populations, and an overall incidence of 1:62,000. It is diagnosed by newborn blood screening programs, except in six of the United States, then treated with milk-free diet *(37)*. A variant mutation described particularly in African-Americans is associated with 10% residual transferase activity and can have milder symptomatology. The Duarte mutation has 50% GALT activity, and is asymptomatic. Two other genetic disorders of galactose metabolism, UDP-galactose-4-epimerase deficiency and galactokinase deficiency do not ordinarily involve liver and are not discussed here *(38)*.

3.2. Pathogenesis

3.2.1. LACTOSE AND THE LIVER

Lactose, the sugar in human and cow milk, is hydrolyzed to glucose and galactose by lactase on the brush border of intestinal mucosal cells, then absorbed. The liver normally transforms this galactose into glucose-1-phosphate through a series of reactions requiring ATP, UTP, and phosphate groups. GALT deficiency blocks normal hepatic galactose to glucose conversion (a source of energy) as well as the glycosylation of various glycolipids and glycoproteins *(39–41)*. Galactitol and galactonate are potentially toxic byproducts which are overproduced. Liver injury is most obvious in infants whose only source of calories is milk, and is probably caused by a combination of factors, including inadequate glucose production, depletion of ATP, and cellular toxicity from galactose metabolites. Jaundice with hepatomegaly and indirect hyperbilirubinemia are the mildest evidences of liver injury. Fulminant hepatic failure may ensue. Liver biopsy reveals steatosis, inflammation, and fibrosis, of which the latter may persist.

3.2.2. CATARACTS

Galactitol, the metabolite implicated in cataract formation, is synthesized in the lens, accumulates and as an osmotically active alcohol, permits water accumulation and lens swelling. The cataracts may be minute, punctate, or filmy and virtually undetectable, requiring sequential skilled ophthalmological examinations *(42)*. They become more obvious with age.

3.2.3. OTHER TISSUES

Galactose metabolism is a property of virtually all tissues. Brain toxicity in GALT deficiency is manifest by diminished IQ and developmental quotient (DQ) as well as perceptual and expressive deficits. Renal toxicity is demonstrated as albuminuria, galactosuria, and aminoaciduria and, in severe cases, with phosphaturia and renal tubular acidosis (Fanconi Syndrome). This toxicity is the basis for a screening test for galactosemia wherein the urine is positive for reducing sugars (Clinitest tablet, Ames) but negative for glucose (Clinistix, Ames). Hypergonadotropic hypogonadism with ovarian failure and amenorrhea in females is virtually universal, although the mechanisms are not well understood *(43–47)*.

3.2.4. FETUS

Endogenous galactose synthesis by maternal tissues, placenta and fetus is unavoidable *(48–50)*. Heterozygous women who comply with milk-free diet during affected pregnancies are unable to fully protect their galactosemic baby from brain toxicity and eventual reproductive failure, although the offspring are spared liver failure.

3.3. Cardinal Symptoms and Signs

An algorithm for diagnosis and treatment of the GALT-deficient individual is shown in Fig. 3. Galactosemic infants can be asymptomatic with abnormal newborn blood screening test for erythrocyte GALT and galactose-1-phosphate. Sick infants, particularly with *E. coli* sepsis,

Table 3
Treatment for Adults with Glycogen Storage Disease

	Type I	*Type III*	*Types VI, IX*
Diet			
Glucose and starch[a]	65% calories	45% calories	unrestricted
Lactose, sucrose	no	yes	yes
Protein	10-15%	25% calories	—
Fat	25% calories	30% calories	—
Multivitamin, calcium			
supplement	yes	yes	yes
Schedule			
Daytime	70% daily calorie requirement Balanced intake every 3-4 hours		
Nocturnal	Up to 30% daily calorie requirement Glucose or glucose polymers, UCS May include some protein and fat		
Expected goals	↓ Hepatic glycogen storage ↓ Xanthomata hyperuricemic gout, and nephropathy Normal hormonal balance (insulin, glucagon, epinephrine, growth hormone)		
Possible results	No chronic renal failure No hepatic tumors Normal life expectancy		

[a]Includes uncooked corn starch (UCS) at initial dose 1.75-2.5 gm/kg/feed. Dose is then adjusted to: a) avoid excess weight gain and b) maintain normal glucose, lactate, triglyceride and hormonal status.
Monitor with glucostat when adjusting diet or if patient develops symptoms of falling blood glucose (weakness, sweating, pallor, tachycardia, irritability).

that are improved or normalized with this regimen include hyperuricemia, hyperlactic acidemia, metabolic acidosis and hypertriglyceridemia. Since this diet's introduction in the 1970s, many individuals have not required allopurinol or supplemental bicarbonate.

Even as adults, type I patients, in particular, require frequent glucose/starch snacks, both day and night *(81)*. A treatment protocol and goals are outlined in Table 3. While providing balanced calories and glucose/starch, the glycogen storage diet for type I disease avoids lactose (galactose) and sucrose (fructose), sugars that are converted to glucose via phosphorylated intermediates and aggravate glycogen deposition. In the past the recommended diet was quite high in protein, often > 4 g/kg/d, which may have contributed to renal complications *(68,82)*. Now a normal protein intake for age is prescribed for type I patients, whereas type III patients receive slightly more protein to support gluconeogenesis. Type VI and IX patients may have received supplemental feeds in childhood, but usually no dietary treatment is necessary thereafter.

Calcium intake should be supplemented, both because the lactose-free diet is frequently associated with suboptimal calcium intake and because osteopenia and osteoporosis, which may be of multifactorial origin, are common in adults with, in particular, type I disease.

Granulocyte-macrophage colony stimulating factor (GM-CSF) injections are effective in treating Ib infectious complications, (e.g., chronic oral ulcers and inflammatory bowel disease) accompanying neutropenia *(83–88)*.

Hepatic lobectomy or orthotopic liver transplantation has been performed when patients developed hepatic tumors. Transplantation also cures the metabolic defect of G6Pase deficiency.

4.5. Potential Complications

Type I patients remain at lifelong risk for life threatening hypoglycemia, metabolic acidosis and electrolyte disturbance with intercurrent stress, particularly febrile illnesses associated with vomiting. They may require support with iv glucose infusions in the emergency room and hospitalization for illnesses which ordinarily are treated in the ambulatory setting.

Gout with nephropathy is preventable with allopurinol and has become less common as nutritional management is successfully implemented from infancy, minimizing hypoglycemia and acidosis. Treatment of chronic renal failure, the etiology of which is not clear, involves lowering the protein intake, avoiding acidosis, and standard treatments, including dialysis and renal transplantation (68,69).

The current dietary regimen also improves hyperglucagonemia, which is thought to be one of the hormonal influences in adenoma formation. Ockner's hypothesis that overstimulation of fatty acid metabolic pathways contributes to adenoma formation (89) may also be a relevant mechanism. Surveillance for adenoma and adenocarcinoma formation begins before adulthood, with physical examination, abdominal ultrasonograms and alpha fetoprotein measurement. Unfortunately these tumors are usually not rich in alpha fetoprotein or other serological tumor markers. When adenomas are diagnosed they should be biopsied and their extent and number determined by CT scan. Then a decision can be made regarding resection or the need for orthotopic liver transplant (67,90,91).

Atherosclerosis is a potential complication of glycogen storage with hypertriglyceridemia and high concentrations of VLDL and LDL. By analogy to unbalanced glucose flux in diabetes mellitus, both the renal lesion of focal glomerulosclerosis and premature atherosclerosis are predictable (92). At present there is little evidence to assume atherosclerosis is a clinical issue (93), but eicosapentaenoic acid supplementation (as fish oil) has been suggested to lower serum triglyceride and cholesterol concentrations while raising HDL concentration (94).

Fertility is another newer clinical issue. The sonographic appearance of polycystic ovaries has been noted in females with glycogenoses I, III and IX, without clinical correlates (95). Case reports of pregnancy in glycogenosis I suggest that aggressive glycemic control and monitoring in a high-risk program with early delivery by caesarian section can be successful (96–98).

Finally, fatal pulmonary hypertension has developed in the context of glycogenosis I, particularly with hepatic adenomata (99).

Medical understanding of the real and potential complications of these diseases is rapidly evolving (100). Achieving and maintaining metabolic homeostasis throughout life is the most powerful clinical tool available at this time to prevent complications.

4.6. Prognosis

Life expectancy statistics for Type I glycogen storage disease are not available. However, in the past, hypoglycemic seizures in infancy and refractory acidosis with intercurrent illnesses were fatal or caused permanent brain damage in the majority of cases. Under those circumstances long term survival was not expected. Improved prospective management has skewed survival into adulthood, and long term survival is anticipated, with description of previously unknown complications and with the focus on early diagnosis and management of renal complications and hepatic tumors. The prognosis for the other types is excellent overall, the presence or absence of muscle involvement being an important variable.

4.7. Prevention

DNA probes for the enzymes involved in types Ia, III (muscle cDNA, not liver), IV and IX have been cloned, making molecular diagnosis from CVS tissue or cultured amniocytes possible. Enzymatic activity assays must be performed on fetal liver to diagnose type Ib and can be performed on chorionic villi or cultured amniocytes for the other types. Since Type VI or IX disease is relatively benign, prenatal diagnosis is not recommended, although available.

4.8. Indications for Consulting the Subspecialist

The subspecialist is a valuable resource in making the specific diagnosis and individualizing a management plan. Because hepatologists or endocrine-metabolism specialists see a broad spectrum of glycogenoses, they can obtain the minimum number of diagnostic tests necessary to type the individual patient, counsel about prognosis, and outline the treatment plan. The diagnostic and treatment algorithms for glycogen storage disease should make sense to and be implemented by the generalist, with periodic consultations by the subspecialist and nutritionist to verify that the patient is responding optimally. Development of renal, cardiac and myopathic complications will require addition of other subspecialists to the team. Adults with both type I and III disease may experience skeletal complications, including kyphosis, scoliosis and fractures which require orthopedic input.

5. ENCEPHALOPATHY AND VOMITING: ORNITHINE TRANSCARBAMYLASE DEFICIENCY

5.1. Introduction

Episodic vomiting with abnormal mental status is a hallmark of genetic metabolic disorders that interfere with hepatic ammonia metabolism. Perhaps the best known, and not rare, example is partial ornithine transcarbamylase (OTC) deficiency in females.

The differential diagnosis of these disorders is always expanding, so OTC deficiency serves as a paradigm as well as a specific diagnosable and treatable cause of recurrent hyperammonemia. The information in this section should be considered applicable to males as well as females who exhibit symptoms and signs of hyperammonemia and must be complemented by information on the specific individual enzymatic disorders (101,102).

5.2. Pathogenesis

The hepatic urea cycle is unique. It processes waste ammonia by converting it to nontoxic, excretable urea and simultaneously synthesizing arginine, which would otherwise be an essential amino acid. Five enzymes move ammonia through this cycle (Fig. 5) which uses four ATP molecules for every ammonia molecule processed. OTC is the second enzyme along this pathway, and whereas the other urea cycle disorders are inherited in autosomal recessive fashion, it exhibits X-linked inheritance with some carrier females developing symptoms of encephalopathy and vomiting under stress (Table 4). Male infants with OTC deficiency usually develop hyperammonemic coma in the first week of life and die or are severely neurologically impaired even if their disease is recognized and treated promptly. Up to 20–25% of carbamyl phosphate synthetase (CPS) and OTC deficient individuals may have later onset of symptoms, including during adulthood (103–113). Mutations of AS (114) and AL (115) also have been diagnosed in adults.

The encephalopathy is due to cerebral edema with increased intracranial pressure. Ammonia accumulates in body tissues and reacts with glutamic acid to form glutamine, an osmotically active intracellular storage pool for ammonia. This event occurring in astrocytes lining the blood-brain barrier diminishes circulation to the swelling brain and represents the major event in developing cerebral edema.

Table 4
Historical Events Correlating with Episodic Hyperammonemia

High protein load.
Catabolic stress, e.g., febrile illness.

Critical times

Infancy:	Transition to meats and protein-containing foods.
	Transition to formula and regular cow milk.
	Protein load: human milk 1.5 gm/dL, formula 2.2 gm/dL, cow milk 3.3 gm/dL.
Childhood:	Aversion to meat, vegetarian preferences.
	Frequent episodes of vomiting.
	Vomiting and abdominal pain with disorientation, abnormal wake/sleep patterns, ataxia or confused speech.
	Emergency room visits with possible encephalitis or meningitis improving with IV therapy.
	Learning disability, clumsiness, hyperactivity.
	Mental retardation and vomiting.
Adolescence:	Bulimia, vegetarianism, behavior disorder, menstrual irregularity.
Adulthood:	Intercurrent metabolic stress, e.g., pregnancy.
	Acute or new medical condition, e.g., peptic ulcer.
	Weight loss.
At any age:	Reye's Syndrome.

5.3. Cardinal Symptoms and Signs

As depicted in Table 4, women developing symptoms of hyperammonemia may have history of a recent illness or catabolic stress (e.g. pregnancy) then over a period of hours or days begin vomiting with lethargy, progress to stupor and incoherence, then uncharacteristic, combative behavior and finally coma.

Although the history and physical examination suggest encephalitis, the patient is afebrile, and the physician may next consider drug ingestions and psychiatric illness. Careful history taking (Table 4) and family history of male infant death, mental retardation or similar episodes in other members of the pedigree are helpful clues if they are positive. The absence of such history is not helpful for two reasons, (a) this may be a new mutation in the family, and (b) it can be difficult to obtain a complete family and patient history in an intensive care setting.

However, accompanying the abnormal mental status is hyperpnea with primary metabolic alkalosis, a consequence of the developing cerebral edema, hyper- then hyporeflexia and sometimes cranial nerve signs, e.g. sixth nerve palsy). And plasma ammonia concentration (actually ammonium, NH_4^+) will be a multiple of the upper limit of normal (35 μm/L).

Plasma ammonia is the critical measurement. An abnormally high value should be confirmed immediately. Falsely abnormal results are common, if the blood is obtained from tourniquet-compressed vein rather than free-flowing arterial or venous blood, if it is not placed immediately in an ice-water slurry and transported to the laboratory for urgent determination, and if the laboratory does not routinely perform this measurement.

The diagnostic algorithm in Fig. 6 should be undertaken simultaneously with clinical management of hyperammonemia. Hyperammonemia may be a sign of primary urea cycle defect or be secondary to other genetic and acquired disorders of intermediary metabolism affecting mitochondrial function (e.g. valproate toxicity). Because the differential diagnosis is extensive, immediate and complete formal analysis of the patient's normal and abnormal biochemical parameters is essential. These measurements include complete blood count, arterial blood

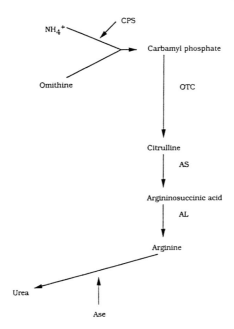

Fig. 5. The urea cycle. Abbreviations: CPS, carbamyl phosphate synthase; AS, argininosuccinic acid synthase; AL, argininosuccinate lyase; Ase, arginase.

gas, electrolytes, bicarbonate, anion gap, liver and renal function tests, coagulation profile, toxicology screen, serum lactate, serum pyruvate, quantitative plasma amino acids, urinalysis including pH and ketones, quantitative urinary organic acids, including orotic acid, urinary carnitine (total and acyl), analysis of cerebrospinal fluid to include glucose, protein, lactate, ammonia and glutamine *(116)* in addition to routine measurements and cultures. Aliquots of the patient's blood, timed urine collection, and CSF should be frozen for later studies as needed.

The results from the above studies which support a diagnosis of OTC deficiency are abnormally high concentrations of blood ammonia and glutamine with low concentrations of citrulline and arginine (products formed downstream of OTC in the urea cycle). Urinary orotic acid excretion will be greatly increased without generalized organic aciduria.

Brain CT is performed, looking for effacement of the ventricles, consistent with cerebral edema, and excluding subdural hematoma or space-occupying lesions. The EEG will have generalized low frequency, high amplitude wave forms and triphasic waves, consistent with a metabolic encephalopathy.

In severe hyperammonemia, tissues other than the brain are saturated with ammonia and glutamine too. The liver can exhibit a toxic hepatitis, with cellular swelling, mitochondrial injury, mildly abnormal serum transaminases, and even liver failure with coagulopathy and mild jaundice. During recovery from an episode, abdominal pain aggravated by meals is common and may reflect not only liver but also bowel smooth muscle recovery from ammonia intoxication. Striated muscle weakness and tremor are notable during the recovery phase.

Liver biopsy should be performed by percutaneous or transjugular approach and a specimen frozen for enzyme analyses. Light microscopy ordinarily reveals some steatosis, no evidence of chronic liver disease, and minimal or no hepatitic component *(117,118)*. Reye's syndrome of encephalopathy and fatty liver is also excluded by liver biopsy *(119,120,121)*. Electron microscopic examination of mitochondria shows minimal abnormalities in individuals with

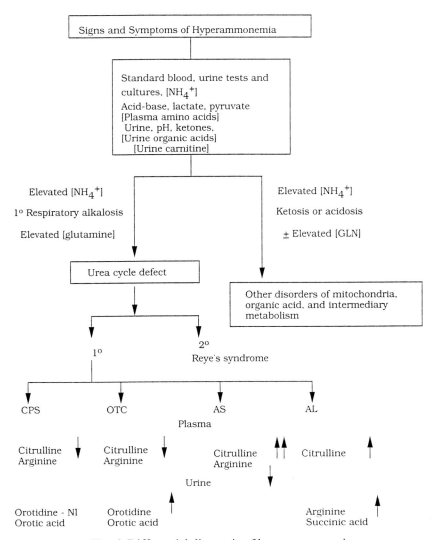

Fig. 6. Differential diagnosis of hyperammonemia.

primary urea cycle defects, whereas drug intoxication or Reye's syndrome is associated with prominent mitochondrial damage *(122,123)*. Enzymatic assay of OTC and a marker enzyme such as CPS will reveal normal CPS activity and profoundly diminished OTC activity rather than a generalized suppression of mitochondrial enzyme activities *(124,125)*.

To confirm the diagnosis, DNA can be extracted from a specimen of peripheral blood, amplified by polymerase chain reaction, and compared with known mutations or sequenced.

5.4. Treatment

The first goal of treatment (Fig. 7) is to remove ammonia and glutamine from tissues, particularly the brain. Hemodialysis is the most efficient emergent treatment since it is performed at the bedside in the intensive care unit, removes approximately 90% of the presented ammonia, and can be continued through multiple passes, then repeated as needed *(126)*.

Ucephan 10% (McGaw Pharmaceuticals) is a fixed formulation of sodium benzoate and sodium phenylacetate which can be given enterally. Buphenyl (Ucyclyd Pharma) is sodium phenylbutyrate, the odorless precursor of phenylacetate. In vivo, benzoate is conjugated with endogenous glycine and the resulting compound, hippurate, is excreted in urine, thus disposing of one potential ammonia molecule for each molecule of benzoate provided. The phenylacetate component similarly combines with glutamine to become phenylacetylglutamine, also excreted in urine and disposing of twice as much ammonia.

The patient with significantly increased intracranial pressure should be intubated with respirator control and may benefit from placement of intracranial monitor and mannitol diuresis.

Metabolic support includes high dose glucose infusion, provision of protein-free nutrition using Intralipid or enteral fat and carbohydrate to prevent catabolism, and restriction of protein intake. Since the patient is demonstrably deficient in arginine and citrulline production, 10% arginine hydrochloride (intravenous, Kabivitrum, Clayton, N.C.) then citrulline (enteral) or arginine free base (enteral) should be given (200 mg/kg/h). HepatAmine (McGaw, Irvine CA) and Hepatic Aid (McGaw, Irvine CA) contain nonessential as well as essential amino acids and are not indicated treatments in spite of the fact that they are used to treat hepatic encephalopathy of other etiologies.

In acutely ill hyperammonemic individuals, all intercurrent complications should be identified and treated promptly. After the episode resolves, the patient can be transferred to a low protein diet and prophylactic Ucephan (2.5 ml/kg/day, maximum 50 mL daily) or Buphenyl. If growth and development have been completed, it is usually not necessary to give supplemental arginine, citrulline or essential amino acid mixtures (EAA).

5.5. Complications

To minimize complications, it is wise to approach the patient's differential diagnosis with an open mind, and to obtain advice from colleagues with special expertise (*see* below). Individuals who have devoted themselves to these uncommon disorders are usually available for consultation, if not directly, certainly by telephone and internet.

It is common for the diagnostic episode of hyperammonemia to be fatal due to brain stem herniation. If the patient survives, structural brain damage with seizure disorder, movement disorder, or irreversible vegetative state are also not rare.

Where the diagnosis and treatment have been prompt and successful, individuals may simply exhibit the signs of attention deficit disorder (ADD) or pervasive deficit disorder (PDD) with left/right reversals, clumsiness, difficulty with numerical concepts, words, or complex motor activities such as driving a car.

Orthotopic liver transplantation and, in the future, hepatocyte transplantation will correct the enzymatic effect and prevent further episodes of hyperammonemia *(127,128)* (Fig. 7).

5.6. Prognosis

The patient remains at lifelong risk for intercurrent hyperammonemia and should be followed at regular intervals for compliance with the medical regimen and verification that plasma ammonia and glutamine are normal.

5.7. Prevention

Identification of affected family members and prenatal diagnosis are possible. Screening adult women with an allopurinol tolerance test, which enhances orotidine and orotic aciduria by inhibiting xanthine oxidase, may reveal other heterozygotes who are asymptomatic *(129)*. The analysis of a 24 hour urine specimen following ingestion of allopurinol 300 mg is a test

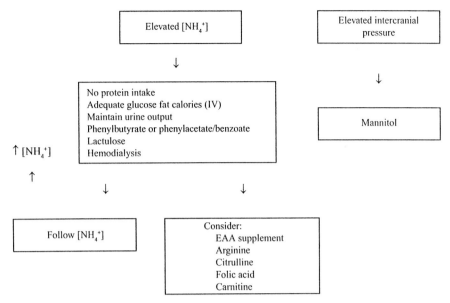

Fig. 7. A scheme for the treatment of hyperammonemia and hepatic coma.

devised by Dr. S. Brusilow and colleagues, which has been standardized only for postmenarchal women. Apparently positive results should be confirmed with DNA analysis so the pregnancies of these women as well as those of the propositus can be monitored with fetal ultrasound to determine if the fetus is male, and assaying OTC activity and DNA in CVS or cultured amniocyte specimens. When infants at risk for urea cycle defects are born, there is a protocol available for prospective treatment to avoid hyperammonemia while confirming or excluding the diagnosis *(101)*.

5.8. Indications for Consulting the Subspecialist

The initial episode will ordinarily require combined input from internist, neurologist, neurosurgeon, hepatologist and subspecialists with special expertise in these disorders. Subsequently supervision can be by the primary physician with assistance as needed from nutritionist, hepatologist and genetic counselor.

6. PATIENT AND PROFESSIONAL INFORMATION SOURCES

1. Cystic Fibrosis Foundation
   6931 Arlington Road
   Bethesda, MD 20814
   (800) FIGHT CF
2. Association for Glycogen Storage Disease
   Box 896
   Durant, IA 52747
   (319) 785-6038
3. National Urea Cycle Disorders Foundation
   1306 45 Avenue North East
   Minneapolis, MN 55421

SUMMARY

Cystic fibrosis, a common autosomal recessive disease, is diagnosed when sweat chloride concentration is > 60 meq/1. More than 600 different mutations are known of which the delta F508 amino acid deletion, is most common. Genotyping is necessary to screen first degree relatives and prevent CF.

Gallstones, biliary cirrhosis and portal hypertension develop in at least 30% of CF patients. As survival improves (current median > 31 yr) CF-associated hepatobiliary disease will become more prevalent.

Survival correlates with severity of pulmonary disease and the quality of medical care, mandating referral to Cystic Fibrosis Centers and coordinated subspecialty management.

Since galactosemia is usually diagnosed by newborn screening for deficient galactose-1-phos phosphate uridyl transferase (GALT) and treatable with milk restriction, life expectancy beyond the neonatal period is normal.

Complications include a toxic hepatitis with residual fibrosis, cataracts, which can be slowly progressive in adulthood, disturbed psychosocial and neurodevelopmental function, and reproductive failure.

The major hepatic glycogenoses are types I, III, IV, VI, and IX. Within each type are multiple subtypes. Types I and III have sequelae of significance to the primary care physician. Type Ib is characterized by neutropenia and risk of recurrent infection. Type IV is fatal in the child unless liver transplantation is performed.

Type I individuals (glucose-6-phosphatase system) require lifelong therapies to maintain glucose homeostasis and surveillance for development of hepatic adenoma and adenocarcinoma. They also are at risk for uric acid nephropathy and chronic glomerulonephritis which can progress to end stage renal disease. Somatic growth and sexual maturation may be delayed in Type I patients.

Type III patients (debranching enzyme) may have liver injury and develop significant portal hypertension. Their hepatic symptoms improve with age; when striated and cardiac muscle are involved, the myopathy may be progressive.

Type VI and IX patients (phosphorylase and phosphorylase kinase deficiencies) are usually asymptomatic or minimally symptomatic with hepatomegaly and short stature, but normal maturation. Rarely cirrhosis, portal hypertension or hepatic tumors can develop in adulthood.

Diminished muscle tone and strength with lax joints, osteoporosis and possibly premature atherosclerosis can complicate the hepatic glycogenoses, especially type I.

Urea cycle enzymopathies (1:30,000 births) are commonly associated with death or profound neurological impairment in infancy due to hyperammonemic coma. Recurrent vomiting with abnormal mental status are symptoms of hyperammonemia in patients with late onset disease (20–25% of cases), particularly female carriers of ornithine transcarbamylase (OTC) deficiency.

Hyperammonemia due to urea cycle disorders is treatable with dietary protein restriction, arginine supplementation, and provision of alternate excretory pathways for ammonia (e.g., phenylacetate).

REFERENCES

1. Welsh MJ, Tsui LC. Boat TF, Beaudet AL. Cystic Fibrosis. In:Scriver CR, Beaudet AL, Sly WS, Valle D, eds. The Metabolic and Molecular Bases of Inherited Disease. 7th ed. New York:McGraw-Hill 1995; 3799–3878.
2. di Sant'Agnese PA, Blanc WA. A distinctive type of biliary cirrhosis of the liver associated with cystic fibrosis of the pancreas. Pediatrics 1956, 18:387-409. Shwachman H, Kowalski M, Khaw K. Cystic fibrosis: a new outlook:75 patients above 25 years of age. Medicine 1977; 56:129–149.

4. di Sant'Agnese PA, Davis PB. Cystic fibrosis in adults: 75 cases and a review of 232 cases in the literature. Am J Med 1979; 66:121–132.

5. Feigelson J, Anagnostopoulos C, Poquet M, Pecau Y, Munck A, Navarro J. Liver cirrhosis in cystic fibrosis— therapeutic implications and long term follow up. Arch Dis Child 1993; 68:653–657.

6. Colombo C, Apostolo MG, Ferrari M, Seia M, Genoni S, Giunta A, Sereni LP. Analysis of risk factors for the development of liver disease associated with cystic fibrosis. J. Pediatr 1994; 124:393–399.

7. Vawter GF, Shwachman H. Cystic fibrosis in adults:an autopsy study. Pathol Ann 1979; 14:357–382.

8. Nagel RA, Westaby D, Javaid A, et al. Liver disease and bile duct abnormalities in adults with cystic fibrosis. Lancet 1989; 2:1422–1425.

9. O'Brien S, Keogan M, Casey M, Duffy G, McErlean D, Fitzgerald MX, Hegarty JE. Biliary complications of cystic fibrosis. Gut 1992; 33:387–391.

10. Waters DL, Dorney SF, Gruca MA, Martin HC, Howman-Giles R, Kan AK, DeSilva M, Gaskin KJ. Hepatobiliary disease in cystic fibrosis patients with pancreatic sufficiency. Hepatology 1995; 21:963-9.

11. Hayes FJ, O'Brien A, O'Brien C, Fitzgerald MX, McKenna MJ. Diabetes mellitus in an adult cystic fibrosis population. Irish Med J 1995; 88:102-104.

12. Lanog S, Thorsteinsson B, Lund-Andersen C, Nerup J, Schiotz PO, Koch C. Diabetes mellitus in Danish cystic fibrosis patients:prevalence and late diabetic complications. Acta Paediatr 1994; 83:72-7.

13. Andersen DH. Cystic fibrosis of the pancreas and its relationship to celiac disease. Am J Dis Child 1938; 56:344–399.

14. Smyth RL, Ashby D, O'Hea U, Burrows E, Lewis P, van Veizen D, Dodge JA. Fibrosing colonopathy in cystic fibrosis:results of a case-control study. Lancet 1995; 346:1247-51.

15. FitzSimmons SC, Burkhart GA, Borowitz D, Grand RJ, Hammerstrom T, Durie PR, Lloyd- Still JD, Lowenfles AB. High-dose pancreatic-enzyme supplements and fibrosing colonopathy in children with cystic fibrosis. N Eng J Med 1997; 336:128–139.

16. Gaffney K, Gibbons D, Keogh B, Fitzgerald MX. Amyloidosis complicating cystic fibrosis. Thorax 1993; 48:949–950.

17. Alvarez-Sala R, Prados C, Sastre Marcos J, Garcia Rio F, Vicandi B, de Ramon A, Vil lamor J. Amyloid goiter and hypothyroidism secondary to cystic fibrosis. Postgrad Med J 1995; 71:307,308.

18. Samuels MH, Thompson N, Leichty D, Ridgway EC. Amyloid goiter in cystic fibrosis. Thyroid 1995; 5:213–215.

19. Grey AB, Ames RW, Matthews RD, Reid IR. Bone mineral density and body composition in adult patients with cystic fibrosis. Thorax 1993; 48:589–593.

20. Bachrach LK, Loutit CW, Moss RB. Osteopenia in adults with cystic fibrosis. Am J Med 1994; 96:27–34.

21. Cotting J, Lentze M, Reichman J. Effects of ursodeoxycholic acid treatment in nutrition and liver function in patients with cystic fibrosis and longstanding cholestasis. Gut 1990; 31:918–921.

22. Colombo C, Castellani MR, Balistreri WF, Seregni E, Assaisso ML, Giunta A. Scintigraphic documentation of an improvement in hepatobiliary excretory function after treatment with ursodeoxycholic acid in patients with cystic fibrosis and associated liver disease. Hepatology 1992; 15:677–684.

23. Colombo C, Crosignami A, Assaisso M, et al. Ursodeoxycholic acid therapy in cystic fibrosis-associated liver disease:a dose-response study. Hepatology 1992; 16:924–930.

24. Colombo C, Bertolini E, Assaisso ML, Bettinardi N, Giunta A, Podda M. Failure of ursodeoxycholic acid to dissolve radiolucent gallstones in patients with cystic fibrosis. Acta Paediatr 1993; 82:562–565.

25. Doershuk CF, Stern RC. Spontaneous bacterial peritonitis in cystic fibrosis. Gut 1994; 35:709–711.

26. Kessler WR, Andersen DH. Heat prostration in fibrocystic disease of the pancreas and other conditions. Pediatr 1951, 8:648–656.

27. Noble-Jamieson G, Valente J, Barnes ND, Friend PJ, Jamieson NV. Rasmussen A, Calne RY. Liver transplantation for hepatic cirrhosis in cystic fibrosis. Arch Dis Child 1994; 71:349–352.

28. Stern RC, Mayes JT, Weber FL Jr, Blades EW, Schulak JA. Restoration of exocrine pancreatic function following pancreas-liver-kidney transplantation in a cystic fibrosis patient. Clin Transplant 1994; 8:1–4.

29. Mack DR, Traystman MD, Colombo JL, Sammut PH, Kaufman SS, Vanderhoof JA, Antonson DL, Markin RS, Shaw BW Jr, Langnas AN. Clinical denouement and mutation analysis of patients with cystic fibrosis undergoing liver transplantation for biliary cirrhosis. J Pediatr 1995; 127:881–887.

30. Rosenfeld M, Davis R, FitzSimmons S, Pepe M, Ramsey B. Gender gap in cystic fibrosis mortality. Amer J Epidemiol 1997; 145:794–803.

31. FitzSimmons SC. Cystic Fibrosis Foundation. Annual Data Report, Bethesda, MD, August 1997.

32. Cloney DL, Sutphen JL, Borowitz SM, Frierson H Jr. Crohn's disease complicating cystic fibrosis. Southern Med J 1994; 87:81–83.

33. Lloyd-Still JD. Crohn's disease and cystic fibrosis. Dig Dis Sci 1994; 39:880–885.

34. Abdul-Karim FW, King TA, Dahms BB, et al. Carcinoma of extrahepatic biliary system in an adult with cystic fibrosis. Gastroenterology 1982, 82:758–762.

35. Sheldon CD, Hodson ME, Carpenter LM, Swerdlow AJ. A cohort study of cystic fibrosis and malignancy. BrJ Cancer 1993; 68:1025–1028.

36. Neglia JP, FitzSimmons SC, Maisonneuve P, Schoni MH, Schoni-Affolter F, Corey M, Lowenfels AB. The risk of cancer among patients with cystic fibrosis. N Engl J Med 1995; 332:494–499.

37. Committee on Genetics. Newborn Screening Fact Sheets. Pediatr 1996;98:473–501.

38. Segal S, Berry GT. Disorders of galactose metabolism. In:Scriver CR, Beaudet AL, Sly WS, Valle D, eds. The Metabolic and Molecular Bases of Inherited Disease. 7th ed. New York:McG raw-Hill 1995; 967–1000.

39. Mason HH, Turner, ME. Chronic galactosemia:report of case with studies on carbohydrates. Am J Dis Child 1935, 50:359–574.

40. Petry K, Greinix HT, Nudelman E, et al. Characterization of a novel biochemical abnormality in galactosemia:deficiency of glycolipids containing galactose or Nacetylgalactosamine and accumulation of precursors in brain and lymphocytes. Biochem Med Metab Biol 1991; 46:93–104.

41. Ornstein KS, McGuire EJ, Berry GT, Roth S, Segal S. Abnormal galactosylation of complex carbohydrates in cultured fibroblasts from patients with galactose-1phosphate uridyl-transferase deficiency. Pediatr Res 1992; 31:508–511.

42. Beigi B, O'Keefe M, Bowell R, Naughten E, Badawi N, Lanigan B. Ophthalmic findings in classical galactosaemia—prospective study. Br J Ophthal 1993; 77:162–164.

43. Hoefnagel D, Wurster-Hili D, Child EL. Ovarian failure in galactosemia. Lancet 1979, 2:1197.

44. Steinmann B, Gitzelmann R, Zachmann M. Hypogonadism and galactosemia. N Engl J Med 1981, 304:464–465.

45. Kaufman FR, Kogut MD, Donnell GN, et al. Hypergonadotropic hypogonadism in female patients with galactosemia. N Engl J Med 1981, 304:994–998.

46. Chen YT, Mattison D, Feigenbaum L, et al. Reduction in oocyte number following prenatal exposure to a high galactose diet. Science 1981, 214:1145–1147.

47. Sauer MV, Kaufman FR, Paulson RJ, Lobo RA. Pregnancy after oocyte donation to a woman with ovarian failure and classical galactosemia. Fert Steril 1991; 55:1197–1199.

48. Irons M, Levy HL, Pueschel S, Castree K. Accumulation of galactose-1-phosphate in the galactosemic fetus despite maternal milk avoidance. J Pediatr 1985, 107:261–263.

49. Jakobs C, Kleijer WJ, Bakker HD, Van Gennip AH, Przyrembel H, Niermeijer MF. Dietary restriction of maternal lactose intake does not prevent accumulation of galactitol in the amniotic fluid of fetuses affected with galactosemia. Prenat Diagn 1988, 8:641–645.

50. Berry GT, Nissim I, Lin Z, Mazur AT, Gibson JB, Segal S. Endogenous synthesis of galactose in normal men and patients with hereditary galactosaemia. Lancet 1995; 346:1073–1074.

51. Levy HL, Sepe SJ, Shih VE, Vawter GF, Klein JO. Sepsis due to Escherichia coli in neonates with galactosemia. N Engl J Med 1977, 297:823-5.

52. Waisbren SE, Norman TR, Schnell RR, Levy HL. Speech and language deficits in early-treated children with galactosemia. J Pediatr 1983, 102:75-7.

53. Nelson CD, Waggoner DD, Donnell GN, TuerckJM, Buist NRM. Verbal dyspraxia in treated galactosemia. Pediatrics 1991; 88:346–350.

54. Koch TK, Schmidt KA, Wagstaff JE, Ng WG, Packman S. Neurologic complications in galactosemia. Pediatr Neurol 1992; 8:217-20.

55. Kaufman FR, Horton EJ, Gott P, WolffJA, Nelson MD, Azen C, Manis FR. Abnormal somatosensory evoked potential in patients with classic galactosemia:correlation with neurologic outcome. J Child Neurol 1995; 10:32–36.

56. Kaufman FR, McBride-Chang C, Manis FR, Wolff JA, Nelson MD. Cognitive functioning, neurologic status and brain imaging in classical galactosemia. Eur J Pediatr 1995; 154(7 suppl 2):52–55.

57. Beutler E, Baluda M, Donnell GN. A new method for the detection of galactosemia and its carrier state. J Lab Clin Med 1964, 64:694–705.

58. Weismann UN, Rose-Beutler B, Schluchter R. Leguminose in the diet:the raffinose stachyose question. Eur J Pediatr 1995; 154(7 suppl 2):S93–96.

59. Kaufman FR, Loro ML, Azen C, Wenz E, Gilsanz V. Effect of hypogonadism and deficient calcium intake on bone density in patients with galactosemia. J Pediatr 1993; 123:365–370.

60. Kaufman FR, Xu YK, Ng WG, Donnell GN. Correlation of ovarian function with galactose-1-phosphate uridyl transferase levels in galactosemia. J Pediatr 1988,112:754–756.

61. Nadler HL, Inouye T, Hsia DYY. Clinical galactosemia:a study of fifty-five cases. In:Hsia DYY, ed. Galactosemia. Springfield, IL:Charles C Thomas, 1969,127–139.

62. Waggoner DD, Buist NRM, Donnell GN. Long-term prognosis in galactosemia:results of a survey of 350 cases. J Inherited Metab Dis 1990; 13:802–818.

63. Waggoner DD, Buist NRM. Long-term complications in treated galactosemia. 175 US cases. Int Pediatr 1993; 8:97–100.

64. Chen YT, Burchell A. Glycogen storage diseases. In:Scriver CR, Beaudet AL, Shy WS, Valle D, eds. The Metabolic and Molecular Bases of Inherited Disease. 7th ed. New York:McG raw-Hill 1995;935–966.

65. Pears JS, Jung RT, Hopwood D, Waddell ID, Burchell A. Glycogen storage disease diagnosed in adults. Quar J Med 1992; 82:207–222.

66. Fellows IW, Lowe JS, Ogilvie AL, Stevens A, Toghill PJ, Atkinson M. Type II glycogenosis presenting as liver disease in adults with atypical histologic features. J Clin Pathol 1983, 36:431–434.

67. Mason HH, Andersen DH. Glycogen disease of the liver (von Gierke's disease) with hepatomata:case report with metabolic studies. Pediatrics 1955, 16:785–799.

68. Chen Y-T, Coleman RA, Scheinman Jl, Kolbeck PC, SidburyJB. Renal disease in type I glycogen storage disease. N Engl J Med 1988, 318:7–11.

69. Chen Y-T, Scheinman Jl, Park HK, Coleman RA, Roe CR. Amelioration of proximal renal tubular dysfunction in type I glycogen storage disease with dietary therapy. N Engl J Med 1990; 323:590–593.

70. Hahn-Ullrich H, Sciuk J, Bartenstein P, Kreysing P, Ullrich K. Effective renal plasma flow in patients with glycogen storage disease type 1. Eur J Pediatr 1993;152:674–676.

71. Labrune P, Trioche P, Duvaltier I, Chevalier P, Odievre M. Hepatocellular adenomas in glycogen storage disease type I and II: a series of 43 patients and review of the literature. J Pediatr Gastroenterol Nutr 1997; 24:276–279.

72. Haagsma EB, Smit GP, Niezen-Konig KE, Gouw AS, Meerman L, Slooff MJ. Type IIIb glycogen storage disease associated with end-stage cirrhosis and hepatocellular carcinoma. Hepatology 1997; 25:537–540.

73. Schwenk WF, Haymond MW. Optimal rate of enteral glucose administration in children with glycogen storage disease type 1. N Engl J Med 1986, 314:682–685.

74. Greene HL, Slonim AK, Burr IM, Moran JR. Type I glycogen storage disease:Five years of management with nocturnal intragastric feeding. J Pediatr 1980, 96:590–595.

75. Slonim AK, Coleman RA, Moses WS. Myopathy and growth failure in debrancher enzyme deficiency:improvement with high-protein nocturnal enteral therapy. J Pediatr 1984, 105:906–911.

76. Smit G PA, Berger R, Potasnick R, Moses SW, Fernandes J. The dietary treatment of children with Type I glycogen storage disease with slow release carbobydrate. Pediatr Res 1984, 18:879–881.

77. Chen Y-T, Cornblath M, Sidbury JB. Cornstarch therapy in type I glycogen storage disease. N Engl J Med 1984, 310:171–175.

78. Chen YT, Bazzarre CH, Lee MM, Sidbury JB, Coleman RA. Type I glycogen storage disease:nine years of management with cornstarch. Eur J Pediatr 1993; 152(suppl 1):S56–59.

79. Wolfsdorf Jl, Keller RJ, Landy H, Crigler JF. Glucose therapy for glycogenosis type 1 in infants:comparison of intermittent uncooked cornstarch and continuous overnight glucose feedings. J Pediatr 1990; 117:384–390.

80. Goldberg T, Slonim AK. Nutrition therapy for hepatic glycogen storage diseases. J Am Dietetic Assoc 1993; 93:1423–1430.

81. Wolfsdorf Jl, Crigler JR Jr. Biochemical evidence for the requirement of continuous glucose therapy in young adults with type 1 glycogen storage disease. J Inherited Metab Dis 1994; 17:234–241.

82. Obara K, Saito T, Sato H, Ogawa M, Igarashi Y, Yoshinaga K. Renal histology in two adult patients with type I glycogen storage disease. Clin Nephrol 1993; 39:59–64.

83. Couper R, Kapelushnik J, Griffiths AM. Neutrophil dysfunction in glycogen storage disease Ib:association with Crohn's-like colitis. Gastroenterology 1991;100:549–554.

84. Schroten H, Roesler J, Breidenbach T, et al. Granylocyte and granulocytemacrophage colony-stimulating factors for treatment of neutropenia in glycogen storage disease type 1 b. J Pediatr 1991; 119:748–754.

85. Roe TF, Coates TD, Thomas DW, Miller JH, Gilsanz V. Brief report:treatment of chronic inflammatory bowel disease in glycogen storage disease type Ib with colony stimulating factors. N Engl J Med 1992; 326:1666–1669.

86. Hurst D, Kilpatrick L, Becker J, Lipani J, Kleman K, Perrine S, Douglas SD. Recombinant human GM-CSF treatment of neutropenia in glycogen storage disease 1b. AmJ Ped Hematol-Oncol 1993; 15:71–76.

87. Ishiguro A, Nakahata T, Shimbo T, et al. Improvement of neutropenia and neutrophil dysfunction by granulocyte colony-stimulating factor in a patient with glycogen storage disease type 1 b. Eur J Pediatr 1993; 152:18–20.

88. McCawley LJ, Korchak HM, Douglas SD, Campbell DE, Thornton PS, Stanley CA, Baker L, Kilpatrick L. In vitro and in vivo effects of granulocyte colony-stimulating factor on neutrophils in glycogen storage disease type 1b:granulocyte colony stimulating factor therapy corrects the neutropenia and the defects in respiratory burst activity and Ca2+ mobilization. Pediatr Res 1994; 35:84–90.

89. Ockner RK, Kaikaus RM, Bass NM. Fatty-acid metabolism and the pathogenesis of hepatocellular carcinoma:review and hypothesis. Hepatology 1993; 18:669–676.

90. LimmerJ, Fleig WE, Leupold D, Bittner R, Ditschuneit H, Beger H-G. Hepatocellular carcinoma in type I glycogen storage disease. Hepatology 1988, 8:531–537.

91. Rosh JR, Collins JC, Groisman GM, Schwersenz AH, Schwartz M, Miller CM, LeLeiko NS. Management of hepatic adenoma in glycogen storage disease la. J Pediatr Gastroenterol Nutr 1995; 20:225–228.

92. Yokoyama K, Hayashi H, Hinoshita F, et al. Renal lesion of type la glycogen storage disease:the glomerular size and renal localization of apolipoprotein. Nephron 1995; 70:348–352.

93. Lee PJ, Celermajer DS, Robinson J, McCarthy SN, Betteridge DJ, Leonard JV. Hyperlipidaemia does not impair vascular endothelial function in glycogen storage d isease type 1 a. Atherosclerosis 1994; 110:95–100.

94. Levy E, Thibault L, Turgeon J, Roy CC, Gurbindo C, Lepage G, Godard M, Rivard GE, Seidman E. Beneficial effects of fish-oil supplements on lipids, lipoproteins, and lipoprotein lipase in patients with glycogen storage disease type 13. Am J Clin Nutr 1993; 57:922–929.

95. Lee PJ, Patel A, Hindmarsh PC, Mowat AP, Leonard JV. The prevalence of polycystic ovaries in the hepatic glycogen storage diseases:its association with hyperinsulinism. Clin Endocrinol 1995; 42:601–606.

96. Farber M, Knuppel RA, Binkiewicz A, Kennison RD. Pregnancy and von Gierke's disease. Obstetr Gynecol 1976, 47:226–228.

97. Johnson MP, Compton A, Drugan A, Evans Ml. Metabolic control of von Gierke disease (glycogen storage disease type la) in pregnancy:maintenance of euglycemia with cornstarch. Obstetr Gynecol 1990; 75:507–510.

98. Ryan IP, Havel RJ, Laros RK Jr. Three consecutive pregnancies in a patient with glycogen storage disease type IA (von Gierke's disease). Am J Obstetr Gynecol 1994; 170:1687–1690.

99. Ohura T, Inoue CN, Abukawa D, et al. Progressive pulmonary hypertension:a fatal complication of type I glycogen storage disease. J Inherited Metab Dis 1995; 18:361,362.

100. Talente GM, Coleman RA, Alter C, et al. G Iycogen storage disease in adults (review). Ann Intern Med 1994; 120:218–226.

101. Brusilow SW, Horwich AL. Urea cycle enzymes. In:Scriver CR, Beaudet AL, Sly WS, Valle D, eds. The Metabolic and Molecular Bases of Inherited Disease. 7th ed. New York:McGraw-Hill 1995; 1187–1232.

102. Brusilow SW. Urea cycle disorders:clinical paradigm of hyperammonemic encephalopathy. Chapter 12. In:Boyer JL, Ockner RK, eds. Progress in Liver Diseases. Philadelphia:WB Saunders 1995; 293–309.

103. Tallan HH, Schaffer F, Taffet SL, Schneidman K, Gaull GE. Ornithine carbamoyltransferase deficiency in an adult male patient:significance of hepatic ultrastructure in clinical diagnosis. Pediatr 1983; 71:224–232.

104. DiMagno EP, Lowe JF, Snodgrass PJ, Jones JD. Ornithine DiMagno EP, Lowe JF, Snodgrass PJ, Jones JD. Ornithine transcarbamylase deficiency - a cause of bizarre behavior in a man. N Engl J Med 1986; 315:744–747.

105. Gilchrist JM, Coleman RA. Ornithine transcarbamylase deficiency:adult onset of severe symptoms. Ann Intern Med 1987; 106:556–558.

106. Call G, Seay AR, Sherry R, Qureshi TA. Clinical features of carbamyl phosphate synthetase-1-deficiency in an adult. Ann Neurol 1984; 16:90–93.

107. Snebold NG, Rizzo JF, Lessel S, Pruett RC. Transient visual loss in ornithine transcarbamylase deficiency. Am J Ophthal 1987, 104:407–412.

108. Arn PH, Hauser ER, Thomas GH, Herman G, Hess D, Brusilow SW. Hyperammonemia in women with a mutation at the ornithine carbamoyltransferase locus. N Engl J Med 1990; 322:1652–1655.

109. Brusilow SW, Finkelstein JE. Restoration of nitrogen homeostasis in a man with ornithine transcarbamylase deficiency. Metabolism 1993; 42:1336–1339.

110. Wong IJC, Craigen WJ, O'Brien WE. Post-partum coma and death due to carbamoylphosphate synthetase I deficiency. Ann Intern Med 1994; 120:216,217.

111. Wilson BE, Hobbs WN, Newmark JJ, Farrow SJ. Rapidly fatal hyperammonemic coma i n adults. U rea cycle enzyme deficiency. West Med J 1994; 161:166–168.

112. Yoshino M, Nishiyori J, Yamashita F, Kumashiro R, et al. Ornithine transcarbamylase deficiency in male adolescence and adulthood. Enzyme 1990; 43:160–168.

113. Felig DM, Brusilow SW, Boyer JL. Hyperammonemic coma due to total parenteral nutrition in an adult woman with heterozygous ornithine transcarbamylase deficiency. Gastroenterology 1995; 109:282–284.

114. Matsudo Y, Tsuji A, Katunuma N. Qualitative abnormality of liver argininosuccinase in a patient with citrullinemia. Adv Exp Med Biol 1982, 153:77–81.

115. Moser HW, Efron ML, Brown H, Diamond R, Neumann CG. Argininosuccinic aciduria:report of two cases and demonstration of intermittent elevation of blood ammonia. Am J Med 1967, 42:9–26.

116. Hourani BT, Hamlin EM, Reynolds TB. Cerebrospinal fluid as a measure of hepatic encephalopathy. Arch Intern Med 1971, 127:1033–1066.

117. LaBrecque DR, Latham PS, Riely CA, Hsia YE, Klatskin G. Heritable urea cycle enzyme deficiency in liver disease in 16 patients. J Pediatr 1979, 94:580–587.

118. Zimmerman A, Bachmann C, Baumgartner R. Severe liver fibrosis in argininosuccinic aciduria. Arch Pathol Lab Med 1986, 110:136–140.

119. Reye RDK, Morgan G, Baral J. Encephalopathy and fatty degeneration of the viscera:a disease entity in childhood. Lancet 1963, 2:749–752.

120. Wigger HJ. Frozen section of liver in the diagnosis of Reye syndrome. Am J Surg Path 1977, 1:271–174.
121. Badizadegan K, Perez-Atayde AR. Focal glycogenosis of the liver in disorders of ureagenesis:its occurrence and diagnostic significance. Hepatology 1997; 26:365–673.
122. Partin JC, Schubert WK, Partin JS. Mitochondrial ultrastructure in Reye's syndrome (encephalopathy and fatty degeneration of the viscera). N Engl J Med 1971, 285:1339–1343.
123. Latham PS, LaBrecque DR, McReynolds JW, Klatskin G. Liver ultrastructure in mitochondrial urea cycle enzyme deficiencies and comparison with Reye's syndrome. Hepatology 1984, 4:404–407.
124. Brown T, Brown H, Hug G. Carbamoylphosphate synthetase and ornithine transcarbamylase in liver of Reye's syndrome. N Engl J Med 1974, 291:797–798.
125. Snodgrass PJ, DeLong GR. Urea cycle enzyme deficiencies and an increased nitrogen load producing hyperammonemia in Reye's syndrome. N Engl J Med 1976, 294:855–860.
126. Neu AM, Christenson MJ, Brusilow SW, Nissenson RA. In:Fine RN, ed. Dialysis Therapy. 2nd ed. Philadelphia:Hanley and Belfus 1992; 371,372.
127. Hasegawa T, Tzakis AG, Todo S., Reyes J, Nour B, Finegold DN, Starzl TE. Orthotopic liver transplantation for ornithine transcarbamylase deficiency with hyperammonemic encephalopathy. J Pediatr Surg 1995; 30:863.
128. Jan D, Poggi F, Jouvet P, Rabier D, Laurent J, Beringer A, Hubert P, Sandlebray JM, Revillon Y. Definitive cure of hyperammonemia by liver transplantation in urea cycle defects:report of three cases. Transplant Proc 1994; 26:188.
129. Hauser ER, Finkelstein JE, Valle D, Brusilow SW. Allopurinol-induced orotidinuria. A test for mutations at the ornithine carbamoyltransferase locus in women. N Engl J Med 1990; 322:1641–1645.

VIII Women and Liver Diseases

26 Pregnancy and Liver Disease

Francis Ruiz and Caroline A. Riely

CONTENTS

1. INTRODUCTION

Liver diseases during pregnancy are particularly important for the primary care physician, because a diagnosis and/or treatment is often required in a timely fashion.

1.1. Normal Physiological Changes During Pregnancy

There are many physiologic changes that occur during pregnancy. The plasma blood volume expands during pregnancy by approx 45–55%. This leads to an increased volume of distribution, with a resultant decrease in hemoglobin, and urea nitrogen. Albumin levels decrease from an average of 4.2 g/dL in the nonpregnant state to 3.1 g/dL near parturition due to the relative increase in plasma volume *(1)*. Also, there is an increase in serum alkaline phosphatase levels beginning around the fifth month of pregnancy and rising to two- to fourfold above normal values by term. This is due to entry of placental alkaline phosphatase into maternal blood *(2)*. Factors VII and IX, fibrinogen, cholesterol, and triglyceride levels rise as well. In contrast, 5'-nucleotidase, GGT, ALT, AST, and bilirubin levels remain normal in the absence of liver disease. The most common characteristics, found in up to two thirds of normal pregnancies, are spider nevi, primarily on the upper trunk and face, and palmar erythema *(3)*. In the individual without liver disease, these findings disappear after delivery.

2. LIVER DISEASES UNIQUE TO PREGNANCY (*SEE* TABLE 1)

2.1. Hyperemesis Gravidarum

In 60%–90% of all normal pregnancies, mild nausea and vomiting occur early in gestation. Hyperemesis gravidarum is a state of severe nausea and vomiting that occurs in approx 1% of pregnancies. It is a common condition that usually presents in the first trimester, and can be lethal.

From: *Diseases of the Liver and Bile Ducts: Diagnosis and Treatment*
Edited by: G. Y. Wu and J. Israel © Humana Press Inc., Totowa, NJ

2.3.1.2. Laboratory. A microangiopathic hemolysis is manifested by low haptoglobin, high LDH levels, and the presence of schistocytes. There is an increase in levels of aminotransferases from 2–20-fold above normal with a mean of 150 IU/L, and mildly elevated bilirubin. Platelets are low (<100,000/mm^3) secondary to increased platelet aggregation. However, the PT and PTT remain normal. This is helpful in differentiating HELLP syndrome from acute fatty liver of pregnancy.

2.3.2. TREATMENT AND PROGNOSIS

The only definitive treatment is delivery of the fetus. If the condition develops after the 36th wk and maturity of the fetal lungs is demonstrated, delivery is recommended. In cases that develop before the 36th wk, the optimal treatment is not clear. There is some evidence to support the benefit of controlling the eclampsia, and postponing delivery to administer corticosteroids for acceleration of fetal lung maturation *(19)*. Because laboratory abnormalities in the mother peak in the first 2 d postpartum, supportive care and especially administration of blood products are required during this period. The maternal mortality rate is 1–3%.

2.3.3. COMPLICATIONS

Spontaneous hepatic rupture, a dreaded complication of the HELLP syndrome, should be suspected when a patient develops abdominal distention, severe abdominal pain, and a sudden drop in hematocrit and blood pressure. Paracentesis reveals hemoperitoneum and the prognosis, at this time, is very poor. CT scan or MRI are useful in demonstrating hepatic rupture *(20)*. Other complications include disseminated intravascular coagulation (20%), abruptio placentae (16%), acute renal failure (7%), and pulmonary edema (6%) *(16)*. The mortality rate for infants born to mothers with HELLP is high, on the order of 35%. However, the mortality rates vary considerably, depending on the maturity of the fetus at the time of delivery and the severity of the syndrome in the mother *(21)*.

2.3.4. PREVENTION

Because HELLP syndrome always presents in patients with pre-eclampsia, standard measures to reduce the risk of developing pre-eclampsia, and prompt treatment when it occurs should reduce the risk of developing HELLP.

2.4. Acute Fatty Liver of Pregnancy

This is a rare and potentially fatal disease that occurs with a frequency of approx 1 in 13,000, usually occurring during the third trimester *(22)* (*see* Chapter 7, this volume). The cause of this disease is unknown, and there may be overlap in laboratory findings between HELLP syndrome and acute fatty liver of pregnancy.

2.4.1. DIAGNOSIS

2.4.1.1. Symptoms and Signs. The patient is often nulliparous, close to term, in the third trimester, and presents with nausea and vomiting, epigastric pain, anorexia, and jaundice. Some patients will have symptoms of liver failure, including hypoglycemia, coagulopathy, and encephalopathy. On physical examination, the patient may have hypotension, peripheral edema, abdominal pain, and the liver is frequently small.

2.4.1.2. Laboratory. Laboratory values usually show an increased PT and PTT, with a decrease in fibrinogen level. Also, aminotransferases are increased in the range of 300 IU/L. Serum ammonia levels, as well as bilirubin and alkaline phosphatase, are usually increased although albumin is decreased. The white cell count is usually increased to >15,000/mm^3 and DIC may be present *(23)*. There may be renal involvement with increased creatinine, proteinuria, and low urine output *(24)*. Pre-eclampsia is present in 50% or more of patients affected with acute fatty liver of pregnancy. Although not usually necessary in typical cases, a liver biopsy can differentiate an atypical presentation of acute fatty liver of pregnancy from many other disorders. Typical histologic features include ballooned pale hepatocytes due to accumulation of microvesicular fat. Frozen sections stained with oil red O can demonstrate the fat *(23,25)*.

2.4.2. TREATMENT AND PROGNOSIS

The treatment is supportive care and delivery. This disease can be complicated by acute pancreatitis, gastrointestinal bleeding, hepatic coma, disseminated intravascular coagulation, and sometimes patients require hemodialysis. Also, the use of lactulose therapy may be required for control of encephalopathy. All attempts should be made to deliver the baby promptly. Despite severe hepatic necrosis, there is no progression to cirrhosis *(26)*.

3. EFFECTS OF PREGNANCY ON USUAL LIVER DISEASES

Women with liver disease do not have an increased risk for having children with congenital anomalies. However, they do have more gestational problems, and an increased risk for prematurity or stillbirth.

3.1. Cirrhosis and Portal Hypertension

There is increased risk of bleeding from esophageal varices in pregnant females with portal hypertension. Portal hypertension due to prehepatic venous obstruction is less often associated with spontaneous abortions, prematurity, and prenatal mortality than is portal hypertension due to cirrhosis. Sclerotherapy is the treatment of choice for bleeding esophageal varices in this setting. Vasopressin is contraindicated because it may induce labor.

3.2. Chronic and Acute Hepatitis

Viral hepatitis is the most common cause of jaundice in pregnancy in the United States.

3.2.1. CHRONIC HEPATITIS B

In general, pregnancy is well-tolerated in patients with hepatitis B (*see* Chapter 9, this volume). The placenta is an excellent barrier for preventing transmission, and only when transplacental leakage occurs, or at amniocentesis, is the fetus at risk for intrauterine transmission. Transmission to the infant takes place during delivery, rather than *in utero*, and occurs in 80% of the cases if the mother is HBeAg-positive, compared to 39% if she is HBeAg-negative. Infants of HBsAg-positive mothers should receive HBIG (0.5 mL) within 12 h of birth, as well as the first dose of hepatitis B vaccine. Also, all infants should receive the vaccine at birth *(27)*.

3.2.2. CHRONIC HEPATITIS C

Hepatitis C virus (HCV) is transmitted from mother to fetus less commonly than hepatitis B (*see* Chapter 10, this volume). Vertical transmission of hepatitis C occurs in 6% of newborns at risk. There is an increased risk of transmission of hepatitis C in women coinfected with HIV due to high levels of HCV viremia. Passive immunoprophylaxis with immunoglobulin is ineffective *(28)*.

3.2.3. ACUTE HEPATITIS A

There is no evidence that infection with hepatitis A (*see* Chapter 8) is more common or more severe in pregnancy. If the mother is viremic at delivery, there is an increased risk to the fetus and passive immunoglobulin prophylaxis for the newborn is indicated *(28)*.

3.2.4. HEPATITIS E

Like hepatitis A, hepatitis E is enterically transmitted (*see* Chapter 8, this volume). Vertical transmission is known to occur. It is associated with an extremely high maternal mortality during pregnancy (up to 20%), with a high rate of fetal loss. Hepatitis E occurs commonly in Asia, Africa, the Middle East, and Mexico. Serologic tests to detect antibodies to HEV and the virus RNA have been developed *(28)* (*see* Chapter 3, this volume).

3.2.5. HERPES SIMPLEX HEPATITIS

This infection may be associated with fulminant hepatic failure in the relatively immunocompromised state of pregnancy. Clinically, patients will have a prodrome of fever, malaise, and upper respiratory symptoms in the third trimester, usually lasting between 4 d and 2 wk. The patient presents with right upper quadrant pain, and may have cutaneous herpetic lesions on physical examination. Laboratory values show normal to moderate increases in bilirubin and very high aminotransferase levels, often >1000 IU/L. Coagulopathy is present in 91% of cases, and the ammonia level may be increased. CT scan has been reported to show multiple low density, nonenhancing areas, consistent with multifocal hemorrhagic necrosis. The risk of infection to infants of affected mothers with a primary episode of HSV at delivery is 33–50% as opposed to 3–5% in cases of recurrent HSV *(29)*. In one study of 14 patients, a maternal mortality rate of 43% has been reported *(29)*. A liver biopsy may be required to make the diagnosis. Typical intranuclear inclusion bodies are characteristic histologic findings. The patient should be started on acyclovir, because the outcome may be fatal. Prompt therapy has been reported to enhance the probability of survival *(29)*.

4. AUTOIMMUNE DISORDERS

4.1. Autoimmune Hepatitis

Autoimmune hepatitis is a clinical syndrome (*see* Chapter 11, this volume) that responds to corticosteroids alone or in combination with azathioprine. Patients should be kept on the same prepregnancy dose of immunosuppression required to maintain remission. Azathioprine has not been shown to be teratogenic in this setting of low-dose therapy. These patients are at increased risk for pre-eclampsia, prematurity, and increased fetal wastage *(30)*.

4.2. Primary Biliary Cirrhosis

Although bilirubin levels can remain unchanged or even decrease in pregnant women with PBC (*see* Chapter 15, this volume), most of the reported cases have shown an increase in cholestasis and its associated itching during the third trimester, resolving after delivery *(31)*.

4.3. Other/Miscellaneous Disorders

4.3.1. HEPATIC NEOPLASIA

Hepatic adenomas are at risk of enlarging under the effects of high levels of sex steroids seen in pregnancy, and rupture into the peritoneum may result.

4.3.2. ACUTE PORPHYRIA

The acute neurologic porphyrias consist of acute intermittent porphyria, variegate porphyria, and hereditary coproporphyria (*see* Chapter 19, this volume). Acute intermittent porphyria is the most common and severe. A female preponderance suggests that hormones may play a role in the phenotypic expression. Pregnancy, through the effects of estrogen, can exacerbate the disease by stimulating delta aminolevulinic acid synthesis. Management consists of avoiding any precipitating agents such as alcohol, starvation, and infection. Treatment of acute episodes involves glucose infusion and high carbohydrate diet, in order to suppress traffic through the blocked enzymatic pathway. In refractory cases, iv administration of hematin is needed (32).

4.3.3. Familial Hyperbilirubinemia

The unconjugated hyperbilirubinemia of Gilbert's syndrome (*see* Chapter 14) is not exacerbated by pregnancy. The Dubin-Johnson syndrome is characterized by chronic, familial jaundice and deposition of a dark pigment inside hepatocytes (*see* Chapter 14, this volume). Eighty percent of patients are asymptomatic during pregnancy, but some may experience symptoms such as fatigue, anorexia, abdominal pain, and progressive jaundice, peaking in the third trimester, then returning to normal after delivery. Alkaline phosphatase and other liver enzyme levels are normal. The diagnosis can be confirmed after delivery by a nuclear medicine scan (HIDA) and liver biopsy. There is increased risk of prematurity, spontaneous abortion, and stillbirth, but the mother's prognosis is excellent *(33)*.

4.4. Liver Transplantation

Pregnancy has frequently been reported after liver transplantation. Patients with allografts have increased risk of hypertension, pre-eclampsia, and premature delivery. Pregnancy does not have an adverse effect on liver function or survival *(34)*.

5. EFFECTS OF ALCOHOL AND LIVER DISEASE ON FERTILITY

5.1. Alcohol

Alcohol-related injury to various organs, including, but not limited to, the liver can impair reproductive function.

5.1.1. Effects in Males

Alcohol affects the normal function of testes, pituitary, hypothalamus, and adrenal glands. Males who are chronic alcoholics are both hypogonadal and feminized, as manifested by testicular atrophy, impotence, and loss of libido. This is related to toxicity of alcohol and acetaldehyde within the testes, suppression of LH, FSH secretion from the anterior pituitary, and decreased testosterone binding affinity for sex hormone-binding globulin. Feminization is manifested by the presence of a female escutcheon and body habitus, palmar erythema, spider angiomata, and gynecomastia, and may be related to high levels of estrogen. Abstinence from alcohol may result in spontaneous recovery of sexual function, but not in men with testicular atrophy. Several therapeutic trials have been conducted with treatments, but only single-dose oral testosterone has been shown to be beneficial in some.

5.1.2. Effects in Females

One of every three alcoholic persons in the United States is a woman. Chronic alcoholic women are not superfeminized, but instead have severe hypogonadism. Failure of the ovaries is manifested by reduced plasma levels of estradiol and progesterone, loss of secondary sexual characteristics, such as breast and pelvic fat, and ovulatory failure. Unlike men, steroid production in the woman is not acutely altered by alcohol *(35)*.

5.2. Chronic Liver Diseases

In general, hypogonadism is less prevalent, and less severe in nonalcoholic liver disease.

5.2.1. Hemochromatosis (*see* Chapter 18)

Gonadal failure is characterized by reduced libido, impotence, reduction in sexual body hair, gynecomastia, and loss of spermatogosis due to testicular atrophy. Serum estrogen levels are normal. Phlebotomy does not improve impotence. However, chronic administration of human chorionic gonadotropin increases testosterone. Alternatively, testosterone itself can be administered. Gonadal effects in female patients have not been reported, because the disease is usually manifested after menopause.

5.2.2. WILSON'S DISEASE (SEE CHAPTER 21)

Copper accumulation does not occur in the gonads or the pituitary. A stimulation of secretion of all anterior pituitary hormones except prolactin occurs, perhaps resulting in normal gonadal function.

5.2.3. AUTOIMMUNE HEPATITIS (SEE CHAPTER 11)

This is a disease of young women who often develop amenorrhea at the onset of the disease. When the disease becomes inactive with corticosteroids, the menses return and the patient may become pregnant (36).

5.3. Portal Hypertension

Patients with noncirrhotic portal hypertension (see Chapter 29, this volume) are more likely to become pregnant than patients with cirrhotic portal hypertension because, in the latter, ovulation is markedly reduced (36).

6. ORAL CONTRACEPTIVES AND THE LIVER

6.1. Cholestasis

Oral contraceptives impair bile excretion by interfering with uptake of bile acids from sinusoidal blood. Cholestasis in patients on oral contraceptives was a clinical problem when these drugs were introduced in the 1960s. The jaundice is characterized as the cholestatic canalicular type. The onset is insidious within 1 wk to 1 mo of treatment. This liver damage, originally associated with high/medium doses, is not seen with low doses now in use (37).

6.2. Hepatic Adenoma

Hepatic adenoma, a benign liver tumor, can present with a painless or painful right upper abdominal mass (vascular), or when ruptured, as hemoperitoneum. Most cases occur in women who are of child-bearing age. However, it can also occur in men taking androgenic steroids. In most instances, hepatic adenomas regress when oral contraceptives use is discontinued. Rarely, hepatic resection by enucleation, combined with hepatic vascular exclusion, is necessary to prevent unpredictable hemorrhage. Malignant transformation to hepatocellular carcinoma can rarely occur (38).

6.3. Focal Nodular Hyperplasia

Focal nodular hyperplasia (FNH) is a benign tumor composed of hepatocytes and Kupffer cells, which occurs in women, usually as an asymptomatic incidental finding. Whereas there is a strong association between oral contraceptives and hepatic adenoma, the association of FNH with oral contraceptive has not been firmly established. A pre-existing FNH lesion may increase in size under the influence of oral contraceptives, and hemorrhage and necrosis can occur in this setting. There is no evidence that FNH can undergo malignant transformation (39,40).

6.4. Fibrolamellar Carcinoma

This liver tumor can be difficult to differentiate from FNH and hepatic adenoma. Electron microscopy is useful in arriving at the correct diagnosis. Simultaneous occurrence of FNH and fibrolamellar carcinoma has been seen.

6.5. Hepatic Vein Thrombosis (Budd-Chiari Syndrome)

Oral contraceptives and pregnancy have been associated with development of a hypercoagulable state. Patients with hepatic vein thrombosis develop ascites, abdominal discomfort, and abnormal serum liver tests. Doppler ultrasound is useful in diagnosis, and liver biopsy is an important adjunct in diagnosis.

6.6. Peliosis Hepatis

Peliosis hepatis consists of large blood-filled cavities of various sizes with sinusoidal dilatation, but no endothelial lining. Most cases are secondary to oral contraceptives and anabolic steroids. However, it has also been associated with cat-scratch disease (*Rochalimaea henselae*) in patients with AIDS, or with the use of tomoxifen, and Danazol. It is seldom diagnosed by liver biopsy.

SUMMARY

During pregnancy many serum values are altered due to normal physiological changes in the mother.

Hyperemesis gravidarum can result in liver dysfunction and occurs in the first trimester.

Intrahepatic cholestasis of pregnancy, acute fatty liver of pregnancy, and the HELLP syndrome usually manifest themselves in the second or third trimester.

REFERENCES

1. Elliott JR, O'Kell RT. Normal clinical chemical values for pregnant women at term. Clin Chem 1971;17:156,157.
2. Zuckerman H, Sadovsky E, Kallner B. Serum alkaline phosphatase in pregnancy and puerperium. Obstet Gynecol 1995;39:819–824.
3. Burroughs AK. Liver disease and pregnancy. In: Mcintyre N, Benhamou J-P, Bircher J, Rizzeto M, Rodes J, eds. Oxford textbook of clinical hepatology. Oxford University Press, New York, 1991, pp. 1321–1332.
4. Abell TA, Riely CA. Hyperemesis gravidarum. Gastroenterol Clin North Am 1992;21:835–849.
5. Adams RH, Gordon J, Combes B. Hyperemesis gravidarum. I. Evidence of hepatic dysfunction. Obstet Gynecol 1968;31:659–664.
6. Wallstedt A, Riely CA, Shaver D, et al. Prevalence and characteristics of liver dysfunction in hyperemesis gravidarum. Clin Res 1990;38:970A.
7. Kallen B. Hyperemesis during pregnancy and delivery outcome: a registry study. Eur J Obstet Gynecol Reprod Biol 1987;26:292–302.
8. Gross S, Librach C, Cecutti A. Maternal weight loss associated with hyperemesis gravidarum: a predictor of fetal outcome. Am J Obstet Gynecol 1989;160:906–909.
9. Holzbach RT, Sivak D, Braun D. Familial recurrent intrahepatic cholestasis of pregnancy: a genetic study providing evidence for transmission of a sex-limited, dominant trait. Gastroenterology 1983;85:175–185.
10. Reyes H. The spectrum of liver and gastrointestinal disease seen in cholestasis of pregnancy. Gastroenterol Clin North Am 1992;21:905–921.
11. Berg B, Helm G, Petersohn L, et al. Cholestasis of pregnancy. Acta Obstet Gynecol Scand1986;65:107–113.
12. Riely CA. The liver in pregnancy. In: Schiff L, Schiff E, eds. Diseases of the liver, 7th ed. Lippincott, Philadelphia, 1993, pp. 1059–1073.
13. Reid R, Ivey K, Rencoret RH, Storey B. Fetal complications of obstetric cholestasis. BMJ 1976;1:870–872.
14. Lunzer M, Barnes P, Byth K, O'Halloran M. Serum bile acid concentrations during pregnancy and their relationship to obstetric cholestasis. Gastroenterology 1986;91:825–829.
15. Steven MM. Pregnancy and liver disease. Gut 1981;22:592–614.
16. Sibai BM, Ramadan MK, Usta I, Salama M, Mercer, BM, Friedman SA. Maternal morbidity and mortality in 442 pregnancies with hemolysis, elevated liver enzymes and low platelets (HELLP syndrome). Am J Obstet Gynecol 1993;169:1000–1006.
17. Sibai BM. The HELLP syndrome: (hemolysis, elevated liver enzymes, and low platelet count): much ado about nothing? Am J Obstet Gynecol 1990;162:311–316.
18. Rolfes DB, Ishak KG. Liver disease in toxemia of pregnancy. Am J Gastroenterol 1986;81:1138–1144.

19. Magann EF, Bass D, Chauhan SP, Sullivan DL, Martin, RW, Martin JN Jr. Antepartum corticosteroids: disease stabilization in patients with the syndrome of hemolysis, elevated liver enzymes, and low platelets (HELLP). Am J Obstet Gynecol 1994;171:1148–1153.
20. Barton JR, Sibai BM. Care of the pregnancy complicated by HELLP syndrome. Gastroenterol Clin North Am 1992;21:937–950.
21. Sibai BM, Taslimi MM, el-Nazer A, Amon E, Mabie BC, Ryan GM. Maternal-perinatal outcome associated with the syndrome of hemolysis, elevated liver enzymes, and low platelets in severe pre-eclampsia and eclampsia. Am J Obstet Gynecol 1986;155:501–509.
22. Riely CA, Latham, PS, Romero R et al. Acute fatty liver of pregnancy: a reassessment based on onservations in nine patients. Ann Int Med 1987;7:55–58.
23. Kaplan MM. Acute fatty liver of pregnancy. N Engl J Med 1985;313:367–370.
24. Bacq Y, Riely CA. Acute fatty liver of pregnancy: the hepatologist's view. Gastroenterologist 1993;1:397–364.
25. Rolfes DB, Ishak KG. Acute fatty liver of pregnancy: a clinicopathologic study of 35 cases. Hepatology 1985;5:1149–1158.
26. Riely CA. Acute fatty liver of pregnancy. Semin Liver Dis 1987;7:47–54.
27. Ayoola EA, Johnson AOK. Hepatitis B vaccine in pregnancy: immunogenicity, safety, and transfer of antibodies to infants. Int J Gynaecol Obstet 1987;39:297–301.
28. Mishra L, Seeff LB. Viral hepatitis, A through E, complicating pregnancy. Gastroenterol Clin North Am 1992;21:873–887.
29. Klein NA, Mabie W, Shaver DC, et al. Herpes simplex virus hepatitis in pregnancy: two patients successfully treated with acyclovir. Gastroenterology 1991;100:239–244.
30. Lee MG, Hanchard B, Donalson EK, et al. Pregnancy in chronic active hepatitis with cirrhosis. J Trop Med Hyg 1987;90:245–248.
31. Nir A, Sorokin Y, Abramovici H, et al. Pregnancy and primary biliary cirrhosis. Int J Gynecol Obstet 1989;28:279–282.
32. Brodie MJ, et al. Pregnancy and the acute porphyrias. Br J Obstet Gynecol 1977;84:726–731.
33. DiZoglio JD, Cardillo E. The Dubin-Johnson syndrome and pregnancy. Obstet Gynecol 1973;42:560–563.
34. Laifer SA, Darby MJ, Scantlebury VP, et al. Pregnancy and liver transplantation. Obstet Gynecol 1990;76:1083–1088.
35. Cicero TJ, Nock B, O'Connor L, et al. Acute alcohol exposure markedly influences male fertility and fetal outcome in the male rat. Life Sci 1994;55:901–910.
36. Navasa M, Rodes J. Liver disease and gynaecology. In: Mcintyre N, Benhamou J-P, Bircher J, Rizzetto M, Rodes J, eds. Oxford textbook of clinical hepatology. Oxford University Press, Oxford, UK, 1991, 1284–1286.
37. Lindgren A, Olsson R. Liver damage from low-dose oral contraceptives. J Int Med 1993;234:287–292.
38. Eckhauser FE, Knol JA, Raper SE, et al. Enucleation combined with hepatic vascular exclusion is a safe and effective alternative to hepatic resection for liver cell adenoma. Am Surg 1994;60:466–472.
39. Bassel K, Lee M, Seymour NE. Focal nodular hyperplasia of the liver. South Med J 1994;87:918–920.
40. Becker T, Raiford DS, Webb L, et al. Rupture and hemorrhage of hepatic focal nodular hyperplasia. Am Surg 1995;61:210–214.

IX Special Management Considerations

27 Ascites/Spontaneous Bacterial Peritonitis

William H. Ramsey

CONTENTS

INTRODUCTION
PATHOGENESIS
CARDINAL SYMPTOMS AND SIGNS
DIAGNOSIS
TREATMENT
POTENTIAL COMPLICATIONS
PROGNOSIS
PREVENTION
INDICATIONS FOR CONSULTING THE SUBSPECIALIST
CONCLUSIONS
REFERENCES

1. INTRODUCTION

Ascites is defined as the pathological accumulation of fluid within the peritoneal cavity occurring as a consequence of hepatic cirrhosis and portal hypertension. Ascites may also occur in the presence of other disease states, such as tuberculosis, nephrotic syndrome, malignancy, congestive heart failure, and noncirrhotic liver disease. This chapter will focus on the approach to patients with cirrhotic ascites.

The development of ascites in a cirrhotic patient should be considered *a priori* evidence that the patient has portal hypertension. The new onset of ascites signals decompensation of previously stable cirrhosis, and ascites may develop in conjunction with esophageal variceal hemorrhage or hepatic encepholopathy. The occurrence of ascites portends a poor prognosis. In most patients, ascites is readily managed with medical therapy, but in a few, the condition becomes refractory to conventional treatment. In these patients more invasive measures may become necessary, such as intermittent large volume paracentesis, peritoneovenous shunting, transjugular intrahepatic portosystemic shunting (TIPS), or even orthotopic liver transplantation.

Spontaneous bacterial peritonitis (SBP) is a not uncommon complication of cirrhotic ascites, occurring in 12–26% of ascitic patients at the time of hospital admission, whether or not symptoms of infection are present. It is defined as an infection of ascitic fluid that occurs in the absence of a local source of infection *(1)*. Whenever a cirrhotic patient with ascites develops fever, abdominal pain, or begins to fail, SBP should be considered, and a diagnostic paracentesis should be performed. Prompt recognition and treatment improve survival, and subsequent

From: *Diseases of the Liver and Bile Ducts: Diagnosis and Treatment*
Edited by: G. Y. Wu and J. Israel ©Humana Press Inc., Totowa, NJ

prophylactic antibiotic therapy reduces the recurrence rate. Nonetheless, the diagnosis of SBP generally implies a poor prognosis.

2. PATHOGENESIS

2.1. Cirrhotic Ascites

The precise mechanism by which cirrhotic ascites occurs is not known, but three hypotheses have been proposed: the underfill hypothesis, the overflow hypothesis, and more recently, the peripheral arterial vasodilation hypothesis. The underfill hypothesis purports that increased sinusoidal pressure leads to increased formation of hepatic lymph, which enters the abdominal cavity. Splanchnic blood volume increases, systemic vascular resistance and effective plasma volume decrease, and avid renal sodium and water retention occur. The overflow hypothesis suggests that the liver disease in some way triggers a reflex renal sodium and water retention, which in time leads to the formation of ascites. The peripheral vasodilation theory combines aspects of both previous theories *(2)*.

2.2. Spontaneous Bacterial Peritonitis

In patients with cirrhotic ascites, several factors may promote the entrance of internal organisms into ascitic fluid: impaired reticuloendothelial cell activity, decreased serum and ascites complement levels, and low ascites protein levels. Although it was once believed that direct transmural bacterial migration from the gut occurred, current theory favors bacterial translocation to the lymphatic system and portal vein. This concept better explains the frequent occurrence of monomicrobial infection in SBP *(3)*.

3. CARDINAL SYMPTOMS AND SIGNS

3.1. Symptoms

3.1.1. CIRRHOTIC ASCITES

The primary symptom in patients with cirrhotic ascites is an increase in abdominal girth. The patient often relates that this is of recent onset, but the laxity of the abdominal wall and the severity of the liver disease suggest a more gradual process *(4)*. Mild to moderate ascites may be regarded as only a cosmetic problem without any significant health risk or urgency. As the ascites becomes more advanced, however, it may be associated with significant limitation of movement and discomfort, related to the sheer weight of the fluid that the patient must bear. Related symptomatology may include heartburn, shortness of breath, peripheral edema, and abdominal wall hernia, that must be repaired.

3.1.2. SBP

Because SBP occurs in the setting of advanced liver disease, most patients (81%) are clinically jaundiced *(5)*. In one series, 87% of patients had signs and symptoms of infection, including fever (68%), abdominal pain (49%), and mental status change (54%) *(6)*. The clinical manifestations may be subtle, however, (e.g., a mild mental status change noted only by a family member), and the diagnosis should be considered whenever a cirrhotic patient deteriorates.

3.2. Physical Examination

3.2.1. CIRRHOTIC ASCITES

The presence of a moderate amount of ascites may be difficult to detect on physical examination and in one study, its overall accuracy rate was only 58% *(7)*. The usual maneuvers to detect ascites include percussion for flank dullness and shifting dullness, which in another study had a 90% negative predictive value *(8)*. The fluid wave, which requires two examiners, and obvious massive ascites to be positive, and the puddle sign, which is sensitive, but often impractical to perform, are less useful. Physical signs of advanced liver disease, including icterus, spider telangiectasias, palmar erythema, gynecomastia and testicular atrophy in males, and caput medusae are frequently seen. Lower extremity edema may be present.

3.2.2. SBP

Fever, direct or indirect abdominal tenderness, or mental status changes are usually present in SBP. Physical examination may be relatively unhelpful in making the diagnosis of SBP, especially in patients whose only abnormality is a subtle mental status change. Again, stigmata of advanced liver disease are frequently present.

4. DIAGNOSIS

4.1. Imaging Studies

If there is doubt about the presence of ascites on physical examination, abdominal ultrasonography should be performed. The smallest amount of fluid detectable by ultrasonography is reported to be 100 mL *(9)*. Ultrasonography is also useful in guiding abdominal paracentesis, and in assessing for underlying organ enlargement. Abdominal CT scan is equally sensitive in detecting ascites. However, imaging studies are not helpful in establishing the diagnosis of SBP.

4.2. Laboratory Findings

4.2.1. SERUM AND URINE

In cirrhotic ascites, baseline serum and urine electrolyte measurements are crucial in determining the aggressiveness of therapy that will be required, and in following the response to therapy. The serum sodium level normally runs slightly low (134 mEq/L) in these patients, despite an increase in total body sodium. Hypokalemia and hypophosphatemia are also common, but hyperkalemia may develop with potassium-retaining diuretic therapy. Urinary sodium excretion is variable, but is very low (<10 mEq/24 h) in severe cases. A reversal in the urinary sodium/potassium ratio is the therapeutic endpoint of diuretic therapy.

Measurement of the serum albumin level is required to determine the serum-ascites albumin gradient (*see* Section 4.2.3.2.). If SBP is suspected, blood cultures are taken. Baseline serum creatinine and blood urea nitrogen levels are drawn prior to initiating diuretic therapy. A serum glucose level should also be obtained.

4.2.2. TECHNIQUE OF DIAGNOSTIC PARACENTESIS

Diagnostic paracentesis should be performed in each patient with new onset of ascites, if SBP is suspected, or if there is a change in clinical status suggesting a perforated viscus or the development of hepatocellular carcinoma. Contraindications to the procedure include disorders of blood coagulation (PT >5 s above control, platelet count <50,000/mm^3), intestinal obstruction, and infection of the abdominal wall. Relative contraindications are an uncooperative patient, and a history of multiple abdominal surgeries. If there is doubt about the presence of ascites, ultrasonographic guidance should be employed.

The patient should have an empty bladder, and should be positioned at a 45–90° angle. The point of aspiration should be in the midline, midway between the umbilicus, and the pubic bone. If surgical scars interfere, the left or right lower quadrants lateral to the rectus muscles are alternative sites *(10)*. Using sterile technique, and 1% xylocaine local anesthetic, a slow Z-tract insertion is made in 5 mm increments with a bare steel needle (1.5-in, 22-gage for diagnostic, 16–18 gage for therapeutic taps, 3.5-in spinal needle for obese patients). During

Table 1

Ascitic Fluid Tests

Mandatory	Optional	Selected Cases
Cell count	Total protein for tuberculosis	Smear and culture
Albumin (1st tap)	Glucose	Cytology
Culture (in blood culture bottles)	Lactic dehydrogenase	Cholesterol
Gram's stain	Amylase	Triglycerides
		Bilirubin

Modified from refs. *2,4.*

insertion of the needle, continuous aspiration should be avoided, as it may cause a falsely dry tap, due to bowel or omentum occluding the needle. Once the peritoneal cavity is entered, 5 cc of air is injected. Then 10 cc of fluid is gently aspirated followed by larger volumes up to 100–200 cc for a diagnostic tap. The needle should first be stabilized. If flow stops, the syringe should be removed from the needle, the needle twisted 90° and inserted in 1–2 mm increments until flow is restored *(4).* After the needle is removed, an adhesive bandage or pressure dressing should be placed over the site. Complications are rare. Abdominal wall hematoma (1%) may necessitate transfusions *(10).* If leakage of ascites occurs at the site, an ostomy appliance may be utilized until flow spontaneously ceases.

4.2.3. Ascitic Fluid

4.2.3.1. Routine. The recommended ascites fluid tests are outlined in Table 1. Screening tests are performed upon the initial tap, and follow-up tests (via repeat tap), if necessary, are based upon the results. Cell count is the most important single test, as the result affects the interpretation of culture results *(4).* The ascites albumin level is important for determination of the serum-ascites albumin gradient. Ascites cultures are critical for the diagnosis of SBP or one of its variants. Blood culture bottles inoculated with 5 cc of ascitic fluid at the bedside should be the method of choice, as these have a higher yield than conventional cultures *(11).* Optional and case-directed ascites fluid tests are listed in Table 1.

4.2.3.2. Serum-Ascites Albumin Gradient. In general, patients with ascites due to cirrhosis and portal hypertension have a low level of ascites fluid protein (<2.0 g/dL). However, because higher values are not infrequently found in uncomplicated cirrhotic ascites, a more reliable indicator is needed. The serum-ascites albumin gradient, calculated by subtracting the ascites value from the serum value (obtained on the same day), is a much more accurate reflection of portal hypertension (97% accurate). If the gradient is >1.1 g/dL, portal hypertension is the etiology of the ascites, whereas a gradient of <1.1 g/dL, suggests it is not *(12).* This gradient has replaced the exudate-transudate concept of ascites, and the classification based on it is outlined in Table 2 *(13).*

4.2.3.3. SBP. The neutrophil (WBC) count in ascitic fluid is the best predictor of SBP. Patients with >500 WBCs/mm^3 are considered to have SBP even without clinical signs and symptoms of peritonitis. If the WBC count is 250–500/mm^3 with clinical signs of infection, presumed SBP exists. However, if the patient is asymptomatic, the tap should be repeated in 24–48 h. A WBC count <250/mm^3 with sterile fluid rules out SBP *(14).* Several subcategories of SBP have been described, including culture-negative neutro-cytic ascites (WBCs >500 mm^3, negative cultures) which should be treated as an SBP equivalent, and bacterascites (WBCs <250/mm^3, positive monomicrobial culture). Symptomatic bacterascites should be regarded as likely (>33% chance) to progress to

Table 2

Types of Ascites by Serum-Ascites Albumin Gradient

High gradient (≥1.1 g/dL)	Low gradient (<1.1 g/dL)
Cirrhosis	Peritoneal carcinomatosis
Alcoholic hepatitis	Peritoneal tuberculosis
Cardiac failure	Pancreatic ascites
Massive liver metastases	Biliary ascites
Fulminant hepatic failure	Nephrotic syndrome
Budd-Chiari syndrome	Serositis
Portal vein thrombosis	Bowel obstruction or infarction
Veno-occlusive disease	
Fatty liver of pregnancy	
Myxedema	
"Mixed" (portal hypertension plus another cause of ascites, e.g., tbc.)	

Modified from ref. *13*.

SBP, whereas asymptomatic bacterascites rarely progresses to peritonitis *(15)*. Figure 1 outlines an algorithm of the usefulness of the ascitic fluid cell count and culture data in the management of these patients.

A very high ascites WBC count (>10,000/mm^3) is diagnostic of secondary bacterial peritonitis (bowel perforation or abscess). A rising ascites WBC count after 48 h on antibiotic therapy should be suggestive of this as well *(3)*. The organisms found to be the most common causes of SBP are outlined in Table 3 *(15)*.

A polymicrobial (neutrocytic >250 WBCs/mm^3) ascitic fluid culture is suggestive of secondary bacterial peritonitis, particularly if anaerobic organisms are cultured. Polymicrobial bacterascites (WBCs <250/mm^3) suggests that bowel contents have been accidentally sampled.

5. TREATMENT

5.1. Dietary Therapy

Sodium restriction and diuretics are the basis of medical therapy of cirrhotic ascites. A baseline urinary sodium excretion (off diuretics) of >25 meq/24 h is suggestive that dietary sodium restriction alone might be effective, whereas, a value of <10 meq/24 h indicates that diuretics will also be required. Since there is little fluctuation in sodium excretion throughout the day, a spot urine sodium determination may be as useful as a 24-h collection (multiply the concentration by the daily volume for the 24-h sodium result).

The degree of diuresis that can be achieved is directly proportional to the amount of dietary sodium restriction in these patients. However, the most effective level of restriction, 500 mg/d of sodium, is not practical, as it is quite unpalatable, and may often preclude sufficient nutritional support for the patient. A reasonable level is 2 g/d of sodium. Fluid restriction below 2 L/d is not necessary in most patients, unless the serum sodium level drops below 120 meq/dL. It is useful to have the person who prepares the patient's meals review the diet with the dietitian *(4)*. Potassium-containing salt substitutes should be avoided if the patient is on a potassium-retaining diuretic agent.

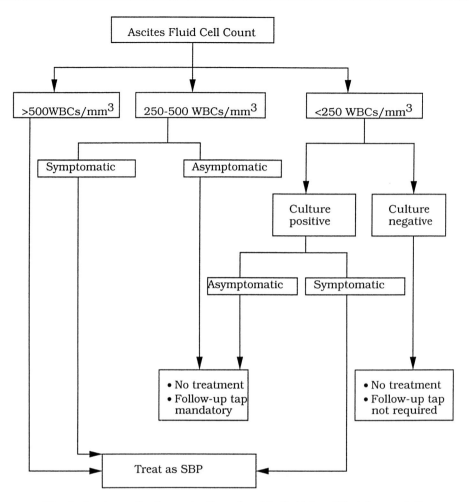

Fig. 1. A scheme for the evaluation of ascitic fluid (modified from ref. *3*).

Table 3

Bacteriology of Subacute Bacterial Peritonitis (SBP)

Organism	Frequency
E. coli	46%
Streptococci/ Group D streptococci	30%
Klebsiella pneumoniae	9%
Other aerobic Gram-negative bacilli	8%
Anaerobes	(<1%)
Other: *Staphylococcus*, diphtheroids	6%

Modified from ref. *15*.

5.2. Diuretics

Spironolactone and furosemide are the primary diuretics employed, starting with doses of 100 mg and 40 mg/d, respectively, and titrating the doses higher according to the response, up to a maximum of 400 and 160 mg/d, respectively. As spironolactone has a long half life, a single daily dose is adequate, and adjustment in dosage should not be considered until at least 2 wk have passed. A target daily weight loss of 0.5–1 lb. is recommended although a faster rate of diuresis is permissible if the patient has peripheral edema (<2 lb/d). If the patient is not responding adequately, then monitoring weight and urinary sodium determinations can help determine whether inadequate dietary sodium restriction is the problem. If a third diuretic is a consideration, hydrochlorothiazide 25–50 mg, or metolazone 5 mg can be added, but often this leads to complications of prerenal azotemia or hyponatremia *(4)*. Refractory ascites is defined as failure to achieve a therapeutic response despite sodium restriction and maximal diuretic therapy, or the development of renal or electrolyte disturbances during treatment. However, more than 90% of cirrhotic ascites respond to salt restriction and diuretics *(16)*.

5.3. Large Volume Paracentesis

Patients with refractory ascites may be treated with intermittent (every 1–6 wk) large volume paracentesis. A maximum paracentesis of 5 L is recommended, despite the fact that larger amounts may be removed safely *(17)*. Intravenous albumin infusion (10 g/L of ascites removed) has been shown to prevent acute changes in cardiac index, femoral blood flow, and renin/aldosterone levels following large volume paracentesis *(18)*. However, the expense of albumin infusion ($100–1250/paracentesis) may not be justified as no difference in the progression to renal failure or death has been demonstrated in those treated with and without albumin infusions *(4)*. If use of a plasma expander is the chosen mode of therapy, albumin has been shown to be superior to a similar dose of dextran or polygeline in preventing hypovolemia after large volume paracentesis *(19)*.

5.4. Antibiotics (SBP)

As noted in Table 3, *E. coli*, streptococci, and *Klebsiella* species are the predominant etiologic agents in SBP, accounting for 80–85% of cases *(15)*. Anaerobes are rare, which is presumed to be due to the high oxygen content of ascitic fluid *(20)*. Therefore, third-generation cephalosporins are the drugs of choice for empirical treatment of SBP. Cefotaxime, 2 g administered intravenously every 8 h has a cure rate of 85% and is more effective and safer than ampicillin and tobramycin *(21)*. Once the causative organism has been identified, the antibiotic may be changed according to the reported susceptibilities. The standard duration of iv antibiotic treatment for such a serious infection is 10–14 d. However, prompt sterilization of the ascitic fluid occurs with treatment, and one study showed no difference in cure rates in patients treated with iv cefotaxime for 5 vs 10 d *(22)*. Therefore, a 5–7-d course of treatment is acceptable if the ascitic fluid WBC count has been documented at <250/mm³ prior to discontinuation of treatment *(3)*. Figure 2 outlines an algorithm for treatment of patients diagnosed with SBP.

5.5. Peritoneovenous Shunts

If a patient with cirrhotic ascites has a poor response to medical measures and therapeutic paracentensis, peritoneovenous (LeVeen or Denver) shunting is one of the third line considerations. This maneuver enjoyed popularity in the 1970s and 1980s, but fell into disuse due to significant complications including shunt malfunctions (30%), sepsis (25% despite antibiotics), peritonitis, endocarditis, postshunt cardiopulmonary congestion, variceal bleeding, and most commonly, disseminated intravascular coagulation. The latter complication has been reduced by the complete removal of ascites with partial replacement by normal saline at the time of surgery *(7)*. One study comparing shunts with medical therapy revealed more complications in the surgical group, and an overall 1-yr mortality in both groups of 75% *(22,23)*. Another study comparing shunts with therapeutic paracentesis was more favorable, citing a 1-yr survival of 50% in both groups. However, there was a significant increase in patient comfort in the shunt group *(24)*. These shunts, therefore, are a viable option, but the potential difficulties

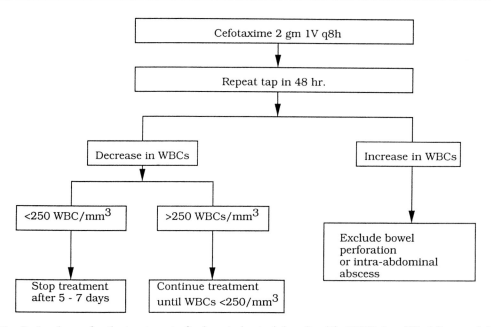

Fig. 2. A scheme for the treatment of subacute bacterial peritonitis (SBP) (modified from ref. *3*).

should be carefully outlined to the patient. Contraindications to the procedure include recent esophageal variceal hemorrhage, intrinsic renal disease, and active alcoholic hepatitis.

5.6. TIPS Procedure

The TIPS procedure is another consideration as a third line measure if conventional therapy and therapeutic paracentesis cannot control cirrhotic ascites adequately (*see* Chapter 6, this volume). Of course, esophageal variceal bleeding is the primary indication for a TIPS procedure, and improvement of refractory ascites is ordinarily regarded as a secondary benefit of the procedure. In an uncontrolled prospective study of the TIPS in 50 patients with cirrhosis and refractory ascites, 37 patients (74%) had complete responses (total remission of ascites within 3 mo), and nine patients (18%) had partial responses, but mortality from underlying diseases was significant. Two patients died within 2 wk of shunt placement. An additional 29 patients died (10 of progressive liver disease and 19 of other causes) during a follow-up of 1.3 yr. After the procedure, 25 patients (50%) had hepatic encephalopathy, as compared with 20 patients (40%) before the procedure. Renal function improved in 28 of 33 patients for more than 6 mo, but did not improve in six patients with organic renal disease *(25)*.

In another study of 42 patients undergoing the TIPS procedure for refractory ascites, predictors of clinical response (>6 mo survival, without hepatic encephalopathy, and not requiring therapeutic paracentesis) were age <65 yr and creatinine clearance >42 ml/min. Overall, the 1- and 2-yr survival rates were 46% and 38%, respectively, and the hepatic encephalopathy rate was 19% *(26)*. A study of the hemodynamics and sodium homeostasis in seven patients undergoing the TIPS procedure for cirrhosis and refractory ascites revealed that the natriuresis associated with TIPS is delayed, and occurs 1 mo after insertion. The conclusion was that in carefully selected patients, TIPS is a safe and effective treatment, but that careful attention to renal and cardiac status is crucial *(27)*. The role for TIPS as a treatment for refractory ascites remains to be established and requires further studies. The data, thus far, suggest that it is a viable option, but carries significant morbidity and mortality, primarily due to the underlying disease in these patients.

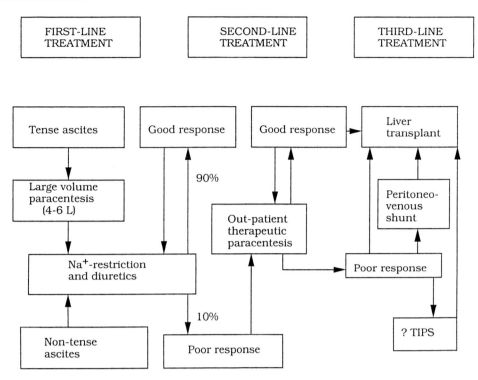

Fig. 3. A scheme for the management of cirrhosis and ascites (modified from ref. *15*).

5.7. Liver Transplantation

Orthotopic liver transplantation is the only treatment that corrects the underlying cause of the portal hypertension that leads to refractory ascites. Patients with ascites should be considered for transplantation when they first present. If they become refractory to dietary and diuretic treatment, develop SBP, hepatorenal syndrome, or hepatic encephalopathy, they should be placed at the top of the transplant selection list. Unfortunately, the availability of donor organs limits the practical usefulness of this procedure. An algorithm for the overall approach to the management of patients with cirrhotic ascites is outlined in Fig. 3 *(13)*.

6. POTENTIAL COMPLICATIONS

In addition to SBP and its variants, complications of cirrhotic ascites include tense ascites, with respiratory compromise and impaired ambulation, abdominal wall hernias, hepatic hydrothorax, and meralgia paresthetica *(4)*. As noted in Fig. 3, tense ascites is an indication for therapeutic paracentesis. Elective surgical treatment should be considered for all cirrhotic ascites patients with hernias, because more than half eventually require surgery for complications. Recurrences are common unless the ascites has been reduced with medical treatment preoperatively. Pleural effusions are common, and are treated best with medical treatment of the ascites *per se*, using the measures outlined in this chapter. Meralgia paresthetica due to pressure injury to the lateral femoral cutaneous nerve is also reversible with medical treatment of the ascites.

Another potential complication of cirrhotic ascites is the hepatorenal syndrome, also called functional renal failure or renal failure of cirrhosis. This syndrome is defined as renal failure that occurs in patients with liver disease in the absence of clinical, laboratory, or anatomical evidence of other known causes *(28)*. Despite intense investigation, the pathogenesis of the hepatorenal syndrome is unknown. Plasma endothelin, a renal vasoconstrictor, is elevated in the hepatorenal syndrome, but it is unclear whether this is a primary or a secondary effect. Excess production of a vasodilator substance is another proposed mechanism. Several candidate agents have been studied, including prostacyclin, bradykinin, substance P, atrial natriuretic protein, and nitric oxide *(29)*.

Efforts to treat the hepatorenal syndrome medically are usually futile, but all patients suspected to have the syndrome should undergo a volume challenge using a solution of 100 g of albumin in 500 mL of isotonic saline. Large-volume paracentesis should then be performed. Other considerations would be the use of renal vasodilators, such as dopamine, a peritoneovenous shunt, or the TIPS procedure *(30)*. Currently, the only definitive therapy for the hepatorenal syndrome is liver transplantation. Without it, the majority of patients with the hepatorenal syndrome die.

7. PROGNOSIS

7.1. Cirrhotic Ascites

The 1-yr survival for medically treated patients with cirrhosis and ascites is 75% *(31)*. Once the ascites has become refractory to diuretic therapy, the 1-yr survival drops to 25% *(32)*. This dismal survival rate holds for all modes of intervention, including intermittent therapeutic paracentesis, peritoneovenous shunts, and the TIPS procedure. The one exception, of course, is for those patients who are fortunate enough to have liver transplantation, in which case the overall 1-yr survival rate exceeds 75% *(33)*.

7.2. SBP

The mortality rate for SBP has improved dramatically during the past several decades, dropping from a mortality rate of 80–90% down to 30–40% *(34)*. Most patients who survive an episode of SBP succumb to liver failure or complications of portal hypertension rather than SBP-related sepsis. Once a patient has had an episode of SBP managed successfully, the expected rate for one or more recurrences is approx 50%, with a 70% chance of recurrence at 1 yr *(35)*. An episode of SBP in a cirrhotic ascitic patient is an indication for liver transplantation.

8. PREVENTION

8.1. Cirrhotic Ascites

In a patient with alcoholic cirrhosis, abstinence from alcohol is the major intervention to stabilize liver function, and to prevent the onset of ascites. Once ascites has occurred, strict compliance with dietary salt restriction and diuretics offers the best chance of prevention. Noncompliance is the most common reason for failure of medical treatment. As noted above, noncompliance with dietary salt restriction can be easily diagnosed by monitoring the patient's weight and urinary electrolytes.

8.2. SBP

Patients with cirrhotic ascites at highest risk for developing SBP are those with a low ascitic protein level, an increased bilirubin level, gastrointestinal bleeding, and acute liver failure *(36)*. The best prevention for SBP is successful medical treatment of the ascites. The use of antibiotics for primary prophylaxis of SBP in high-risk patients has been shown to reduce the occurrence rate significantly, but no reduction in mortality has been demonstrated. This raises the issue of the cost-effectiveness of primary prophylaxis vs waiting to implement aggressive treatment of SBP when it does occur *(1)*. Similarly, secondary prophylaxis with oral quinolone antibiotics has reduced recurrences of SBP after an initial episode, but has not reduced mortality.

Norfloxacin 400 mg/d for up to 1 yr in one study *(37)*, and Ciprofloxacin 750 mg/d for up to 6 mo *(38)*, in another reduced recurrences significantly (20 vs 68% and 3.6 vs 22%, respectively).

9. INDICATIONS FOR CONSULTING THE SUBSPECIALIST

If a patient with cirrhotic ascites truly develops refractory ascites, then a subspecialist should be consulted, as more invasive interventions will become necessary. As noted above, however, most patients (90%) respond to medical therapy *(16)*, and noncompliance with diet or medications should be ruled out before a patient is deemed to be refractory. The development of SBP should also indicate the need for referral to a subspecialist, as assessment for possible liver transplantation becomes an issue in these patients.

10. CONCLUSIONS

Most patients with cirrhotic ascites can be successfully managed with dietary measures and diuretics. As noncompliance and continuing alcohol ingestion are frequent causes for failure of treatment, the family should be intimately involved in the patient's care and management. Once truly refractory ascites or SBP occurs, the prognosis worsens significantly, and consideration of liver transplantation becomes relevant. Second-line and third-line interventions such as intermittent therapeutic paracentesis, peritoneovenous shunts, the TIPS procedure, and in the case of SBP, antibiotics, may maintain the patient for a limited period of time, but more realistically should be viewed as bridges to liver transplantation, should the patient be an acceptable transplant candidate and a donor organ become available.

SUMMARY

Ascites is the accumulation of fluid within the peritoneal cavity in patients with cirrhosis and portal hypertension.

Abdominal ultrasound is a sensitive indicator of the presence or absence of ascites.

Diagnostic paracentesis is essential for the evaluation of the patient with new onset of ascites.

The serum-ascites albumin gradient is more useful than the ascites fluid protein level for categorizing ascites.

The majority of patients with cirrhotic ascites respond to treatment with dietary sodium restriction and oral diuretics.

Noncompliance is a common reason for medical treatment of ascites to "fail."

Spontaneous bacterial peritonitis should be a diagnostic consideration when a patient with cirrhosis and ascites develops fever, abdominal pain, mental status changes, becomes encephalopathic, or otherwise deteriorates.

Refractory ascites, defined as failure to respond to or intolerable side effects from medical therapy, suggests a poor prognosis, the need for specialty care, and consideration of liver transplantation.

Invasive measures for refractory ascites, including intermittent therapeutic paracentesis, peritoneovenous shunting, and the transjugular intrahepatic portosystemic shunt (TIPS) procedure may often sustain the refractory patient for a limited period of time.

REFERENCES

1. Garcia-Tsao G. Spontaneous bacterial peritonitis. Gastro Clin North Am 1992;21:257–273.
2. Rustgi AK, Friedman LS. Ascites and its complications. In: Bayless TM, ed. Current therapy in gastroenterology and liver disease, 4th ed. Mosby, St. Louis, 1994, pp. 516–524.
3. Gilbert JA, Kamath PS. Spontaneous bacterial peritonitis; an update. Mayo Clin Proc 1995;70:365–370.

4. Runyon BA. Approach to the patient with ascites. In: Yamada T, ed. Textbook of gastroenterology, 2nd ed. Lippincott, Philadelphia, 1995, pp. 927–952.

5. Hoefs JC, Runyon BA. Spontaneous bacterial peritonitis. Dis Mon 1985;31:1–48.

6. Runyon BA. Monomicrobial non neutrocyte bacterascites: a variant of spontaneous bacterial peritonitis. Hepatology 1990;12:710–715.

7. Herlong HF. Hepatorenal syndrome and ascites. In: Bayless TM, ed. Current therapy in gastroenterology and liver disease, 2nd ed. Mosby, St. Louis, 1986, pp. 361–365.

8. Cattau EL, Benjamin SB, Knuff TC, Castell DO. The accuracy of physical exam in the diagnosis of suspected ascites. JAMA 1982;247:1164–1166.

9. Goldberg BB, Goodman, GA, Clearfield HR. Evaluation of ascites by ultrasonography. Radiology 1970;96:15–22.

10. Lesesne, HR. Abdominal paracentesis. In: Drossman, DR, ed. Manual of gastroenterologic procedures, 3rd ed. Raven, New York; 1993, pp. 94–98.

11. Runyon, BA. Ascitic fluid culture technique. Hepatology 1988;8:983–985.

12. Runyon BA, Montaro AA, Akriviadis, EA, et al. The serum-ascites albumin gradient is superior to the transudate exudate concept in the differential diagnosis of ascites. Ann Int Med 1992;117:215–220.

13. Runyon, BA. Care of patients with ascites. New Engl J Med 1994;330:337–342.

14. Kline MM, McCallum RW, Guth PH. The clinical value of ascites fluid culture and leukocyte count studies in alcoholic cirrhosis. Gastroenterology 1976;70:408–412.

15. Bhuva M, Ganger D, Jensen D. Spontaneous bacterial peritonitis: an update on evaluation, management, and prevention. Am J Med 1994;97:169–175.

16. Gines P, Arroyo V, Quintero E, et al. Comparison of paracentesis and diuretics in the treatment of ascitics with tense ascites: results of a randomized study. Gastroenterology 1987;93:234–241.

17. Tito L, Gines P, Arroyo V, et al. Total paracentesis associated with intravenous albumin management of patients with cirrhosis and ascites. Gastroenterology 1990;98:146–151.

18. Luca A, Garcia-Pagan JC, Bosch J, et al. Beneficial effects of intravenous albumin infusion on the hemodynamic and humoral changes after total paracentesis. Hepatology 1995;22:753–758.

19. Gines A. Albumin plasma expander preferred for cirrhotic patients with ascites treated with large volume paracentesis. Liver Update: American Liver Foundation 1996:10:5.

20. Scheckman P, Onderdonk AB, Bartlett JG. Anaerobes in spontaneous bacterial peritonitis. (Letter) Lancet 1977;2:1223.

21. Felisart J, Rimola A, Arroyo V. et al. Cefotaxime is more effective than is ampicillin tobramycin in cirrhotics with severe infections. Hepatology 1985;5:457–462.

22. Runyon BA, McHutchison JG, Antillon MR et al. Short course versus long course antibiotic treatment of spontaneous bacterial peritonitis: a randomized controlled study of 100 patients. Gastroenterology 1991;100:1737–1742.

23. Stanley MM, Ochi S, Lee KK et al. Peritoneovenous shunting as compared with medical treatment in patients with alcoholic cirrhosis and massive ascites. N Engl J Med 1989;321:1632–1638.

24. Gines P, Arroyo V, Vargas C et al. Paracentesis with intravenous infusion of albumin as compared with peritoneovenous shunting in cirrhosis with refractory ascites. N Engl J Med 1991;325:829–835.

25. Ochs A, Rossle M, Haag K, et al. The transjugular intrahepatic porto systemic stent-shunt procedure for refractory ascites. N Engl J Med 1995;332:1192–1197.

26. Deschenes M, Spahr L, Martinet JP, et al. Predictors of clinical response to transjugular intrahepatic portosystemic shunt (TIPS) in cirrhotic patients with refractory ascites. (Abstract) Gastroenterology 1996;110:A1180.

27. Wong F, Sniderman K, Liu P, et al. Tranjugular intrahepatic portosystemic stent shunt: effects on hemodynamics and sodium hemostasis in cirrhosis and refractory ascites. Ann Int Med 1995;122:816–822.

28. Epstein, M. Hepatorenal syndrome. In: Epstein M, ed. The kidney in liver disease, 3rd ed. Williams and Wilkins, Baltimore, 1988, pp. 89–118.

29. Epstein M. The hepatorenal syndrome—newer perspectives. (Editorial) N Engl J Med 1992;327:1810–1811.

30. Roberts LR, Kameth PS. Ascites and hepatorenal syndrome: pathophysiology and management. Mayo Clin Proc 1996;71:874–881.

31. D'Amico G, Morabito A, Pagliaro L et al. Survival and prognostic indicators in compensated and decompensated cirrhosis. Dig Dis Sci 1986;31:468.

32. Bories P, Garcia-Compeau Q, Michel H. The treatment of refractory ascites by the LeVeen shunt: A multicenter controlled trial. J Hepatol 1986;3:212.

33. Starzl TE, Demetris AJ, Van Thiel D. Liver transplantation. N Engl J Med 1989;321:1014–1022, 1092–1099.

34. Runyon BA. Spontaneous bacterial peritonitis: an explosion of information. Hepatology 1988;8:171–175.

35. Tito L, Rimola A, Gines P, et al. Recurrence of spontaneous bacterial peritonitis in cirrhosis. Hepatology 1988;8:27–31.

36. Andreu M, Sola R, Sitges-Serra A, et al. Risk factors for spontaneous bacterial peritonitis in cirrhotic patients with ascites. Gastroenterology 1993;104:1133–1138.
37. Soriano G, Guaraer C, Tomas A, et al. Norfloxacin prevents bacterial infection in cirrhosis with gastrointestinal hemorrhage. Gastroenterology 1992;103:1267–1272.
38. Rolacbon A, Cordier L, Bacq Y, et al. Ciprofloxacin and long term prevention of spontaneous bacterial peritonitis: results of a prospective controlled trial. Hepatology 1995;22:1171–1174.

28 Hepatic Encephalopathy

Karen K. Kormis and George Y. Wu

CONTENTS

1. INTRODUCTION

Hepatic encephalopathy is a reversible decrease in the level of consciousness occurring as a consequence of liver disease. The manifestations of hepatic encephalopathy vary, and this diagnosis should be considered in any critically ill patient with altered mental status and evidence of liver disease. Prompt diagnosis and treatment may prevent further complications in severely ill patients, and improve the quality of life in patients with more subtle disease.

The most common type of hepatic encephalopathy is portal-systemic encephalopathy, classically associated with increased blood ammonia levels. This occurs in patients with cirrhosis and portal hypertension with portal-systemic shunting, or in patients with spontaneous or surgical portal-caval anastomosis. In addition, the recently developed transjugular intrahepatic portosystemic shunt (TIPS) procedure for the control of variceal bleeding caused by portal hypertension, appears to be associated with increased frequency of encephalopathy (*see* Chapter 6). Syndromes of hepatic encephalopathy may also be seen in patients with fulminant hepatic failure, urea cycle enzyme deficiencies, and Reye's syndrome *(1)*.

Hepatic encephalopathy may also be classified according to the type of presentation. Acute hepatic encephalopathy can present as a single episode or as recurrent episodes. Chronic hepatic encephalopathy may occur as recurrent episodes of mental status changes or as irreversible hepatocerebral degeneration. Subclinical encephalopathy can be detected by abnormalities in neuropsychological examination in the absence of clinical manifestations *(2)*.

From: *Diseases of the Liver and Bile Ducts: Diagnosis and Treatment*
Edited by: G. Y. Wu and J. Israel © Humana Press Inc., Totowa, NJ

2. PATHOGENESIS

The exact pathogenesis of hepatic encephalopathy remains unclear. Although serum ammonia levels are often elevated in patients with hepatic encephalopathy, some patients have normal levels. Studies using positron emission tomography show a significant increase in the cerebral metabolic rate for ammonia associated with an increased blood-brain barrier permeability. This finding may explain the increased sensitivity of cirrhotic patients to ammonia-producing conditions *(3)*. There are many possible explanations for a lack of correlation of serum ammonia levels and the degree of hepatic encephalopathy. First, venous ammonia levels do not reflect the intracellular ammonia concentration. Arterial and cerebrospinal levels correlate more closely. The brain is almost entirely dependent upon glutamine synthesis as means for ammonia removal. Glutamine concentrations have been found to be increased in patients with hepatic encephalopathy in autopsy brain samples *(4)*, and cerebrospinal glutamine levels were shown to correlate with the degree of hepatic encephalopathy *(5)*.

Potassium depletion is often seen in cirrhotic patients. The resultant acid-base abnormalities favor the shift of ammonia into cells, increasing the difference between the degree of hepatic encephalopathy and serum ammonia level. Blood ammonia levels rise after meals and, therefore, may not be meaningful unless fasting levels are consistently obtained. Finally, there may be a temporal dissociation in which the clinical symptoms of hepatic encephalopathy lag behind the peak ammonia levels by 24 h or more. Despite the disparities, it is likely that ammonia plays a role in the pathogenesis of hepatic encephalopathy, probably by inhibition of neurotransmission in the central nervous system.

γ-Aminobutyric acid (GABA), the principal inhibitory neurotransmitter of the brain, has been proposed as a cause of hepatic encephalopathy, but its role has been debated. GABA and the benzodiazepine class of drugs bind to adjacent sites of a common receptor complex. Substances that bind to these receptors, known as "endogenous" benzodiazepines, have been found in the CSF of patients with hepatic encephalopathy *(6)*, and in brain autopsy specimens of patients who died of fulminant hepatic failure *(7)*. This discovery led to the use of the benzodiazepine antagonist flumazenil in patients with hepatic encephalopathy.

The amino acid imbalance hypothesis of hepatic encephalopathy is based on the observation that aromatic amino acids are increased, whereas branched-chain amino acids (BCAA) are decreased in the plasma of patients with hepatic encephalopathy *(8)*. This finding has led to the use of branched chain amino acid supplementation as therapy for hepatic encephalopathy with mixed results.

Finally, it has been suggested that ammonia, mercaptans, and short chain fatty acids together may cause hepatic encephalopathy by suppressing hepatic regeneration *(9)*.

3. CARDINAL SYMPTOMS AND SIGNS

3.1. Physical Examination

The diagnosis of hepatic encephalopathy is made clinically, and is characterized by various degrees of mental impairment, recurrent disturbances of consciousness, and neuromuscular abnormalities. The alteration in mental status may range from subtle changes in personality and sleep pattern to somnolence, confusion, and coma. Patients with mild hepatic encephalopathy often speak slowly in a dull and monotonic tone. Those with subclinical hepatic encephalopathy may have difficulty performing tasks that require mental and neuromuscular coordination *(10)*.

Patients with encephalopathy from fulminant liver failure may have a normal physical examination. Patients with decompensated cirrhosis often display jaundice, scleral icterus, ascites, spider angiomata, palmar erythema, muscle wasting, gynecomastia, and testicular atrophy *(11)*. Fetor hepaticus is a sweetish, musty odor on the breath of some patients with chronic liver disease that is a common, but is not a consistent finding in patients with hepatic encephalopathy.

Asterixis, or flapping tremor, is the most characteristic physical finding of hepatic encephalopathy. The sign is elicited by dorsiflexion of the wrist while extending the arm. When asterixis is present, the hand falls forward followed by brisk recovery to the dorsiflexed position. It may also be tested for by having the patient squeeze two of the examiner's fingers tightly. Alternating relaxation and tightening of the hand grip can be felt by the examiner.

A patient with subclinical hepatic encephalopathy may not demonstrate asterixis. In this case, more subtle changes should be elicited. Impaired handwriting is usually present in milder degrees of hepatic encephalopathy *(12)*. The Number Connection Test (NCT) is fast, simple, and reliable *(13)*. In this test, the patient is timed as he connects numbers that are randomly scattered on a piece of paper. Although the NCT time increases with age and decreases with years of formal education *(14)*, it has been used to objectively detect intellectual impairment in patients with cirrhosis, who appear normal by conventional evaluation. This test also is useful for serial assessments of the same patient.

Since the neurological examination in patients with hepatic encephalopathy is variable, grading systems have been devised to classify the degree of neurological impairment. This is useful for comparing patients in clinical trials and for monitoring response to treatment. Table 1 lists a common grading system *(15)*.

3.2. EEG

Patients with hepatic encephalopathy have an EEG characterized by a progressive decrease in frequency accompanied by an increase in the amplitude of the brain waves as the encephalopathy progressively worsens *(16)*. Triphasic waves are suggestive of hepatic encephalopathy, but are not specific. These waves consist of a high-amplitude positive deflection preceded and followed by low-amplitude negative deflections *(17)*.

3.3. Evoked Potentials

Evoked potentials are electrical signals generated by excitable tissues stimulated by light, sound, or electricity. Endogenous evoked potentials are considered closely related to cognitive processes and may represent a marker for patients with early subclinical hepatic encephalopathy *(18)*.

3.4. Imaging Studies

3.4.1. CT SCAN

Computed tomography (CT) scans are not helpful in making the diagnosis of hepatic encephalopathy. Their primary role is in eliminating other causes of altered mental status, such as cerebral infarction or subdural hematoma. In hepatic encephalopathy, a normal scan is characteristic.

3.4.2. PROTON MAGNETIC RESONANCE SPECTROSCOPY (MRI)

Proton magnetic resonance spectroscopy of the brain has detected metabolic disorders in patients with chronic hepatic encephalopathy. Specific changes in the brain of hepatic encephalopathic patients include elevated cerebral glutamine and myoinositol levels, and decreased choline metabolites. This technique may be useful in monitoring both overt and subclinical hepatic encephalopathy *(19)*.

3.5. Laboratory Findings

Patients with decompensated cirrhosis often have laboratory findings of decreased hepatic function, including a low serum albumin and increased prothrombin time. Hyponatremia, hypokalemia, and hypophosphatemia are the most common electrolyte disturbances.

Table 1
Grading of Hepatic Encephalopathy

Grade of encephalopathy	Level of consciousness	Intellectual function	Personality/ behavior	Neuromuscular abnormalities
0 Normal	Normal	Normal	Normal	None
1 Mild impairment	Alterations of sleep pattern	Subtly impaired computations Short attention span	Euphoria or depression Irritability	Impaired handwriting Slight tremor
2 Moderate impairment	Lethargy Inappropriate behavior	Grossly impaired computations Loss of time	Overt personality change Inappropriate behavior	Asterixis Abnormal reflexes Ataxia
3 Severe impairment	Somnolence Confused when awake	Loss of place Inability to compute Loss of meaningful communication	Bizarre behavior Paranoia or anger	Asterixis Abnormal reflexes Babinski Rigidity
4 Coma	Unconscious	Absent	None	Decerebrate Dilated pupils

An elevated blood ammonia concentration is suggestive of hepatic encephalopathy. Although it is rarely elevated in the absence of hepatic encephalopathy, it has been shown repeatedly that some patients with hepatic encephalopathy have normal blood ammonia levels. Fasting venous ammonia levels do not correlate well to the stage of encephalopathy, but serial levels in an individual patient may be followed to assess response to therapy (*see* Fig. 1).

4. TREATMENT

4.1. Identification and Correction of Precipitating Causes

The goal of treating hepatic encephalopathy is to return the patient to normal neurological function and maintain that function. Other causes of altered mental status, including CNS infection, trauma, hypoxia, and drug intoxication or overdose, should be eliminated first by appropriate tests. An elevated serum ammonia level may be helpful in order to follow an individual patient's response to treatment, but is not diagnostic. If the diagnosis of hepatic encephalopathy is made by clinical findings, as well as exclusion of other causes, the next step in treatment is to determine the precipitating causes (*see* Table 2).

Azotemia, sedating medications, and gastrointestinal hemorrhage all can precipitate hepatic encephalopathy. Other less common causes include increased dietary protein, infection, constipation, and hypokalemic alkalosis.

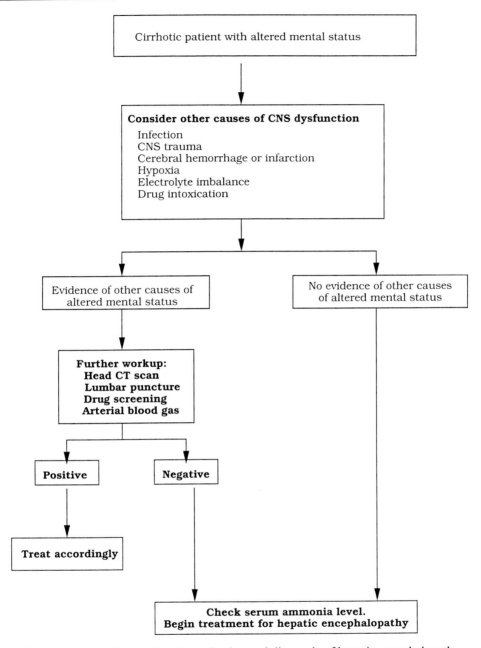

Fig. 1. A schematic plan for the evaluation and diagnosis of hepatic encephalopathy.

4.2. General Medical Measures

The precipitating cause of hepatic encephalopathy should be actively pursued if it is not clinically apparent. If ascites is present, a diagnostic paracentesis should be performed to exclude spontaneous bacterial peritonitis. A nasogastric tube may be needed to detect possible gastrointestinal hemorrhage. Urinalysis, blood, and sputum cultures should be obtained if there are other signs of infection, such as fever or leukocytosis. Serum electrolytes should be checked, especially potassium and magnesium, and deficiencies corrected. The possibility of hypoxemia should be addressed with arterial blood gases or pulse oximetry, and iv fluids started, if indicated. Glucose and phosphate levels should be determined and, finally, thiamine should be administered.

Table 2
Causes of Hepatic Encephalopathy

Azotemia
Medications
   Sedatives
   Analgesics
   Tranquilizers
   Diuretics
Gastrointestinal hemorrhage
Increased dietary protein
Infection
Hypokalemic alkalosis
Constipation
Hepatic necrosis
Noncompliance with therapy

4.3. Dietary Therapy

In acutely encephalopathic patients, nutritional support should be supplied by iv dextrose solutions. An intragastric route may also be employed if the patient is in a coma *(20)*. If the patient is able to tolerate oral intake, a protein-restricted diet should be started. Vegetable protein is preferred over meat protein, because it is less likely to produce encephalopathy in cirrhotic patients. This may be due to its high content of branched-chain amino acids and low content of aromatic amino acids. Patients should not be restricted to less than 0.5 g/kg body weight. The usual starting diet is 40 g/d protein. However, this should be individualized, because many patients will be able to tolerate higher protein loads.

There have been multiple studies using iv or oral branched-chain amino acids (BCAA) in the treatment of hepatic encephalopathy. A meta-analysis suggests that these solutions may be of some benefit, but the results of different trials are difficult to compare, because of their heterogeneity *(21)*. BCAAs are not routinely recommended, due to the equivocal results of clinical trials. They are also extremely expensive. There are two situations in which these formulas may be of benefit: in the rare patient who is unable to tolerate standard protein diets without becoming encephalopathic, and in cirrhotic patients with high protein requirements resulting from sepsis, trauma, or burns.

4.4. Specific Treatment

4.4.1. Nonabsorbable Disaccharides

4.4.1.1. Lactulose. The most dramatic improvement in hepatic encephalopathy is seen with the use of nonabsorbable disaccarides. Lactulose, a synthetic carbohydrate, is the drug of choice in the treatment of both acute and chronic hepatic encephalopathy. It lowers serum ammonia levels in patients with hepatic encephalopathy by multiple mechanisms: Lactulose is degraded by bacteria in the colon to lactate, causing acidification of the luminal contents. The acidification inhibits coliform bacterial growth and ammonia production, and favors the passage of ammonia into the colon from the bloodstream. Lactate and unmetabolized lactulose have laxative effects. Lactulose also appears to stimulate the incorporation of ammonia into protein by intestinal bacteria *(22)*.

If the patient is awake, lactulose may be administered orally, 15–45 mL 2–4 times daily, titrated to reach the goal of 2–3 loose bowel movements per day. For chronic therapy, patients may be instructed to titrate the doses on their own.

For patients in Stage IV hepatic encephalopathy (coma), lactulose may be administered via nasogastric tube. The usual dose is 30 mL of lactulose hourly until a loose bowel movement is obtained, followed by 30 mL every 6 h. If the oral route is contraindicated, lactulose enemas (300 mL in 700 mL of water) may be substituted. The enemas should be retained over 1–2 h with the patient in Trendelenberg position.

Lactulose has also been shown to improve psychometric performance tests in patients with chronic hepatic encephalopathy. The major side-effects of lactulose therapy are flatulence and abdominal cramping. Hypernatremia may occur with resultant dehydration and altered mental status (23), emphasizing the importance of taking an accurate history in cirrhotic patients.

Lactose has been shown to be an effective agent for treatment of hepatic encephalopathy in lactase-deficient patients (24). Its use may be considered in patients who are lactase deficient or who belong to population groups with a high incidence of lactase deficiency.

4.4.1.2. Lactitol. Lactitol is a disaccharide analog of lactulose that can be prepared in a tablet form. It has the same mechanism of action as lactulose and is equally effective. Most studies show that patients find the tablet form more palatable and associated with fewer side-effects (25). Unfortunately, this medication is not currently available in the United States.

4.4.2. ANTIBIOTICS

4.4.2.1. Neomycin. Nonabsorbable antibiotic agents have been used to reduce the population of urease-containing organisms in the colonic lumen. Neomycin is an effective therapy for acute episodes of hepatic encephalopathy (26). The usual dose is 2–4 g/d in divided doses. It also may be given as a 1% retention enema, (1 g in 100 mL normal saline). Although neomycin is poorly absorbed, approx 1–3% of the drug reaches the systemic circulation. Therefore, it should not be used in patients with renal failure. Other side-effects include diarrhea, fungal infections, and malabsorption. Unlike lactulose, which may be used long-term, neomycin is usually recommended for short-term therapy (less than 1 mo). If long-term therapy is instituted, regular monitoring of renal function and yearly audiograms should be performed because of the risk of toxicity.

Although lactulose requires activation of intestinal bacteria, it may be used simultaneously with neomycin with additive effects (27). In theory, neomycin may prevent the degradation of lactulose, and lactulose may interfere with the effects of neomycin, because the antibiotic activity of aminoglycosides is decreased as the pH falls. The stool pH of a patient receiving lactulose should decrease from 6.0–7.0 to 5.0–6.0 if the lactulose is being degraded. This may be tested in patients also receiving neomycin and, if the characteristic pH drop is seen, the two agents may be used together.

4.4.2.2. Metronidazole. Metronidazole appears as effective as neomycin in the treatment of hepatic encephalopathy (28). The usual dose in cirrhotic patients is 250 mg twice daily. Side-effects include diarrhea, nausea, peripheral neuropathy, and an Antabuse-like reaction if alcohol is ingested.

4.4.2.3. Other Antibiotics. Other antibiotics useful in the treatment of hepatic encephalopathy include rifaximin (29), and paromomycin (30). Although these agents are usually considered second-line therapy, they are useful in cases of hypersensitivity reactions to first-line agents.

4.4.3. FLUMAZENIL

Flumazenil, a benzodiazepine antagonist, has been used in patients with hepatic encephalopathy. The major indication for the use of flumazenil is reversal of the effects of benzodiazepine drugs that are commonly used, have a long half-life, and precipitate hepatic encephalopathy in susceptible patients. Flumazenil may also improve cognitive function in patients with subclinical hepatic encephalopathy (31), but how this may be useful clinically remains to be seen.

4.4.4. OTHER MEDICAL THERAPIES

Oral zinc supplementation, as zinc sulfate or acetate (600 mg/d), has been shown to improve the results of neuropsychological testing in patients with subclinical hepatic encephalopathy *(32)*. Sodium benzoate is a drug that bypasses the urea cycle, permitting the excretion of ammonia as hippuric acid in the urine. It is effective in reversing acute hepatic encephalopathy in cirrhotics *(33)*. However, care must be taken in patients with ascites due to the sodium load of the drug.

4.4.5. SURGERY

Surgical options are usually reserved for patients with chronic or recurring hepatic encephalopathy. Patients with surgical portacaval shunts may respond to ligation of the shunt or embolic occlusion of the anastomosis *(34)*. Hepatic encephalopathy caused by transjugular portosystemic shunts in cirrhotic patients is usually readily treated by conventional means, although some patients may require the diameter of the shunt to be narrowed *(35)*. Finally, refractory hepatic encephalopathy is a clear indication for liver transplantation. Patients with severe hepatic encephalopathy have shown improvement in quality of life after transplantation *(36)* (*see* Fig. 2).

5. POTENTIAL COMPLICATIONS

Hepatic encephalopathy is often considered a complication of chronic liver disease. Patients with chronic hepatic encephalopathy may exhibit personality changes and excessive sleepiness that interfere in job performance. Coordination may be impaired and patients may have difficulty driving or operating dangerous equipment.

6. PROGNOSIS

The prognosis of hepatic encephalopathy is dependent upon the patient's underlying liver disease. Patients with hepatic encephalopathy due to fulminant hepatic failure have a worse prognosis than those with chronic liver disease. The overall survival for patients with fulminant hepatic failure has improved from 15 to 50% in certain patient groups *(37)*. The degree of encephalopathy is a strong predictor of outcome with less than 20% of patients in grade 4 coma spontaneously recovering *(38)*.

Patients undergoing liver transplantation for fulminant hepatic failure have a 1-yr survival rate that depends largely upon the grade of hepatic encephalopathy at transplantation; 71% 1-yr survival for patients in grade 1 and 2 hepatic encephalopathy, 80% for grade 3, and 48% for those in grade 4 coma. This is a reflection of the severity of the patient's liver disease at the time of transplantation *(39)* (*see* Chapter 30).

In patients with compensated chronic liver disease, recovery from an episode of hepatic encephalopathy is likely, especially if a precipitating cause can be identified. Those patients with markedly depressed hepatic synthetic function, manifested by ascites, hypoalbuminemia, and prolonged prothrombin time, have an overall poor prognosis. In one study, cirrhotic patients presenting with a first episode of hepatic encephalopathy and gastrointestinal bleeding were found to have only a 15% 1-yr survival without liver transplantation *(40)*. Hepatic encephalopathy is also a poor prognostic variable in patients who receive transjugular intrahepatic portosystemic shunts for variceal hemorrhage *(41)*.

7. PREVENTION

To prevent recurrent episodes of hepatic encephalopathy, patients should be instructed to completely abstain from alcohol, and other hepatotoxins. Patients with a history of hepatic

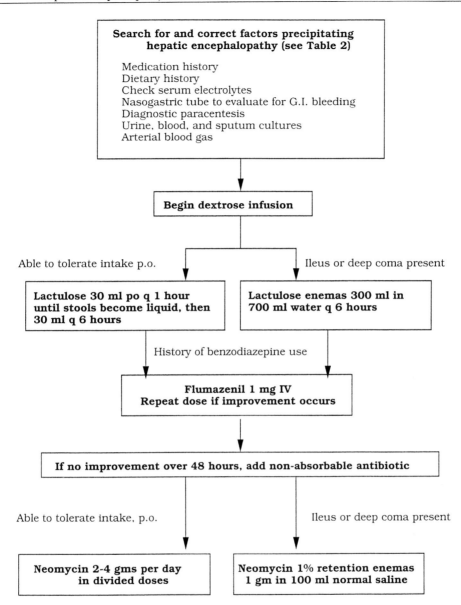

Fig. 2. A schematic plan for initial treatment of hepatic encephalopathy.

encephalopathy should not be given prescriptions for sedative medications, and should be counseled to avoid over-the-counter medications with sedating side effects, such as antihistamines.

Adherence to a protein-restricted diet is mandatory, with an emphasis on vegetable protein. However, patients should not be restricted to below 0.5 g of protein per kilogram of body weight. Finally, chronic lactulose therapy may be instituted with the patient titrating the dose, depending on their bowel habits.

8. INDICATIONS FOR CONSULTING THE SUBSPECIALIST

Patients with previous episodes of hepatic encephalopathy, who present with a recurrence from an easily identifiable cause such as noncompliance, are often managed by primary care physicians. The initial episode of hepatic encephalopathy in a patient warrants a referral to a gastroenterologist or hepatologist for further evaluation of the patient's underlying liver disease. Depending on the individual patient, future workup may include abdominal ultrasound, laboratory testing, and endoscopy to evaluate for esophageal varices. Sudden worsening of previous chronic encephalopathy is also cause for concern, and may herald the development of hepatocellular carcinoma or deterioration of the patient, leading to the possibility of liver transplantation.

9. CONCLUSIONS

Most patients with hepatic encephalopathy can lead normal productive lives. Abstaining from alcohol and sedative medications, along with protein restriction and the use of lactulose, can help prevent recurrences of hepatic encephalopathy. The patient's spouse or close family member should be educated about the symptoms of impending hepatic encephalopathy, such as change in personality or excessive sleepiness. Patients exhibiting such signs should be brought in for medical evaluation immediately.

SUMMARY

Hepatic encephalopathy is a reversible alteration in mental status that occurs in patients with chronic liver disease.

Serum ammonia levels are often elevated in patients with hepatic encephalopathy, but may be normal.

The most characteristic physical examination finding in patients with hepatic encephalopathy is asterixis.

The first step in treatment of hepatic encephalopathy is to identify and treat the precipitating cause.

Protein restriction and use of lactulose is the treatment of choice for both acute and chronic hepatic encephalopathy.

Flumazenil may be useful in patients who have received benzodiazepine drugs.

REFERENCES

1. Conn HO. Hepatic encephalopathy. In: Schiff L, Schiff ER, eds. Diseases of the liver, 7th ed. Lippincott, Philadelphia, 1993, pp. 1036–1060.
2. Blei AT, Finn B. Hepatic encephalopathy. In: Bayless TM, ed. Current therapy in gastroenterology and liver disease, 4th ed. Mosby, St. Louis, MO, 1994, pp. 524–28.
3. Lockwood AH, Yap EWH, Wong WH. Cerebral ammonia metabolism in patients with severe liver disease and minimal hepatic encephalopathy. J Cerebr Blood Flow 1991;11:337–341.
4. Lavoie J, Giguere JF, Pomier Layrargues G, Butterworth RF. Amino acid changes in autopsied brain tissue from cirrhotic patients with hepatic encephalopathy. J Neurochem 1987;49:692–697.
5. Oei LT, Kuys J, Lombarts AJ, Goor C, Endtz LJ. Cerebrospinal fluid glutamine levels and EEG findings in patients with hepatic encephalopathy. Clin Neurol Neurosurg 1979;81:59–63.
6. Mullen KD, Szauter KM, Kaminsky-Russ K. "Endogenous" benzodiazepine activity in body fluids of patients with hepatic encephalopathy. Lancet 1990;1:81–83.
7. Basile AS, Huges RD, Harrison PM, et al. Elevated brain concentrations of 1,4-benzodiazepines in fulminant hepatic failure. N Engl J Med 1991;325:473–478.
8. Rosen HM, Yoshimura N, Hodgman JM, Fischer JE. Plasma amino acid patterns in hepatic encephalopathy of differing etiology. Gastroenterology 1977;72:483–487.
9. Zieve L, Shekleton M, Lyftogt C, Draves K. Ammonia, octanoate and a mercaptan depress regeneration of normal rat liver after partial hepatectomy. Hepatology 1985;5:28–31.
10. Schomerus H, Hamster W, Blunck H, et al. Latent portosystemic encephalopathy. I. Nature of cerebral function defects and their effect on fitness to drive. Dig Dis Sci 1981;26:622–630.
11. Schafer DF, Jones EA. Hepatic encephalopathy. In: Zakim D, Boyer TD, eds. Hepatology. A textbook of liver disease, 2nd ed. Saunders, Philadelphia, 1990, pp. 447–460.
12. Mas A, Salmeron JM, Rodes J. Diagnosis and therapy of hepatic encephalopathy. Ad Exp Med Biol 1994;368:119–123.

13. Conn HO. The trailmaking and number connection tests in assessing mental state in portosystemic encephalopathy. Am J Dig Dis 1977;22:541–550.
14. Finlayson MAJ, Johnson KA, Reitan RM. Relationship of education to neurophysiological measures in brain-damaged and non-brain-damaged adults. J Consult Clin Psychol 1977;45:536–542.
15. Conn HO, Lieberthal MM. The hepatic coma syndromes and lactulose. Williams & Wilkins, Baltimore, 1979.
16. Conn HO, Leey CM, Vlahcevic ZR, et al. Comparison of lactulose and neomycin in the treatment of chronic portal-systemic encephalopathy: a double-blind controlled trial. Gastroenterology 1977;72:573–583.
17. Aguglia U, Gambardella A, Oliveri RL, Lavano A, Quattrone A. Nonmetabolic causes of triphasic waves: a reappraisal. Electroencephalogr 1990;21:120–125.
18. Kullmann F, Hollerbach S, Holstege A, Scholmerich J. Subclinical hepatic encephalopathy: the diagnostic value of evoked potentials. J Hepatology 1995;22:101–110.
19. Kreis R, Ross BD, Farrow NA, Ackerman Z. Metabolic disorders of the brain in chronic hepatic encephalopathy detected with H-1 MR spectroscopy. Radiology 1992;182:19–27.
20. Teran JC, McCullough AJ, Mullen KD. A three-step nutritional approach to patients with hepatic encephalopathy. J Crit Illness 1995;10:309–316.
21. Naylor CD, O'Rourke K, Detsky AS, Baker JP. Parental nutrition with branched-chain amino acids in hepatic encephalopathy. A meta-analysis. Gastroenterology 1989;97:1033–1042.
22. Weber FL Jr. The effect of lactulose on urea metabolism and nitrogen excretion in cirrhotic patients. Gastroenterology 1979;77:518–523.
23. Nelson DC, McGrew WR, Hoyumpa AM. Hypernatremia and lactulose therapy. JAMA 1983;249:1295–1298.
24. Uribe M, Marquez MA, Garcia-Ramos G, et al. Treatment of chronic portal-systemic encephalopathy with lactose in Lactase-deficient patients. Dig Dis Sci 1980;25:924–928.
25. Camma C, Fiorello F, Tine F, Marchesini G, Fabbri A, Pagliaro L. Lactitol in treatment of chronic hepatic encephalopathy: a meta-analysis. Dig Dis Sci 1993;38:916–922.
26. Orlandi F, Freddara U, Candelaresi MT, et al. Comparison between neomycin and lactulose in 173 patients with hepatic encephalopathy: a randomized clinical study. Dig Dis Sci 1981;26:498–506.
27. Weber FL Jr, Fresard KM, Lally BR. Effects of lactulose and neomycin on urea metabolism in cirrhotic subjects. Gastroenterology 1982;82:213–217.
28. Morgan MH, Read AE, Speller DC. Treatment of hepatic encephalopathy with metronidazole. Gut 1982;23:1–7.
29. Bucci L, Palmieri GC. Double-blind, double-dummy comparison between treatment with rifaximin and lactulose in patients with medium to severe degree hepatic encephalopathy. Curr Med Res Opin 1993;12:109–118.
30. Parini P, Cipolla A, Ronchi M, Salzetta A, Mazzella G, Roda E. Effect of rifaximin and paromomycin in the treatment of portal-systemic encephalopathy. Curr Ther Res 1992;52:34–39.
31. Gooday R, Hayes PC, Bzeizi K, O'Carroll RE. Benzodiazepine receptor antagonism improves reaction time in latent hepatic encephalopathy. Psychopharmacology 1995;119:295–298.
32. Reding P, Duchateau J, Bataille C. Oral zinc supplementation improves hepatic encephalopathy. Results of a randomized controlled trial. Lancet 1984;2:493–495.
33. Sashimi S, Dasarathy S, Tandon RK, Jain S, Gupta S, Bhist M. Sodium benzoate in the treatment of acute hepatic encephalopathy: a double-blind randomized trial. Hepatology 1992;16:138–144.
34. Uflacker R, Silva A de O, d'Albuquerque LA, Piske RL, Mourao GS. Chronic portal-systemic encephalopathy: embolization of portal-systemic shunts. Radiology 1987;165:721–725.
35. Hauenstein KH, Haag K, Ochs A, Langer M, Rosse M. The reducing stent: treatment for transjugular intrahepatic portosystemic shunt-induced refractory hepatic encephalopathy and liver failure. Radiology 1995;194:175–179.
36. Tarter RE, Switala J, Plail J, Havrilla J, Van Thiel DH. Severity of hepatic encephalopathy before liver transplantation is associated with quality of life after transplantation. Arch Intern Med 1992;152:2097–2101.
37. Atillasoy E, Berk PD. Fulminant hepatic failure: pathophysiology, treatment, and survival. Annu Rev Med 1995;46:181–191.
38. Hoofnagle JH, Carithers RL, Shapiro C, Ascher N. Fulminant hepatic failure: summary of a workshop. Hepatology 1995;21:240–252.
39. Williams R, Wendon J. Indications for orthotopic liver transplantation in fulminant liver failure. Hepatology 1994;20:5S–10S.
40. Christensen E, Krintel JJ, Hansen SM, Johansen JK, Juhl E. Prognosis after the first episode of gastrointestinal bleeding or coma in cirrhosis. Survival and prognostic factors. Scand J Gastroenterol 1989;24:999–1006.
41. Jalan R, Elton RA, Redhead DN, Finlayson NDC, Hayes PC. Analysis of prognostic variables in the prediction of mortality, shunt failure, variceal rebleeding and encephalopathy following the transjugular intrahepatic portosystemic stent-shunt for variceal hemorrhage. J Hepatol 1995;23:123–128.

SUGGESTED READING

1. Conn HO. Hepatic encephalopathy. In: Schiff L, Schiff ER, eds. Diseases of the liver, 7th ed. Lippincott, Philadelphia, 1993, pp. 1036–1060.
2. Blei AT, Finn B. Hepatic encephalopathy. In: Bayless TM, ed. Current therapy in gastroenterology and liver disease, 4th ed. Mosby, St. Louis, MO, 1994, pp. 524–528.

29 Portal Hypertension/GI Bleeding

Maram Zakko and Roberto Groszmann

1. INTRODUCTION

In portal hypertension, the increase of portal pressure is due to both an increase in vascular resistance and splanchnic blood flow *(1–3)*. Prehepatic, intrahepatic, and posthepatic sites of increased resistance to portal venous blood flow may result in portal hypertension *(1)*. Prehepatic and posthepatic portal hypertension are caused by obstruction of the portal and hepatic veins, respectively. Intrahepatic portal hypertension may be the result of anatomic alterations of the hepatic lobule with secondary compression of portal venules, sinusoids, and hepatic venules, and functional derangement of the intrahepatic microcirculation.

Portal hypertension is initiated by increased resistance to portal venous flow, and is maintained, in part by, an increase in portal venous flow (a hyperdynamic splanchnic circulation) *(2,3)*. The hyperdynamic circulation is the result of vasodilatation and plasma volume expansion. The initial event in the development of portocollateral circulation in cirrhotic patients appears to be a build up in portal pressure. The portocollateral circulation develops in portal hypertensive states in an attempt to decompress the portal circulation and restore it to normal levels. However, whereas the pressure in this portocollateral vascular bed is lower than the obstructed portal circulation, it is still higher than the normal portal pressure. Hence, portal decompression and normalization of the portal pressure is not accomplished. Portal pressures greater than or equal to 12.0 mmHg have been found to be necessary, but not sufficient, for the development of esophageal varices and for variceal rupture *(4)*. Varix wall tension, a concept that integrates local factors, variceal or portal pressures, and varix size may be the decisive factor that determines rupture *(5)*.

From: *Diseases of the Liver and Bile Ducts: Diagnosis and Treatment*
Edited by: G. Y. Wu and J. Israel © Humana Press Inc., Totowa, NJ

Table 1

Causes of Portal Hypertension

Prehepatic portal hypertensive syndromes
1. Splanchnic arteriovenous fistula: splenic and splanchnic vascular bed.
2. Splenic vein thrombosis: pancreatic disease is a common cause, gastric varices may be present in the absence of esophageal varices. It is treatable by splenectomy.
3. Portal vein thrombosis: mainly in the pediatric population; less than 1% in patients with cirrhosis. Causes include coagulopathy, hepatocellular carcinoma, compression or invasion by pancreatic carcinoma, trauma, pancreatic disease, abdominal sepsis, or a complication of endoscopic sclerotherapy.

Posthepatic portal hypertensive syndromes
1. Inferior vena cava obstruction.
2. Cardiac disease.

Intrahepatic causes of portal hypertension (presinusoidal, sinusoidal, and post sinusoidal)[a]
1. Schistosomiasis (presinusoidal).
2. Sarcoidosis (early, presinusoidal; late, sinusoidal as well as presinusoidal).
3. Myeloproliferative diseases (systemic mastocytosis, leukemias, lymphomas, and myelosclerosis may cause presinusoidal and sometimes sinusoidal portal hypertension).
4. Malignant disease of the liver (a variety of sites have been described).
5. Nodular regenerative hyperplasia (not a frequent cause; can do so at multiple sites).
6. Primary biliary cirrhosis (presinusoidal early in the disease, transforms into sinusoidal later when cirrhosis develops).
7. Chronic active hepatitis (presinusoidal).
8. Idiopathic portal hypertension (presinusoidal in early stages).
9. Wilson's disease (mainly presinusoidal).
10. Acute and fulminant viral hepatitis (severe cases has been associated with portal hypertension).
11. Hepatic cirrhosis (mainly sinusoidal).
12. Peliosis hepatis (sinusoidal, but portal hypertension rarely predominates in the clinical picture).
13. Alcoholic hepatitis (postsinusoidal).
14. Budd-Chiari syndrome (postsinusoidal hepatic vein thrombosis).
15. Veno-occlusive disease (postsinusoidal).
16. Hepatic toxins (vinyl chloride, arsenic, vitamin A excess, mercaptopurine, azathioprine, and thioguanine, and others).

[a]At later stages of the pathological process the disease may affect more than one sinusoidal site.

2. CLASSIFICATION

One way to classify the etiology of portal hypertension is according to the site of presumed increased resistance to flow of portal venous blood. The main categories of portal hypertension locations include: prehepatic, intrahepatic (classified according to the predominant anatomic site of increased resistance relative to the hepatic sinusoid), and posthepatic. Examples of common etiologies are listed on Table 1.

3. CARDINAL SIGNS AND SYMPTOMS

In any patient suspected of having portal hypertension, the clinician should look for the physical signs of liver disease, of which the best recognized are jaundice, spider angiomas, testicular atrophy, gynecomastia, and clues to the presence of portosystemic encephalopathy, such as altered mental status, asterixis, and fetor hepatis. Splenomegaly is a helpful clue that is present in most patients with portal hypertension. The spleen is best palpated with the patient lying on his or her right side and inhaling deeply while the examiner applies light pressure to the left upper quadrant. Spleen size correlates poorly with portal venous pressure. Moreover, splenomegaly may be present in many disease states in the absence of portal hypertension. Portal hypertensive patients may have findings suggestive of hyperdynamic circulatory state, including bounding pulses, warm, well perfused extremities, and arterial hypotension.

The presence of dilated abdominal veins supports a diagnosis of portal hypertension. Umbilical vein-epigastric vein shunts result in dilated collaterals on the anterior abdominal wall, whereas portal vein-parietal peritoneal shunts may result in a venous pattern on the flanks. The caput medusae represent tortuous collateral veins around the umbilicus and can be a dramatic finding.

Dilated abdominal collaterals must be distinguished from collaterals due to obstruction in the inferior vena cava. The latter syndrome causes dilated flank veins and prominent veins of the back. A collateral venous pattern on the back is never due to portal hypertension alone. In rare instances, the patient with portal hypertension may present with dilated back veins due to pressure of a large regenerative nodule on the inferior vena cava.

Ascites is a complication that indicates poor prognosis in portal hypertensive liver disease. The presence of ascites supports a diagnosis of portal hypertension, if conditions such as malignancy, congestive heart failure, and peritoneal inflammatory disease are excluded.

There are no laboratory diagnostic tests for portal hypertension. Pancytopenia is frequently encountered in patients with hypersplenism, but it is neither specific nor sensitive for this diagnosis. The cytopenias that result from hypersplenism rarely are a cause of clinical complications in themselves.

4. DIAGNOSIS OF PORTAL HYPERTENSION

Diagnosis of portal hypertension often starts with a suspicion for the condition through the history and physical examination (see Fig. 1). This is usually followed by investigative procedures to confirm the diagnosis, and assess the extent of portal hypertension, which will aid in the short- and long-term management of the patient. Portal hypertension is characterized by alterations in splanchnic and hepatic blood flow, as well as development of portosystemic collateral blood flow, which is responsible for many of the clinical features and complications of portal hypertensive liver disease.

4.1. Portal Pressure Measurements

There are many methods to measure the portal pressure (see Fig. 2). Although these methods are routinely used in academic settings, they are also being increasingly utilized in some clinical situations, with the increasing interest in therapeutic modalities to prevent variceal hemorrhage. The most commonly used method is the indirect measurement of the hepatic vein pressure gradient (HVPG). This is the gradient between the wedged hepatic vein pressure (WHVP) and the free hepatic vein pressure (FHVP). These values are obtained by catheterization of the hepatic vein, usually by a balloon-tipped catheter (1,6–8). A fluid-filled catheter is introduced into an antecubital or femoral vein and advanced under fluoroscopic guidance into a hepatic vein. The direct measurement of the hepatic vein pressure through this catheter is called the free hepatic vein pressure. The wedged hepatic vein pressure is measured by inflating the balloon-tipped catheter until it completely occludes a hepatic vein branch and forms a continuous column of fluid between the catheter and the blood in the vein, the sinusoid, and the portal vein. The WHVP works by the same principle as the wedged pulmonary artery pressure, which is obtained by balloon catheterization of the pulmonary artery, and which is used as an index of left atrial pressure. The rate of successful hepatic vein catheterization is greater than 95%, and the procedure is shown to be extremely safe (8,9).

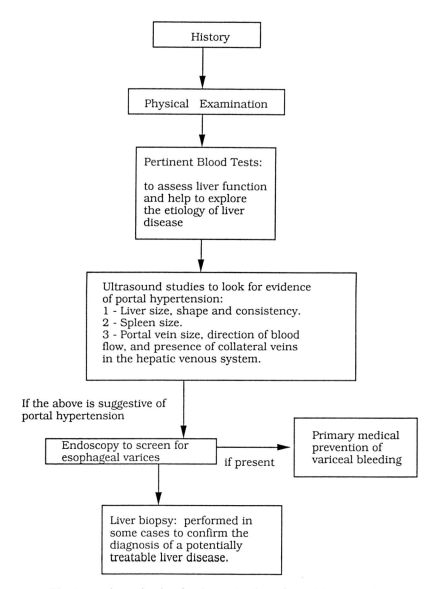

Fig. 1. A schematic plan for the evaluation of portal hypertension.

The technique is indirect because HVPG usually is a measure of the hepatic sinusoidal pressure and not the portal vein pressure. However, it usually reflects the portal vein pressure when the cause of portal hypertension is sinusoidal or postsinusoidal, as in alcoholic liver cirrhosis. In a normal liver, the connections between sinusoids dissipate some of the pressure from the wedged catheter, which results in a static pressure reading slightly lower than actual portal pressure (*see* Fig. 2).

The HVPG underestimates portal pressure in diseases in which obstruction to the flow of portal blood is presinusoidal, and in which connections between sinusoids are preserved. In pure presinusoidal disease, HVPG is normal (*see* Fig. 2).

4.2. Upper Gastrointestinal Endoscopy

It is important to look for esophageal varices, gastric varices or portal gastropathy in patients suspected of having portal hypertension, both for diagnosis and long-term management of these varices. Their

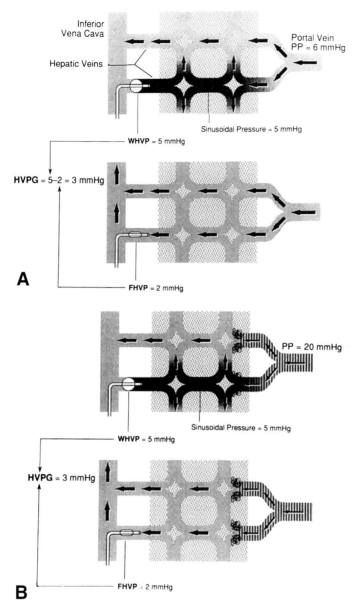

Fig. 2. Principles involved in measuring hepatic vein pressures (pressure levels are provided as examples). Stripes indicate hypertensive area; dark areas indicate stasis. **(A)** The normal liver: Due to normal dissipation of pressure through the sinusoids when the hepatic vein is occluded (top), the measured pressure in the hepatic vein is slightly lower than the normal portal venous pressure. This difference is usually insignificant. **(B)** Presinusoidal portal hypertension wedged venous pressure (WHVP) and hepatic vein pressure gradient (HVPG) are normal in presinusoidal portal hypertension because the intersinusoidal communications are normal and permit decompression of the static column of blood formed by the occluding balloon (top). The site of the obstruction is depicted with twisted lines.

presence confirms the diagnosis of portal hypertension, but their absence does not rule it out. Furthermore, the presence of other complications of portal hypertension, such as encephalopathy and ascites, do not reliably predict the presence of varices. Patients with portal hypertension may develop portosystemic collaterals that are predominantly caudad (below the level of the gastroesophageal circulation).

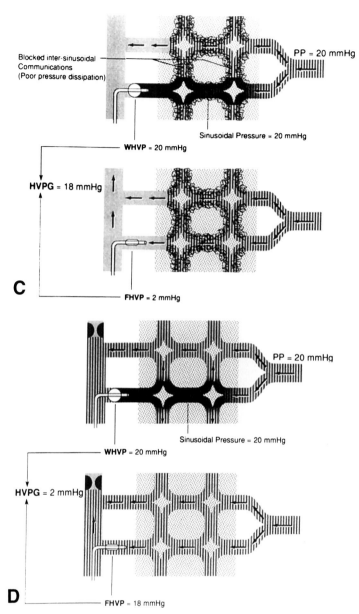

Fig. 2. *(continued)* **(C)** Portal hypertension caused by alcoholic cirrhosis. The portal venous pressure and the WHVP are elevated equally in sinusoidal portal hypertension; effective decompression of the static column of blood created by the occluding balloon (top) can not occur at the sinusoidal level due to disruption of the normal intersinusoidal architecture. In this situation wedged hepatic venous pressure gives an excellent approximation of actual portal pressure. **(D)** Posthepatic portal hypertension: WHVP is elevated, but HVPG is normal in syndromes such as right-sided cardiac failure. The normal HVPG reflects the normal liver architecture present in these syndromes unless permanent liver injury supervenes. (Reprinted by permission from Lippincott-Raven publication: Genecin P, Groszmann RJ. Portal hypertension. In: Schiff L, Schiff ER, eds. Diseases of the Liver, 7th ed., vol. 2, 1993, pp. 935–973.).

4.3. Ultrasonography

Ultrasonography is the method of choice in assessing the portal system in the patient in whom portal hypertension is suspected. This noninvasive test can be used to screen the portal vein for patency, which is vital information in any portal hypertensive patient. Ultrasonography can also identify portal vein collaterals around the azygous system, stomach, spleen, retroperitoneal, and left renal vein. Other useful findings include a congested and enlarged spleen, which is suggestive of portal hypertension, although other causes of splenomegaly must also be considered. The measurement of the portal vein caliber by ultrasound is also helpful. Portal vein diameter in excess of 15 mm is very suggestive of portal hypertension, although the presence of a normal caliber portal vein does not rule it out *(10)*. Inability to visualize the portal vein by ultrasonography is suggestive of portal vein thrombosis.

4.3.1. ECHO-DOPPLER

Echo-Doppler flowmetry measures the direction and velocity of red blood cell flow. B-mode ultrasound can be used to measure cross-sectional areas of a blood vessel and the volume of flow can be estimated by multiplying the velocity by area. The superior mesenteric artery provides 75% of the blood flow entering the portal system and may be used as a representation of portal flow.

4.3.2. COLOR-DOPPLER

Color-Doppler is another ultrasound modality that has been applied to the splanchnic circulation. It applies the B-mode imaging of the blood vessel in addition to the two dimensional flow signals that are converted into colors. This technique permits determination of the presence of blood flow, and can distinguish flow direction as well as the difference between turbulent and laminar flow.

4.4. Liver Spleen Scan

Liver-spleen scan is another method of assessing the presence of portal hypertension (*see* Chapter 5, this volume). Visualization of radioactive colloid shift to the spleen and bone marrow is highly suggestive of increased portal pressure. Its absence, however, does not eliminate the possibility of portal hypertension.

4.5. Computed Tomography

Computed tomography is less useful than ultrasonography in the assessment of the portal venous system. It should not be relied on to diagnose the presence of esophageal varices *(11)*, and is less accurate than ultrasonography in diagnosing some vascular details, such as a thrombus in the portal venous system.

4.6. Magnetic Resonance Imaging (MRI)

MRI is mainly utilized as a more accurate method in visualizing collaterals and in diagnosing portal vein thrombosis and patency of surgical shunts. This technique does not have some of the limitations of ultrasonography, such as difficulties in visualizing the portal vein due to obesity or presence of intestinal gas.

5. COMPLICATIONS OF PORTAL HYPERTENSION

5.1. Esophageal Varices

Esophageal varices are seen in 24–81% of patients with chronic liver disease, with an average of 60% *(12)*. Only 25–30% of patients with varices will experience variceal bleeding *(12,13)*, and the risk of bleeding appears to be greatest within the first year after diagnosis. No single factor has been shown to accurately identify patients with esophageal varices who will suffer variceal hemorrhage. However, the occurrence of esophageal variceal hemorrhage has been shown to correlate with some clinical observations. Some of these observations are specific endoscopic signs, such as large varices, and red color signs, the presence of gastric varices, alcoholic etiology of liver disease, and continued alcohol abuse, the degree of liver dysfunction, and history of prior variceal hemorrhage (12,14,15). Higher portal pressures have been observed to be associated with an increase in early mortality and risk of recurrent hemorrhage. However, it has not been shown that an increase in portal pressure even beyond the threshold value is a predictor of variceal hemorrhage (16).

Mortality from esophageal variceal bleeding is greatest with the initial bleeding episode, and is directly correlated to the degree of hepatic decompensation. Additional poor prognostic factors include cirrhosis complicated by coexistent alcoholic hepatitis, hepatocellular carcinoma, or portal vein thrombosis (17,18). In general, there is a 40% chance of mortality associated with esophageal variceal bleeding.

Recurrence is a significant risk for variceal hemorrhage. Roughly, two thirds of patients will experience recurrent hemorrhage, half of them occurring within the first 6 wk of the index bleed (19). Risk factors predictive of early rebleeding include the degree of hepatic decompensation, age more than 60, severity of the initial bleed, renal insufficiency, large varices, the level of portal pressure, and active bleeding at the time of the initial endoscopy. The risk of recurrent bleeding returns to that of an initial bleed beyond 6 wk of an index bleed.

5.2. Gastric Varices

Gastric varices arise from the short gastric and posterior gastric venous system (20), and they are rarely present in the absence of esophageal varices. Their prevalence in patients with portal hypertension is between 6–78% (20,21). This variability is probably due to two main reasons: the difference in the etiology of portal hypertension between the different studies, because gastric varices were more frequently observed in portal hypertension caused by extrahepatic portal venous occlusion than with cirrhosis, and limitations of the commonly used diagnostic imaging techniques (22). Endoscopic ultrasonography is probably superior to routine endoscopy for detection of gastric varices (23), but good studies are still lacking.

The hemodynamic derangements that trigger gastric variceal rupture are most likely similar to those that are responsible for esophageal variceal rupture. However, gastric varices are less likely to bleed than esophageal varices (21). The reason may be partial decompression of the portal venous system through spontaneous gastrorenal shunts (20).

Following sclerotherapy, junctional varices distal to the gastroesophageal junction without extension to the fundus have lower incidence of rebleeding and improved survival, compared to fundal varices (24). Whereas gastric variceal hemorrhage occurs less frequently than esophageal variceal hemorrhage, the severity of bleeding and mortality, especially with fundal varices, is greater (21,24).

5.3. Portal Hypertensive Gastropathy

Portal hypertensive gastropathy may occur in portal hypertension of any etiology. Gastric mucosal lesions in cirrhotic patients have been recognized for decades, and (25) they are the second most common cause of upper gastrointestinal bleeding in cirrhosis. Bleeding from these sources may rarely present as acute hemorrhage, or more commonly as chronic bleeding. The latter usually reveals itself as iron deficiency anemia. Recurrent gastrointestinal hemorrhage may occur in 62–75% of cases. The risk of bleeding is greatest in those patients with the most severe mucosal disease (26).

Studies of the gastric microcirculation in portal hypertension have shown arteriolar changes and dilation of the submucosal and subserosal veins (25,27,28). Increases in gastric mucosal blood flow have been documented in portal hypertensive gastropathy by hemodynamic studies, in animal models and cirrhotic patients (29–31).

Portal hypertensive gastropathy is associated with the presence of large varices, and prior history of sclerotherapy. It is independent of the magnitude of portal pressure elevation or the presence of *Helicobacter pylori* infection.

Most recent studies agree that portal hypertensive gastropathy occurs at a rate of 50–60% of patients with established cirrhosis *(26–28)*. This is in contrast to earlier reports which tend to estimate it at lower rates. The higher recent values may be due to more advanced technology in endoscopic equipment, increased observer awareness, and more frequent use of sclerotherapy. Portal hypertensive gastropathy may be endoscopically classified as mild or severe *(26,28)*. Mild disease refers to mosaic pattern of the gastric mucosa with multiple erythematous areas surrounded by a fine, white reticulin network. More severe gastropathy has discrete red spots that may become confluent *(28,31)*. The "watermelon stomach" in cirrhosis may represent a more severe form of portal hypertensive gastropathy.

6. TREATMENT OF PORTAL HYPERTENSIVE HEMORRHAGE

6.1. Initial Management

The initial management is similar to that of upper gastrointestinal bleeding due to other causes. However, there are certain aspects specific to portal hypertension that, if attended to, may enhance the probability of a favorable outcome (*see* Fig. 3).

6.2. Gastric Lavage and Bowel Preparation

Gastric lavage is a diagnostic and therapeutic technique. It confirms the diagnosis of upper gastrointestinal bleeding, gives an impression of the magnitude of bleeding, helps prevent the risk of aspiration, and enhances the endoscopic view in diagnosing and treating the bleeding source. Experimental studies in portal hypertensive rat models suggest that blood in the stomach increases blood flow in the superior mesenteric artery and, consequently, also increases portal vein pressure *(32)*. Clinical studies on patients in this regard are not available. However, there are studies that show meal-induced increases in gastro-collateral blood flow and portal pressure in cirrhotic patients. Studies are needed to determine whether gastric lavage in the setting of upper portal hypertensive bleeding may prevent increases in gastro-collateral flow and portal pressure.

There is no evidence that tube-induced mucosal trauma or aspiration of clot predisposes to recurrent hemorrhage. Bowel cleansing by lactulose or neomycin enemas may prevent portosystemic encephalopathy precipitated by hemorrhage and posthemorrhage infections (*see* Chapter 28, this volume).

6.3. Endotracheal Intubation

Patients with active esophageal variceal hemorrhage are at significant risk for aspiration. Aspiration is mainly due to massive hematemesis, encephalopathy, induced pharmacological sedation, and various therapeutic maneuvers. Endotracheal intubation for airway protection is mandatory with the use of balloon tamponade. In the other clinical situations, the decision to intubate depends on each individual case. It is advisable to have a low threshold for intubation to protect from a potentially life threatening aspiration pneumonia.

6.4. Volume Resuscitation

Intravascular volume has an important role in the maintenance of portal hypertension, and is a factor in variceal hemorrhage. In rat models of portal hypertension, hypervolemia is required for full development of the hyperdynamic circulation *(33)*. In other studies conducted on cirrhotic and noncirrhotic portal hypertensive patients, hypervolemia has been documented *(34,35)*. It has also been observed that variceal hemorrhage in pregnancy often

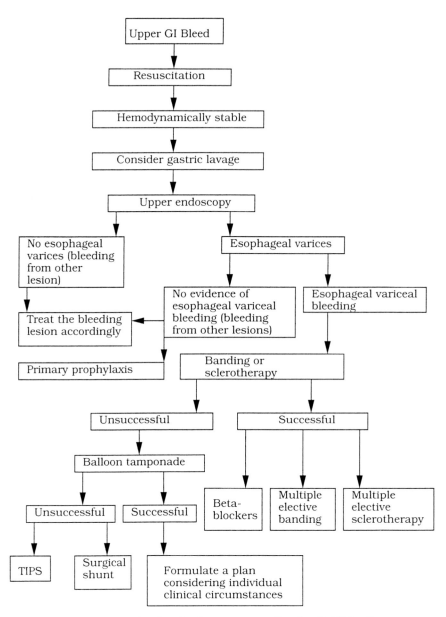

Fig. 3. A schematic plan for the treatment of variceal GI bleeding.

occurs toward the third trimester. This timing coincides with maximal blood volume expansion in pregnancy, which suggests a causative relation between volume expansion and variceal bleeding *(36)*.

Intravascular volume expansion with dextran was accompanied by a prolonged increase in portal pressure in a study with patients with stable portal hypertension *(35)*. Upper GI bleeding was precipitated during volume expansion in two patients. Angiographic studies with its volume expansion was associated with increased incidence of early rebleeding from esophageal varices when it was performed within 7 d of the acute variceal hemorrhage *(37)*.

It is frequently difficult to assess the intravascular volume status in hemorrhaging patients. A Swan-Ganz catheter may be needed for pressure monitoring. The baseline arterial blood pressure of patients with cirrhosis is usually lower than normal. This is due to the persistent vasodilatation related to cirrhosis. Cirrhotic patients also frequently have chronic anemia. Consequently, it is not advisable to raise the arterial pressure to normal, or to normalize the hematocrit, as these maneuvers may lead to overhydration and increased tendency to variceal bleeding. It is always advisable to keep the central venous pressure on the low side of normal to prevent this complication. Volume replacement should be performed cautiously with colloid and blood products to maintain organ perfusion.

6.5. Diagnostic Endoscopy

Upper panendoscopy should be performed urgently, and as soon as the patient is hemodynamically stabilized. Approximately 30% of patients with portal hypertension and upper gastrointestinal bleeding will be found to be bleeding from nonvariceal lesions (38). Variceal hemorrhage is confirmed by the presence of actively bleeding varices, varices with an overlying clot (the white nipple sign), or varices with blood in the upper gastrointestinal tract in the absence of another bleeding site. If the bleeding is diagnosed to be from esophageal varices, endoscopic therapy should be instituted at the time of initial endoscopy.

6.6. Pharmacologic Therapy

6.6.1. VASOPRESSIN/NITROGLYCERIN

Vasopressin (VP) is a splanchnic and systemic vasoconstrictor. The vasoconstriction of the splanchnic arteries results in a decreased portal venous flow leading to decrease in portal venous pressure, variceal pressure, and esophagogastric collateral blood flow. Vasopressin may also decrease esophagogastric collateral blood flow by increasing the lower esophageal sphincter tone and compression of the submucosal collateral vessels (39–41). Significant side-effects caused by systemic vasoconstriction limits its use and it is contraindicated in patients with coronary artery disease and alcoholic cardiomyopathy. Adding nitroglycerin to vasopressin enhances the reduction in portal pressure due to a decrease in portal venous resistance, and opposes the adverse effects of vasopressin on systemic hemodynamics (39).

Three trials have compared vasopressin to vasopressin plus nitroglycerin (42–44). Meta-analysis showed combination therapy was more effective than vasopressin alone in control of variceal hemorrhage. However, it did not show important reduction in mortality. Significant reduction in side-effects with the combined therapy was demonstrated in two of the trials (42,43).

As part of the management of acute esophageal variceal bleeding, vasopressin should be administered as a continuous iv infusion through a central venous line at an initial dose of 0.4 U/min. The dose can be increased gradually to a maximum of 1.0 U/min. Doses greater than 1.0 U/min are associated with increased toxicity without significant further decrease in portal pressure. Nitroglycerin may be started after initiation of vasopressin, and when the patient has a reasonably stable arterial pressure. It is probably best to administer NTG intravenously with an initial dose of 40 mg/min with 40 mg/min increments every 15 min to a maximum of 400 mg/min to maintain systolic arterial blood pressure approx 100 mmHg. Nitroglycerin can also be administered sublingually in this setting at a dose of 0.6 mg every 30 min.

Tapering of vasopressin before discontinuation is not required, because it does not prevent rebleeding, and is not associated with a rebound increase in portal pressure (45). Nitroglycerin should not be used alone in the treatment of variceal hemorrhage. Thus, if nitroglycerin is used, it should be in combination with another agent.

6.6.2. SOMATOSTATIN/OCTREOTIDE

Somatostatin (ST) and octreotide (OT), its synthetic analog, have been shown to be as effective as vasopressin and comparable to other therapies in the control of acute variceal bleeding without significant side-effects. ST and OT were shown to have variable effects on portal vein pressure in stable cirrhotic patients. On the other hand, they were consistently shown to decrease the azygous blood flow that correlates with the collateral and variceal pressures. A number of studies have compared the use of ST with placebo and with other treatment modalities in the treatment of acute bleeding varices. They have found it at least as effective as the other modalities in most studies, and superior to placebo in some studies *(46–48)*. In a recent study, bleeding in an octreotide group was significantly better controlled than the placebo group (87 vs 71%, respectively) *(48)*. In another study, octreotide was found not to be superior to placebo for the control and prevention of early rebleeding from varices, whether associated with sclerotherapy or not *(49)*. These results indicate that more studies are needed in this respect, and that there are not enough data yet to recommend the routine use of octreotide for the treatment of portal hypertensive gastrointestinal bleeding.

ST and OT have only modest systemic hemodynamic effects and were associated with a significantly lower complication rate than vasopressin *(50–52)*.

6.7. Balloon Tamponade

Balloon tamponade is utilized as a temporary measure to control bleeding from esophageal varices in patients who have failed pharmacologic and/or endoscopic therapy, or in whom endoscopic therapy is precluded by massive bleeding. It controls bleeding temporarily and provides time for resuscitation and definitive treatment.

There are three types of balloons available for clinical use. The Sengstaken-Blakemore tube has a gastric balloon with a 250-cc capacity, an esophageal balloon, and a single gastric suction port. The Linton-Nachlas tube has a single gastric balloon with a 600-cc capacity. It has been shown to be superior to the Sengstaken-Blakemore for control of gastric variceal hemorrhage *(53)*. The Minnesota tube is a modified Sengstaken-Blakemore tube. It has a suction port above the esophageal balloon. When the Sengstaken-Blakemore tube is used, a nasogastric tube attached to intermittent suction should be placed with the distal end above the esophageal balloon in order to minimize the risk of aspiration of esophageal secretion. Endotracheal intubation should be performed prior to balloon tamponade.

Application and maintenance of these tubes should be done by experienced medical staff. Following placement of the tube, the gastric balloon is inflated, gentle traction is applied, and tube position is confirmed radiologically. Inflation of the gastric balloon alone will often control the bleeding. If bleeding continues, the esophageal balloon is inflated. The gastric balloon may be inflated for 48–72 h. The esophageal balloon should not be inflated for more than 24 h. Periodic deflation of the esophageal balloon every 8 h may minimize the risk of necrosis to the esophageal mucosa *(54)*. Once bleeding is controlled, the esophageal balloon is deflated, followed by deflation of the gastric balloon. The deflated tube may be then left for 24 h while the patient is observed for recurrent hemorrhage. Techniques on placement and use of these tubes have been previously reviewed *(54–56)*.

Initial control of variceal hemorrhage with balloon tamponade is approx 78%. It varies from 33–90% in different series *(55,57–60)*. This variability is most likely a consequence of patient selection and the experience of the staff performing the procedure. Early rebleeding occurs in approx 30% of cases when balloon tamponade is used as a sole therapy *(57,58)*.

Complications of balloon tamponade therapy are significant. Esophageal rupture is a lethal complication, and occurs at an average of 3%. Major complications have been observed in 14% of cases. Complications are more frequent in series in which tubes were placed by inexperienced staff *(57)*. Special precautions should be taken in patients with hiatus hernia. The gastric balloon should be inflated below the diaphragm, not within the hernia sac, and gentle traction is applied. The esophageal balloon is not inflated. In the presence of a large diaphragmatic defect, the Linton-Nachlas tube may be utilized. Traction with weights should not be used because they increase the complication rate of the procedure.

6.8. Endoscopic Therapy

6.8.1. Endoscopic Sclerotherapy

Endoscopic sclerotherapy (ES) effectively controls acute variceal hemorrhage without affecting portal pressure or portal perfusion. Although described initially with rigid endoscopes, ES is now performed with flexible fiberoptic endoscopes. A dual channel therapeutic endoscope with a disposable single use injector is preferable.

Various sclerosing agents are available. In the United States, sodium tetradecyl (0.5–3.0% concentration) and sodium morrhuate (5% concentration) are the most commonly used agents. Absolute ethanol has also been shown to be effective. The mechanism of action of all these agents is to generate an intense inflammatory response, with resultant fibrosis and thrombosis that obliterates the variceal column. These agents do not appear to have much difference in their efficacy, although studies are limited in this regard.

Varices are usually injected by the injector, a long catheter with a retractable needle at its tip, that can pass through the endoscope channel and be aimed at the site to be injected. Almost all variceal bleeding arises 4–5 cm proximal to the gastroesophageal junction. Therefore, regardless of the sclerosant or technique used, injections should be directed to this area. If not precluded by massive hemorrhage, ES should be performed at the time of initial endoscopy. In patients who continue to bleed or have early recurrent bleeding, repeat endoscopy may be performed within the subsequent 24 h. A failure of sclerotherapy is defined as the presence of further bleeding after two ES sessions during the same hospitalization for variceal hemorrhage (61). Alternative therapy should be pursued at this point.

Control of bleeding is achieved in 75–90% of cases with ES (45,62). ES is superior to vasopressin and balloon tamponade in control of hemorrhage. There was no difference in comparison to somatostatin or octreotide in rebleeding or in-hospital mortality. This was shown by meta-analysis of multiple studies (62). Rebleeding may occur in 30–50% of cases prior to variceal obliteration. The incidence of rebleeding following sclerotherapy is greater than that observed with TIPS or surgical therapy (62,63). However, mortality seems to be comparable or even lower than TIPS.

The incidence of serious complications are approx 20%, with a procedure related mortality of 2–5%. The most frequent severe complication is esophageal ulceration at the site of the injection that may result in bleeding in 20% of cases (54,62). Omeprazole may help to heal these ulcers more rapidly (64). ES is associated with bacteremia in 3–8% of cases. Bacterial peritonitis has been reported in 3–8% of patients undergoing sclerotherapy (65). Many clinicians routinely use antibiotics prior to ES in patients with ascites to prevent this complication, or for prophylaxis of infective bacterial endocarditis if indicated.

6.8.2. Endoscopic Variceal Ligation

Endoscopic variceal ligation (EVL) is placing ligation bands at 4–7 cm proximal to the gastroesophageal junction. In the setting of active variceal bleeding, the bands are placed at or around the variceal site oozing or spurting blood. Later, a maximum of eight bands are placed electively at weekly sessions to achieve obliteration.

A large, controlled trial showed EVL and sclerotherapy achieved comparable results in the initial control of variceal bleeding, which was 77–91% (66–69). However, sclerotherapy is preferable over EVL in this regard, mainly due to technical reasons, better visualization, and no need to use an overtube (70,71). In achieving variceal obliteration, both EVL and sclerotherapy have comparable results. Nevertheless, trials have shown EVL to be more rapid *(72)*. This may account for the decreased rate of rebleeding from esophageal varices with EVL. Both methods failed to achieve variceal obliteration in approx 35% of patients.

Complications are fewer with EVL compared with sclerotherapy mainly due to fewer numbers of postprocedure strictures *(72)*. Both therapies induce esophageal ulceration, which usually heal within 3 wk *(73,74)*. Bacteremia occurs less frequently in EVL than with sclerotherapy, probably because of overtube placement in the esophagus as part of the EVL procedure *(66,75,76)*. Subsequent reports have documented instances of major complications caused by overtube placement like esophageal laceration or perforation, esophageal obstruction from ligation bands and massive bleeding from postligation ulcers *(77–79)*.

6.9. Radiologic Therapy

6.9.1. Transjugular Intrahepatic Portosystemic Shunt (TIPS)

TIPS involves the placement of an expandable metal stent within the intrahepatic tract, bridging the hepatic and portal venous system with resultant prolonged portal decompression (*see* Chapter 6, this volume) *(80–82)*. The splanchnic hemodynamic alterations following TIPS are similar to those observed with a side-to-side nonselective portosystemic shunts. There is marked diversion of portal venous flow through the low resistance shunt and an associated decrease in hepatic perfusion *(81,82)*. This may result in elevated liver enzymes and bilirubin, impaired quantitative tests of hepatic function, decrease in liver volume, portosystemic encephalopathy, and acute liver failure. Systemic hemodynamic alterations, including increased cardiac output and elevated right atrial pressure caused by increased venous return to the right heart, may result in congestive heart failure in susceptible individuals.

TIPS is successfully performed in 94% of cases in experienced centers *(81,82)* and, based on limited data, control of active variceal bleeding is achieved in 96–100% of cases *(81–84)*. Rebleeding is observed in 7–19% of cases, and is usually associated with shunt stenosis or occlusion *(81–85)*. Mortality is low, but may increase if the procedure is done as an emergency.

Thus, at present, TIPS is best reserved for selected cases in whom pharmacological and/or endoscopic therapy failed to control acute bleeding or failed to prevent recurrent variceal hemorrhage *(86)*.

6.10. Surgical Therapy

Surgical decompressive shunts are the most effective therapy for control of acute variceal bleeding and to prevent rebleeding. It was the primary mode of therapy available prior to 1970. However, the high rate of early postoperative mortality, and the high frequency of liver failure and portosystemic encephalopathy following this surgery were major limitations. With the advances in the medical and radiological treatment modalities, surgical therapy is left with a minor role, and is only indicated in specific circumstances.

Portosystemic shunts may be divided mainly into nonselective and selective shunts. All forms of shunts have been used to prevent variceal rebleeding. Nonselective shunts decompress the portal venous system or the portal system and hepatic sinusoids in the case of side-to-side shunts. They are highly effective in controlling variceal hemorrhage, but have a higher rate of portosystemic encephalopathy that is observed in 15–45% of patients *(87)*. Shunt failure in 10–18% of cases is mainly due to thrombosis and occlusion. Operative mortality is 30–50% in patients with Child's C grade liver disease, many of which are performed emergently *(85)*.

In the selective shunts (distal splenorenal shunt DSRS) and (left gastric caval shunt), the main goal is to minimize portosystemic encephalopathy. They selectively decompress the gastroesophageal collateral circulation while maintaining a hypertensive superior mesenteric circulation and portal venous perfusion. Contraindications to the DSRS include refractory ascites, incompatible anatomy (small splenic vein, prior splenectomy), and an emergency situation *(87)*. DSRS failure is 10%, mainly related to shunt thrombosis or transient renal vein hypertension, which may preclude decompression of the collaterals *(88,89)*. Portal vein thrombosis has been reported in 10% of cases *(87)*. The incidence of portosystemic encephalopathy is 10% after DSRS. However, it may increase over time because of development of collaterals from the high resistance portal circulation to the low resistance shunt. Meta-analysis of the trials comparing nonselective shunts and DSRS in patients with primarily alcoholic cirrhosis showed a significantly lower incidence of encephalopathy in the DSRS patients *(90)*. However, there does not appear to be any survival advantage of DSRS over non-selective shunts *(87)*. Shunts are as effective as other therapies (endoscopic or pharmacological), and, therefore, should be considered as an option.

7. PREVENTION

7.1. Primary Prophylaxis

All patients with high variceal bleeding risk should receive prophylaxis for the prevention of the first variceal bleeding. At the moment, beta-blockers are the recommended treatment *(91)*. One randomized controlled clinical trial suggested that long-acting organic nitrates may be an alternative to beta-blockers. There is no justification at the present time to use endoscopic therapy for this indication.

7.2. Secondary Prophylaxis

Endoscopic therapy, beta-blockers, or surgery can be used. Withholding treatment is not justified. If the first choice of therapy fails, one of the other options can be used. First choice for the prevention of gastric variceal rebleeding is beta-blockers. A recent study suggests that the combination of beta-blockers plus isosorbide mononitrate is superior to sclerotherapy in the prevention of rebleeding *(92)*. If this study is confirmed, this therapeutic option will become the first choice option for the prevention of rebleeding.

8. INDICATIONS FOR CONSULTING THE SUBSPECIALIST

Patients suspected of having portal hypertension should be evaluated and then endoscopically screened for the presence of esophageal varices by the subspecialist. In secondary prevention of variceal bleeding, the subspecialist, aided by diagnostic studies, should be involved in deciding whether a specific patient should be managed pharmacologically by performing series of elective endoscopic banding or sclerotherapy or both. The subspecialist should be involved in cases of acute upper gastrointestinal bleeding to perform endoscopy, and sclerotherapy or banding of the esophageal varices, as the first line of intervention. Another role for the subspecialist is determining if and when the patient may need TIPS, or, in some cases, a surgical shunt procedure.

SUMMARY

Portal hypertension can occur with or without liver damage.

Esophageal varices may or may not be found in patients with portal hypertension.

Confirmation of the presence of esophageal varices should be pursued with upper endoscopy in every patient suspected of having portal hypertension.

If present, the patient should take beta-adrenergic blockers, or other pharmacological therapy, as a preventive measure to decrease the likelihood of variceal bleeding.

Bleeding from esophageal varices is one of the most formidable and dramatic life threatening events in medicine.

In acute bleeding from esophageal varices, care should be taken not to over-replace the intravascular volume, as it may elevate the portal pressure and exacerbate bleeding.

Endoscopic therapy is the first line of interventional therapy in acute bleeding from esophageal varices, and has to be performed by an experienced subspecialist.

REFERENCES

1. Groszmann RJ, Atterbury CE. Portal hypertension classification and pathogenesis. Semin Liver Dis 1982;2:177–186.
2. Vorobioff J, Bredfeldt JE, Groszmann RJ. Hyperdynamic circulation in portal hypertensive rat model. A primary factor for maintenance of chronic portal hypertension. Am J Physiol 1983;244:G52–G57.
3. Benoit JN, Wormack WA, Hernandez I, et al. "Forward" and "backward" flow mechanisms of portal hypertension. Relative contributions in the rat model of portal vein stenosis. Gastroenterology 1985;89:1092–1096.
4. Garcia-Tsao G, Groszmann RJ, Fisher RL, et al. Portal pressure, presence of gastroesophageal varices and variceal bleeding. Hepatology 1985;5:419–424.
5. Polio J, Groszmann RJ. Hemodynamic factors involved in the development and rupture of esophageal varices. A pathophysiologic approach to treatment. Semin Liver Dis 1986;6:318–331.
6. Friedman EW, Weiner RS. Estimation of hepatic sinusoid pressure by means of venous catheters and estimation of portal pressure by hepatic vein catheterization. Am J Physiol 1951;165:527.
7. Groszmann RJ. Reassessing portal venous pressure measurements. Gastroenterology 1984;80:1611.
8. Groszmann RJ, Glickman M, Blei AT, et al. Wedged and free hepatic venous pressure measured with a balloon catheter. Gastroenterology 1979;76:253.
9. Bosch J, Mastai R, Kravetz D, et al. Hemodynamic evaluation of patients with portal hypertension. Semin Liver Dis 1986; 6:309.
10. Bolondi L, Gandolfi L, Arienti V, et al. Ultrasonography in the diagnosis of portal hypertension: diminished response of portal vessels to respiration. Radiology 1982;142:167.
11. Balthazar EJ, Naidich DP, Megibow AJ, et al. CT evaluation of esophageal varices. Am J Radiol 1987;148:131.
12. Pascal JP, Cales P, Desmorat H. Natural history of esophageal varices. In: Bosch J, Rodes J, eds. Recent advances in the pathophysiology and therapy of portal hypertension. Serono Symposia Review, Rome, 1987, pp. 127–142.
13. Kleber G, Sauerbrach T, Ansari H, et al. Prediction of variceal hemorrhage in cirrhosis: a prospective follow-up study. Gastroenterology 1991;100:1332–1337.
14. The North Italian Endoscopic Club for the Study and Treatment of Esophageal Varices. Prediction of the first variceal hemorrhage in patients with cirrhosis of the liver and esophageal varices. N Engl J Med 1988;319:983–989.
15. Beppu K, Inokuchi K, Koyanagi N, et al. Prediction of variceal hemorrhage by esophageal endoscopy. Gastrointest Endosc 1982;27:213–218.
16. Vinel JP, Cassigneul J, Levade M, et al. Assessment of short term prognosis after variceal bleeding in patients with alcoholic cirrhosis by early measurement of portohepatic gradient. Hepatology 1986;6:116,117.
17. Schichting P, Christensen E, Faurholdt L, et al. Main causes of death in cirrhosis. Scan J Gastro 1983;18:881–889.
18. McCormick PA, Burroughs AK. Relation between liver pathology and prognosis in patients with portal hypertension. World J Surg 1994;18:171–175.
19. Graham DY, Smith JL. The course of patients after variceal hemorrhage. Gastro 1981;80:800–809.
20. Watanabe K, Kimura K, Matsutami S, et al. Portal hemodynamics in patients with gastric varices: a study in 230 patients with esophageal and/or gastric varices using portal vein catheterization. Gastro 1988;95:434–440.
21. Sarin SK, Lahoti D, Saxene SP, et al. Prevalence, classification and natural history of gastric varices: a long term follow-up study in 568 portal hypertension patients. Hepatology 1992;16:1343–1349.
22. Mathur SK, Dalvi AN, Someshwar V, et al. Endoscopic and radiologic appraisal of gastric varices. Br J Surg 1990;77:432–435.
23. Caletti GC, Brocchi E, Zani L, et al. Assessment of portal hypertension by endoscopic ultrasonography. Gastrointest Endosc 1988;36:S21–S27.
24. Korula J, Chin K, Ko Y, et al. Demonstration of two distinct subsets of gastric varices. Dig Dis Sci 1990;36:303–309.
25. Palmer ED. Erosive gastritis in cirrhosis: influence of portal hypertension on the gastric mucosa. Am J Dig Dis 1957;2:31–36.
26. D'Amico G, Montalbano L, Traina M, et al. Natural history of congestive gastropathy in cirrhosis. Gastroenterology 1990;99:1558–1564.
27. Hashizume M, Tanaka K, Inokuchi K. Morphology of gastric microcirculation in cirrhosis. Hepatology 1987;3:1008–1012.
28. McCormack TT, Sims J, Eyre-Brook I, et al. Gastric lesions in portal hypertension: inflammatory gastritis or congestive gastropathy. Gut 1985;26:1226–32.
29. Groszmann RJ, Colombato LA. Gastric vascular changes in portal hypertension. Hepatology 1988;8:1708–1710.
30. Panes J, Bordas JM, Pique JM, et al. Increased gastric mucosal perfusion in cirrhotic patients with portal hypertensive gastropathy. Hepatology 1992;103:1875–1882.
31. Albillos A, Colombato LA, Enriquez R, et al. Sequence of morphological and hemodynamic changes of gastric microvessels in portal hypertension. Gastro 1992;102:2066–2072.

32. Chen L, Groszmann RJ. The presence of blood in the stomach lumen increases splanchnic blood flow and portal pressure in portal hypertensive rats. Hepatology 1995;22:259A.

33. Colombato LA, Albillos A, Groszmann RJ. Vasodilatation and sodium retention in prehepatic portal hypertension. Gastro 1992;102:931–935.

34. Murray JF, Dawson AM, Sherlock S. Circulatory changes in chronic liver disease. Am J Med 1958;24:358–367.

35. Boyer JL, Chatterjee C, Iber FL, et al. Effect of plasma volume expansion in portal hypertension. N Engl J Med 1966;275:750–755.

36. Britton RC. Pregnancy and esophageal varices. Am J. Surg 1982;143:421–425.

37. Bredfeldt JE, Bosch J, Groszmann RJ. Splanchnic angiography increases portal pressure in portal hypertensive patients. Hepatology 1982;2:684A.

38. Terblanche J, Yakoub HI, Bornman PC, et al. Acute bleeding varices. A five year prospective evaluation of tamponade and sclerotherapy. Ann Surg 1981;194:521–530.

39. Groszmann RJ, Kravetz D, Bosch J, et al. Nitroglycerin improves the hemodynamic response to vasopressin in portal hypertension. Hepatology 1982;6:757–762.

40. Bosch J, Kravetz D, Rodes J. Effects of somatostatin on hepatic and systemic hemodynamics in patients with cirrhosis of the liver. Comparison with vasopressin. Gastro 1981;80:518–525.

41. Nusbaum M, Conn HO. Arterial vasopressin infusion: science or seance. Gastro 1975;69:263–267.

42. Tsai YT, Lay CS, Lai KH, et al. Controlled trial of vasopressin plus nitroglycerin vs vasopressin alone in the treatment of bleeding esophageal varices. Hepatology 1986;6:406.

43. Gimson AES, Westaby D, Hegarty J et al. A randomized trial of vasopressin and vasopressin plus nitroglycerin in the control of acute variceal hemorrhage. Hepatology 1986;6:410.

44. Bosch J, Groszmann RJ, Garcia-Pagan JC, et al. Association of transdermal nitroglycerin to vasopressin infusion in the treatment of variceal hemorrhage: a placebo controlled clinical trial. Hepatology 1989;10:962.

45. Ready JB, Robertson AD, Rector WG. Effects of vasopressin on portal pressure during hemorrhage from esophageal varices. Gastroenterology 1991;100:1411.

46. Burroughs AK, McCormick DA, Hughes MD, et al. Randomized, double blind, placebo controlled trial of somatostatin for variceal bleeding. Gastroenterology 1990;99:1388–1395.

47. Valenzuela JE, et al. A multicenter, randomized, double blind trial of somatostatin in the management of acute hemorrhage from esophageal varices. Hepatology 1989;10(6):958–961.

48. Besson I, Ingrand D, et al. Sclerotherapy with or without octreotide for acute variceal bleeding. N Engl J Med 1995;9:555–600.

49. Burroughs AK, et al. Double blind RCT of 5 day octreotide versus placebo, associated with sclerotherapy for trial/failures. Hepatology 1996;24(4:2):352A (abstract 901).

50. Bosch J, Kravetz D, Bruix J, et al. Azygous blood flow in cirrhosis. Effects of balloon tamponade, vasopressin, somatostatin and propranolol. Hepatology 1983; 3:855A.

51. Sung JJY, Chung SCS, Lei CW, et al. Octreotide infusion or emergency sclerotherapy for variceal hemorrhage. Lancet 1993; 141:637-41.

52. Hwang JS, Lon CH, Chang CF, et al. A randomized controlled trial comparing octreotide and vasopressin in the control of acute esophageal variceal bleeding. J Hepatol 1992; 16:320-25.

53. Teres J, Cecilia A, Bordas JM, et al. Esophageal tamponade for bleeding varices. Controlled trial between Sengstaken-Blakemore tube and the Linton-Nachlas tube. Gastroenterology 1978;75:566–569.

54. Matloff DS. Treatment of acute variceal bleeding. In: Groszmann RJ, Grace ND, eds. Gastro clinics of North America. Saunders, New York, 1992, pp. 103–118.

55. Pitcher JL. Safety and effectiveness of the modified Sengstaken-Blakemore tube: a prospective study. Gastroenterology 1971;61:291–298.

56. Terblanche J. Esophagogastric varices. In: Taylor MD, Gollan JL, Steer ML, Wolfe MM, eds. Gastrointestinal emergencies. Williams and Wilkins, Baltimore, 1992, pp. 33–44.

57. Chojkier M, Conn HO. Esophageal tamponade in the treatment of bleeding varices. A decadal progress report. Dig Dis Sci 1980;25:267–272.

58. Hunt PS, Korman MG, Hansky J, et al. A eight year prospective experience with balloon tamponade in emergency control of bleeding esophageal varices. Dig Dis Sci 1992;27:413–416.

59. Fort E, Sautereau D, Silvain C, et al. A randomized controlled trial of terlipressin plus nitroglycerin vs balloon tamponade in the control of acute variceal hemorrhage. Hepatology 1990;11:678–681.

60. Paquet KJ, Feussner H. Endoscopic sclerosis and esophageal balloon tamponade in acute hemorrhage from esophageal varices: A prospective controlled randomized trial. Hepatology 1985;5:580–583.

61. Terblanche J, Krige JEJ. Emergency sclerotherapy. In: Bosch J, Groszmann RJ, eds. Portal hypertension: pathophysiology and treatment. Blackwell Scientific Publications, London, 1994, pp. 140–153.

62. D'Amico G. The treatment of portal hypertension: a meta-analysis review. Hepatology 1995;22:3432–3454.

63. Groupe dieted des Anastomoses Intra-Hepatiques TIPS vs sclerotherapy + propranolol in the prevention of variceal rebleeding: preliminary results of a multi-center randomized trial. Hepatology 1995;22:297A.

64. Gimson A, Polson R, Westaby D, et al. Omeprazole in the treatment of intractable oesophageal ulceration following injection sclerotherapy. Gastroenterology 1990;99:1829–1831.
65. Schembre D, Bjorkman DJ. Post-sclerotherapy bacterial peritonitis. Am J Gastro 1991;86:481–486.
66. Stiegmann GV, Goff JS, Michaletz-Onody PA, et al. Endoscopic sclerotherapy as compared with endoscopic ligation for bleeding esophageal varices. N Engl J Med 1992;326:1527–1532.
67. Laine L, El-Newihi HM, Migikovsky B, et al. Endoscopic ligation compared with sclerotherapy for the treatment of bleeding esophageal varices. Ann Int Med 1993;119:1–7.
68. Lo GH, Lai KH, Cheng JS, et al. A prospective, randomized trial of sclerotherapy in the management of bleeding esophageal varices. Hepatology 1995;22:466–471.
69. Gimson AES, Ramage JK, Panox MZ, et al. Randomized trial of variceal banding versus injection sclerotherapy for bleeding esophageal varices. Lancet 1993;342:391–394.
70. Jensen DM, Kovacs TOG, Randall GM, et al. Initial results of a randomized study of emergency banding vs. sclerotherapy for bleeding gastric or esophageal varices. Gastrointest Endosc 1993;39:279A.
71. Laine L. Ligation: Endoscopic treatment of choice for patients with bleeding esophageal varices? Hepatology 1995;22:663–665.
72. Laine L, Cook D. Endoscopic ligation compared with sclerotherapy for treatment of esophageal variceal bleeding. Ann Int Med 1995;123:280–287.
73. Young MF, Sanowski RA, Rasche R. Comparison and characterization of ulcerations induced by endoscopic ligation of esophageal varices versus endoscopic sclerotherapy. Gastrointest Endosc 1993;39:119–122.
74. Nijhawan S, Rai RR, Nepalia S, et al. Natural history of post-ligation ulcers. Am J Gastro 1994;89:2281.
75. Tweng CC, Green RM, Burke SK, et al. Bacteremia after endoscopic band ligation for esophageal varices. Gastrointest Endosc 1992;38:336–337.
76. Cohen LB, Korsten MA, Scherf EJ, et al. Bacteremia after endoscopic injection sclerosis. Gastrointest Endosc 1983;29:198–200.
77. Johnson PA, Campbell DR, Antonson CW, et al. Complications associated with endoscopic band ligation of esophageal varices. Gastrointest Endosc 1993;39:181–184.
78. Saltzman JR, Arora S. Complications of esophageal variceal band ligation. Gastrointest Endosc 1993;39:185,186.
79. Earnest ML, Bohorfoush AG, Sethi A, et al. Evidence of proximal esophageal injury after variceal band ligation. Gastrointest Endosc 1993;39:274.
80. Palmaz JC, Sibbett RR, Reuter SR, et al. Expandable intrahepatic portacaval shunt stents: early experience in the dog. Am J Radiol 1985;145:821–825.
81. Rossle M, Hoage K, Ochis A, et al. The transjugular portasystemic stent-shunt procedure for variceal bleeding. N Engl J Med 1994;330:165–171.
82. Laberge JM, Ring EJ, Gordon RL, et al. Creation of transjugular intrahepatic portosystemic shunts with the wallstent endoprosthesis: results in 100 patients. Radiology 1993;187:413–420.
83. Martin M, Zajko AB, Orons PD, et al. Transjugular intrahepatic portosystemic shunt in the management of variceal bleeding: indications and clinical results. Surgery 1993;114:719–727.
84. Ring EJ, Lake JR, Roberts JP, et al. Using transjugular intrahepatic portosystemic shunts to control variceal bleeding before liver transplantation. Ann Int Med 1992;116:304–309.
85. Cello JP, Grendell JH, Crass RA, et al. Endoscopic sclerotherapy versus portacaval shunt in patients with severe cirrhosis and acute variceal hemorrhage. N Engl J Med 1987;316:1589–1600.
86. Shiffren ML, Jeffers L, Hoofnagle JH, et al. The role of transjugular intrahepatic portosystemic shunt for therapy of portal hypertension and its complications: a conference sponsored by the national digestive disease advisory board. Hepatology 1995;22:1591–1597.
87. Rikkers LF, Sorrell T, Gongliang J. Which portosystemic shunt is best? Gastroenterol Clin North Am 1992;21:179–196.
88. Mehigan DG, Zuidema GD, Cameron JL. The incidence of shunt occlusion following portosystemic decompression. Surg Gynecol Obstet 1980;150:661.
89. Eckhauser FE, Pomerantz RA, Knol JA, et al. Early variceal rebleeding after successful distal splenorenal shunt. Arch Surg 1986;121:547.
90. Spina GP, Galeotti F, Opocher E, et al. Selective distal splenorenal shunt versus side to side portacaval shunt. Am J Surg 1988;155:564.
91. D'Amico G, Pagliaro L, Sorensen TIA, et al. Prevention of first bleeding in cirrhosis. A meta-analysis of randomized trials of nonsurgical treatment. Ann Intern Med 1992;117:59–70.
92. Villanueva C, Balanzo J, et al. Nadolol plus isosorbide mononitrate compared with sclerotherapy for the prevention of variceal bleeding. N Eng J Med 1996;25:1624–1629.

30 Acute Hepatic Failure

Kiran Sachdev and Jonathan Israel

CONTENTS

1. INTRODUCTION

Acute hepatic failure is the rapid onset of severe hepatocellular dysfunction, often accompanied by encephalopathy, and, frequently, in the absence of prior liver disease. Loss of hepatocellular function from a variety of possible etiologies can lead to a constellation of metabolic derangements, including defective protein and clotting factor synthesis, gluconeogenesis, ureagenesis, plasma detoxification, as well as neurologic complications (often associated with cerebral edema). The culmination of these derangements not infrequently leads to multiorgan failure and death.

Although some improvements in management, such as improved critical care medicine and orthotopic liver transplantation, have increased survival, mortality from all causes of acute liver failure is still 50% and its prognosis remains much worse than for chronic liver diseases *(1)*.

Acute liver failure can be separated into two separate syndromes, including: fulminant hepatic failure (FHF), which refers to hepatic failure occurring within 8 wk of the onset of symptoms including jaundice *(2)*; and subfulminant hepatic failure (sub-FHF), in which liver failure occurs over more than an 8-wk period, but within 2–3 mo of the onset of jaundice *(3)*.

More recently, a proposal to further narrow the time of onset of FHF to less than 2 wk from the onset of symptoms has been made. These authors also suggest that sub-FHF be redefined as the onset of hepatic encephalopathy 2 wk to 3 mo after the onset of jaundice *(4)*. The distinction between these different variants of liver failure is more than semantics, and may have therapeutic implications. Late-onset hepatic failure, i.e., hepatic encephalopathy 8–24 wk

From: *Diseases of the Liver and Bile Ducts: Diagnosis and Treatment*
Edited by: G. Y. Wu and J. Israel © Humana Press Inc., Totowa, NJ

from the onset of jaundice, tends to occur in older patients and often leads to the formation of ascites. It is almost never associated with cerebral edema and has a higher mortality rate. In contrast, FHF may occur at any age, cerebral edema is frequently seen, ascites is rare, and mortality is closely related to the etiology *(5,6)*.

2. CARDINAL SIGNS AND SYMPTOMS

Patients with FHF often have no prior evidence of liver disease. Illness usually begins with malaise and jaundice. The onset of hepatic encephalopathy occurs in a progressive fashion, and acute liver failure ensues rapidly. Early signs and symptoms may include changes in personality, episodes of antisocial behavior, impaired mental status, and character disturbances. Violent behavior and convulsions may eventually occur. Prominent motor abnormalities include asterixis, flapping tremor, paratonia, hyperactive stretch reflexes and decerebrate posturing. With progression of encephalopathy, consciousness becomes impaired. Characteristic neuro-ophthalmologic findings include intact pupillary reflexes and brisk ocular responses. Fetor hepaticus (fishy odor on the breath) is invariably present. Routine serum chemistries and hematologic data suggest hepatic injury. The most important index of hepatocellular necrosis is markedly elevated serum aminotransferase levels. They are often greater than 10 times normal values. An important parameter of hepatocellular dysfunction is a markedly prolonged prothrombin time (PT) that is not corrected with parenteral vitamin K.

3. PATHOGENESIS

There are numerous causes of FHF (*see* Table 1) that can be divided into four basic categories. These include infections, toxins, ischemia, and metabolic.

3.1. Infections

The most common infectious agents that precipitate FHF are hepatitis viruses A, B, C, D, and E. Other as yet uncharacterized hepatitis viruses may also be involved. Less than 1% of hepatitis A patients develop FHF. The risk increases when the illness is contracted in older patients. Prolonged PT in these patients identifies those at increased risk for developing FHF, whereas absolute values of aminotransferases are not necessarily a prognostic factor. Diagnosis is made by the presence of IgM anti-hepatitis A antibodies in the setting of acute liver failure. The risk of FHF is higher with hepatitis B virus (HBV) infection and occurs in 1–4% of hospitalized patients with HBV. Thirty to 60% of all patients with fulminant viral hepatitis have hepatitis B surface antigen. People who clear the HBV have a better prognosis. In these patients, the hepatitis B surface antigen is negative. However, IgM anti HBV core antibody is positive. Serum HBV DNA suggests active viral replication, but can be negative in the blood despite being present in liver cells. Such rapid viral clearance indicates a favorable response, because it implies a good immune response against the hepatitis B virus *(7)*. HBV mutants with defects in the hepatitis B surface antigen gene have been identified, and may account for some cryptogenic cases of FHF. Outbreaks of FHF due to the hepatitis Be antigen mutants (mutation in the precore region that prematurely terminates the synthesis of hepatitis Be antigen) have been reported in several areas of the world, including Japan and Israel *(8,9)*. Reactivation of viral replication in carriers of hepatitis B may lead to fulminant hepatitis. This can lead to FHF, and has been reported in association with antitumor chemotherapy and in renal transplant patients after cessation of immunosuppressive treatment *(10,11)*. There have been rare case reports of hepatitis C causing FHF *(12)*. HDV coinfection with hepatitis B increases the likelihood of the development of fulminant viral hepatitis. Coinfection may occur coincident with the acquisition of acute HBV infection, or may occur shortly after the initial HBV infec-

Table 1

Some causes of FHF

Viruses A-E, CMV, HSV
Toxins/drugs
Vascular
Tumor infiltration
Wilson's disease
Reye's syndrome
Acute fatty liver of pregnancy

tion and present clinically as a relapse of acute viral hepatitis *(13)*. The presence of hepatitis D viral antigen in the liver, or IgM anti-delta virus antibodies in the serum, would support this diagnosis. Similar to hepatitis A, hepatitis E virus is an enterically transmitted agent that is responsible for water-borne acute viral hepatitis. It is not known to cause chronic disease, but is implicated in causing FHF in pregnant women, and the mortality rate in this group of patients is as high as 40% *(14)* *(see* Chapter 8, this volume). The virus is endemic in India, northern and sub-Saharan Africa, Mexico, and parts of southeast Asia. It is occasionally seen in travelers returning from these endemic regions to North America and Europe. Among five Western studies in patients with FHF, hepatitis E was identified in only two, and accounted for only 6/97 (6%) of the total cases. Other viruses that can cause fatal hepatic necrosis, especially in the immunocompromised host, include herpes simplex, cytomegalo-, Epstein-Barr, and varicella viruses *(15)*.

3.2. Drugs and Toxins

Two patterns of hepatic injury can result from exposure to chemical agents (see Table 2). Intrinsic toxins cause injury in a predictable and reproducible fashion that is often dose related. Idiosyncratic hepatotoxins, on the other hand, can result in FHF from short-term exposure in an unpredictable fashion *(see* Chapter 13, this volume).

Intrinsic hepatoxic effects depend upon the interplay between intrinsic toxicity and host vulnerability. Carbon tetrachloride causes zone 3 fulminant necrosis.

There are certain direct toxins to the liver such as fluorinated hydrocarbons, including trichlorethylene and tetrachlorethylene, that have been employed as solvents. Toxicity often develops after inhalation or by percutaneous exposure. Acetaminophen ingestion has become a common method of suicide *(6,16)*. Hepatotoxicity associated with overdoses is well described. However, in the setting of alcoholism, even therapeutic doses can cause fatal hepatic necrosis *(17)*. Renal failure is often associated as well. Treatment with enteral acetylcysteine helps ameliorate hepatotoxicity, and can be given even up to 36 h after ingestion.

Idiosyncratic hepatotoxic drugs cause hepatic injury that occurs unpredictably, independent of the intrinsic properties of the drug, and is a function of an individual's susceptibility to the drug. Idiosyncratic hepatotoxic drugs act by one of two mechanisms *(see* Chapter 13, this volume; *1)* in hypersensitivity reactions, liver injury usually develops after an initial sensitization period of 1–5 wk. The clinical hallmarks of this type of injury are fever, rash, and serum eosinophilia. Histologically an eosinophilic infiltrate is seen in the liver. Drugs that can cause damage by this mechanism include sulfonamides, dapsone, sulindac, and other NSAIDS. Hepatotoxins that cause injury by metabolic means lack the clinical and histologic hallmarks, as well as the prompt recurrence of the hepatic injury after 1–2 challenge doses of the drug that is seen with hypersensitivity reactions. This latter characteristic suggests the production of hepatotoxic metabolites *(18)*. All commonly used inhaled anesthetic agents have a potential

Table 2

Examples of Some Drugs that Cause FHF

Intrinsic	Idiosyncratic
Acetaminophen	Halothane
CCl$_4$	NSAIDs
Trichloroethylene	INH
Aspirin	Methyldopa
	Amiodarone
	Valproic acid

of decreasing hepatic blood flow at the level of the portal vein and the hepatic artery, and are examples of idiosyncratic hepatotoxins. In addition, volatile anesthetics decrease cardiac output in a dose-dependent fashion. Of the three volatile anesthetics (halothane, enflurane, isoflurane), halothane is the commonest cause of hepatitis accounting for 5% of cases of FHF [19]. FHF develops 5–15 d after a second exposure to halothane, and has a predilection for middle-aged, obese, atopic females [20]. Twenty percent of halothane is metabolized and excreted, compared to 2% and 0.2% of enflurane and isoflurane, respectively [21–23]. Therefore, halothane generates more toxic byproducts that may account for its higher hepatotoxicity [24].

3.3. Vascular Injuries

Vascular injuries precipitating FHF occur due to deficient oxygen delivery to the liver. There are two distinct syndromes. The first is cardiac-related hepatic ischemia producing marked aminotransferase elevation, centrilobular necrosis, and acute liver failure. Etiologies include myocardial infarction, cardiac arrest, cardiomyopathy, and pulmonary embolism. The second is occlusion of the hepatic venous outflow. This condition may be seen with the Budd-Chiari syndrome, or in venocclusive disease in the setting of intensive chemotherapy and bone marrow transplantation (25).

3.4. Miscellaneous

Amanita phylloides mushroom poisoning occurs predominantly in continental Europe between September and November. Hepatic failure is preceded by muscarinic effects like profuse vomiting, sweating, and diarrhea. With early identification, antidotes like penicillamine are very effective [26]. Wilson's disease, also called hepatolenticular degeneration, is discussed in greater detail in Chapter 21. Although it may present as FHF, it usually causes chronic progressive hepatitis leading to cirrhosis. Serum copper and urinary copper excretion may be increased, but serum ceruloplasmin levels are decreased.

Acute fatty liver of pregnancy is seen in the third trimester of pregnancy and may present with sudden onset of jaundice (*see* Chapter 7). In some, preceding hypertension, peripheral edema, and proteinuria suggest toxemia of pregnancy. In severely affected women, the course is complicated by coma, renal failure, and hemorrhage. Finally, unusual conditions that can present as FHF include malignancy (especially myeloproliferative disorders), sepsis, disseminated TB, and amebic liver abscesses [27,28].

4. CLINICAL FEATURES

Patients developing FHF undergo a rapid onset of mental status changes, progressing from being healthy to near death in a matter of a few days. In addition to jaundice and mental status changes, there is a decreased hepatic dullness to percussion that reflects loss of liver cell mass.

4.2. Hepatic Encephalopathy

One of the most prognostically significant symptoms is hepatic encephalopathy (*see* Chapter 28). Onset of encephalopathy can be sudden, and precede the onset of jaundice. Once the patient has progressed to grade 3–4 encephalopathy, the prognosis is poor. One of the earliest signs of encephalopathy is a change in personality. Nightmares, headaches, and dizziness are other inaugural nonspecific symptoms. Delirium, nausea, and seizures indicate reticular system stimulation *(29)*. Uncooperative, violent behavior often continues, even when consciousness is clouded. Asterixis may be transient and *fetor hepaticus* is usually present.

4.2. Cerebral Edema

Cerebral edema develops in 75–80% of patients with grade 4 encephalopathy, and is the leading cause of death in patients with FHF *(30)*. Irrespective of etiology, cerebral edema is a major cause of death in patients with FHF. Earliest clinical signs may include paroxysmal or sustained muscle tone with teeth grinding, systolic hypertension, decerebrate posturing, and hyperventilation. Late signs include abnormal pupillary reflexes, and, ultimately, impairment of brain stem function. The cause of cerebral edema in FHF is not well understood and is likely multifactorial. Some authors suggest that it is caused by disruption of the blood-brain barrier *(17)* with direct leakage of plasma into CSF (vasogenic mechanism), whereas others have hypothesized cellular alterations that allow increased water uptake into brain cells (cytotoxic mechanisms) *(31)*. Cerebral edema in the confinement of the cranial vault increases intracranial pressure and decreases intracerebral perfusion. Cerebral ischemia occurs if cerebral perfusion pressure (CPP), systolic blood pressure (SBP)-intracerebral pressure (ICP) is not maintained above 40–50 mmHg. This occurs when ICP exceeds 30 mmHg. Full recovery of cerebral function is the rule in those patients in whom liver function returns, although permanent brain damage has been reported in a few cases *(32)*.

4.3. Coagulopathy

FHF is invariably associated with a coagulopathy that may predispose to hemorrhage if hemostasis is challenged by damage to blood vessels *(19)*. Two factors that contribute to coagulopathy are thrombocytopenia, and decreased levels of liver clotting factors. The platelet count decreases to less than 80,000/mm^3 in as many as half of patients with FHF *(33)*. Causes of thrombocytopenia include bone marrow depression, hypersplenism, and consumption of platelets by intravascular coagulation. Not only are circulating platelets reduced in number, but platelet lipids are altered as well, resulting in abnormalities in platelet function *(34)*. Platelet function appears to be normal in patients with liver failure when encephalopathy is not present, and the acquired platelet defect found in FHF subsides with patient recovery *(35)*.

The clotting factors synthesized in the liver include factors I (fibrinogen), II (prothrombin), V, VII, IX, and X. Defective protein synthesis results in prolongation of both prothrombin time (PT) and partial thromboplastin time (PTT). The extent of prolongation of PT is regarded as a sensitive index of severity of hepatocellular protein synthetic insufficiency, provided that vitamin K has been administered parenterally *(36)*. Prolongation of PT may precede clinical deterioration, including the development of encephalopathy. The half-life of factor VII is only 1–5 h, and, hence, its plasma concentration decreases earlier and to a greater extent than other liver-produced clotting factors. Decreased levels of factor V imply that hepatic damage has occurred independent of vitamin K-dependent factors II, VII, IX, and X. Measurements of factor V and PT are the two most widely used tests to follow the clinical course of patients with FHF. Disseminated intravascular coagulation (DIC) may occur because of reduced clearance of activated clotting factors. Antithrombin 3 and plasminogen levels are decreased, and increased levels of fibrin degradation products are noted.

5. COMPLICATIONS

5.1. Acid-Base Disturbances

A wide spectrum of acid-base disturbances can be associated with FHF. Hyperventilation is a common feature of FHF, and produces a low pCO_2 that may lead to respiratory alkalosis *(37)*. Hypokalemia, if it occurs, is associated with an increased concentration of plasma HCO_3 and metabolic acidosis. Extensive tissue damage caused by massive hepatic necrosis, especially in the presence of hypotension, may result in accumulation of lactic acid, pyruvate, and free fatty acids, leading to metabolic acidosis. Finally, depression of the respiratory center in the brain, possibly as a result of circulating toxins and cerebral edema, can result in hypercapnia and respiratory acidosis *(29)*.

5.2. Electrolyte Changes

Abnormal concentrations of serum electrolytes may contribute to altered neurologic and cardiac function. Hyponatremia is often present due to impaired renal excretion of free water despite renal retention of sodium *(38)*. Hypokalemia often occurs with the increased renal retention of sodium. Other factors contributing to hypokalemia in patients with FHF are inadequate potassium intake, vomiting, secondary aldosteronism, and the use of diuretics. Severity of hypokalemia does not correlate with the extent of liver failure, but can exacerbate encephalopathy *(39)*.

5.3. Hypoglycemia

Severe hypoglycemia (blood glucose <40mg/dL) occurs in approx 40% of the patients with FHF *(40)*. It results mainly from impaired hepatic glucose release. Massive necrosis of hepatocytes leads to depletion of the glycogen content of the liver and impaired gluconeogenesis. Accompanying changes in the serum concentration of hormones, such as insulin, glucagon, and growth hormone, may also contribute to hypoglycemia. Plasma insulin concentration is increased due to impaired catabolism of this hormone by the diseased liver *(41)*.

5.4. Circulatory Changes

The circulatory changes in FHF resemble those of septic shock. There are decreased systemic vascular resistance and decreased blood pressure secondary to severe peripheral shunting from plugging of small vessels by platelets. Other contributory factors to these vascular changes include interstitial edema and abnormal vasomotor tone. Tissue hypoxia at the microcirculation level occurs due to decreased tissue oxygen extraction leading to lactic acidosis. Later, brain stem depression leads to failure of the autonomic vasomotor mechanism, and may worsen circulatory failure. Cardiac dysrhythmias are noted in later stages of FHF *(42)*.

5.5. Infections

In a study of 50 patients with acute liver failure, 90% had clinical or bacteriologic evidence of infection *(43)*. The risk of infection is increased in patients with FHF because of decreased opsonic activity of polymorphonuclear leukocytes and macrophages *(44)*. Also, alterations in cell-mediated and humoral immunity have been noted *(45)*. Infections in blood and the respiratory tract are often detected within 3 d of admission. Typical manifestations of infections, such as fever and leukocytosis, may be absent. More than two thirds of infections are caused by Gram-positive organisms such as staphylococcus aureus *(46)*.

Other complications of fulminant hepatic failure include upper gastrointestinal tract bleeding, pancreatitis, bacterial and fungal sepsis, renal failure, and cardiopulmonary abnormalities.

6. TREATMENT OF FULMINANT HEPATIC FAILURE

6.1. General Measures

Care of patients who develop FHF is centered around management of the complications until either the liver recovers or a graft is found for transplantation (*see* Fig. 1). Numerous trials with corticosteroids to charcoal hemoperfusion have been attempted. Although several bioartificial devices are currently undergoing clinical evaluation and are in various stages of development, unlike dialysis for renal failure patients, an artificial hepatic device to substitute for the liver remains elusive. Another area of investigation involves the use of partial auxiliary hepatic grafts or cellular transplants to supplement the patient's critically ill native liver *(47,48)*. These types of techniques are not yet readily available, but may hold some hope for the future.

In recent years, survival of patients with fulminant hepatic failure has improved because of improvements in intensive supportive care, combined with the availability of liver transplantation *(49)*. Soon after a patient with FHF is admitted, and continuously thereafter, the appropriateness of liver transplantation should be assessed, because transfer to a specialized center is best accomplished when the patient has early (grade 1 or 2) encephalopathy. Neurologic changes can occur in patients with FHF in an unpredictable fashion. Sudden rapid rises in ICP can result in midbrain herniation and death. If a patient meets stringent transplant criteria, he or she should be transferred via a helicopter to a transplant center, rather than in a pressurized aircraft or prolonged ground transport. The depressurization changes associated with the former and the centrifugal forces associated with the latter may have a deleterious effect on cerebral edema (50). If the patient progresses to grade 3 or 4 encephalopathy, transfer to an ICU in a tertiary referral center is imperative. Initial evaluation in patients with fulminant hepatic failure should include measurement of blood glucose, acetaminophen, and serum ceruloplasmin (patients less than 50 yr of age) levels. In addition, prothrombin time, serologic tests for hepatitis viruses, and toxicologic screening should all be performed.

A minority of patients with FHF may benefit from specific and generally highly effective therapies. In FHF due to acetaminophen overdose, therapy with acetylcysteine (loading oral dose of 140 mg/kg, followed by 70 mg/kg every 4 h for 68 hours for a total of 17 doses) to restore glutathione stores, clearly improves prognosis. Administration of acetylcysteine has maximum efficacy if performed within 15 h of the overdose, but can be given up to 36 h later *(51)*. Herpes zoster or cytomegalovirus may cause FHF, and may respond to specific therapy with acyclovir and ganciclovir, respectively *(50)*. The few patients that present with Budd-Chiari syndrome and FHF may dramatically improve with portal vein decompression by an emergency mesocaval or mesoatrial shunt. Finally, if discovered early, antidotes like penicillamine for mushroom poisoning can be highly effective *(26)*.

6.2. Cerebral Edema

Patients with FHF are at risk for developing cerebral edema, and should be kept in a quiet environment with their trunks at a 45° incline and subjected to minimum tactile stimulation. Direct measurement of ICP using subdural or extradural transducers is a valuable guide to treatment. The goal is to maintain CPP greater than 50 mmHg and ICP less than 20 mmHg. Although placement of a monitor is invasive and bleeding is a potential complication, it is used in most transplant centers because it permits rapid detection and appropriate treatment of cerebral edema. Monitors are also useful in avoiding worsened ICP with manipulation of the patient, such as suctioning or changing body position. Acute hyperventilation is effective in early cerebral edema, but is not recommended when intracerebral blood flow is reduced *(52)*.

Mannitol is the mainstay of treatment throughout, and is administered as a rapid bolus (0.3–0.4 mg/kg) *(30)*. If diuresis does not ensue, then plasma osmolality should be measured,

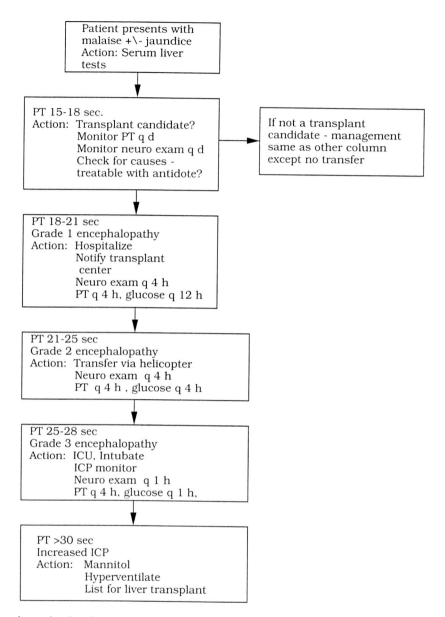

Fig. 1. A schematic plan for the management of fulminant hepatic failure. ICP, Intracranial pressure.

and the mannitol dose repeated if osmolality is less than 320 milliosm. In patients with coex-isting renal failure, the administration of mannitol needs to be coupled with the removal of three times the administered volume by ultrafiltration after 15 min *(53)*.

Cerebral edema refractory to these measures may respond to thiopental. The initial bolus is 185–500 mg over 15 min, followed by infusion of 50–250 mg/h *(54)*. This infusion may mask signs of raised ICP, and should only be used when there is ICP monitoring. Prophylactic use of dexamethasone is not effective in reducing cerebral edema *(55)*. CT scan of the brain is insensitive for the diagnosis of cerebral edema *(56)*. Only one third of patients with FHF demonstrate evidence of brain swelling on CT scan *(57)*. However, CT scans on admission to exclude intracerebral hemorrhage, after placement of ICP monitor, have been found useful to exclude structural lesions.

6.3. Hepatic Encephalopathy

The use of lactulose in chronic liver failure is well established. It has been used in the treatment of FHF-associated encephalopathy, although its value in this condition is unconfirmed. Indeed, there has never been a controlled trial demonstrating a beneficial effect of lactulose in treatment of hepatic encephalopathy complicating FHF. Lactulose may be administered orally via nasogastric tube or as a high-volume, retention enema. However, in the presence of a coagulopathy, rectal administration may cause colonic bleeding, whereas oral administration may be ineffective in the presence of ileus. Lactulose usually does not prevent deepening of coma because of underlying hepatic necrosis.

6.4. Glucose Monitoring

Capillary blood glucose should be measured every 4 h in conscious, and hourly in comatose, patients with FHF. Glucose is administered as 10% dextrose by continuous infusion. If blood glucose falls below 100 mg\dL, 100 mL of 50% dextrose solution boluses should be admin-istered immediately with an upward adjustment of the 10% dextrose infusion rate.

6.5. Gastrointestinal Bleeding

In an attempt to reduce gastrointestinal bleeding from gastric or duodenal ulceration, intragastric pH should be monitored every 3–4 h and maintained greater than 5 with regular doses of an H_2-receptor antagonist and or antacids.

6.6. Coagulopathy

The clinical impact of coagulopathy has been reduced by the use of fresh frozen plasma (FFP), cryoprecipitate, and platelet concentrate. However, the use of fresh frozen plasma has not been shown to be of any value in the absence of acute bleeding *(58)*. As mentioned earlier, deficiency of clotting factors is not the only cause of bleeding. Hemorrhage is more likely in the presence of an associated thrombocytopenia and DIC. FFP and platelet transfusions should be given to maintain platelet levels greater than 60,000, if invasive procedures are to be performed or the patient is bleeding. Vitamin K should be given early in the course of hepatic failure, but usually has little effect on PT. DIC in these patients is suggested by a more rapid decrease in the clotting factors than anticipated, due to impaired hepatic synthe-sis, thrombocytopenia, and is characterized by the presence of fibrin degradation products in the blood, the absence of plasminogen activators, and schistocytes on peripheral smear. This process may be fueled by the administration of FFP or clotting factors. It should be noted that the added salt and water load present in these products may precipitate cerebral edema.

6.7. Renal Failure

Renal failure occurs in greater than 50% of patients with FHF. Urea production may be decreased in FHF, so azotemia may not be pronounced despite low creatinine clearance. Infusion of dopamine (2–4 mg/kg/h) may reverse deterioration in renal function by increasing renal blood flow in patients who are oliguric *(53)*. Dialysis is indicated for the treatment of severe metabolic acidosis, hyperkalemia, and fluid overload. As mentioned earlier, in patients treated with mannitol for cerebral edema, who become oliguric, urgent hemodialysis or hemofiltration is indicated.

6.8. Cardiovascular Status

Initial hemodynamic abnormalities in FHF are similar to those in septic shock and are characterized by high cardiac output with decreased systemic vascular resistance (SVR) and diastolic blood pressure. Swan-Ganz monitoring is critical in these patients. Volume replacement is carried out with appropriate combinations of blood products and crystalloid solutions, while maintaining the pulmonary capillary wedge pressure (PCWP) less than 12 mmHg to avoid precipitating cerebral and pulmonary edema. Persistent hypotension, despite adequate volume replacement, is associated with a poor prognosis. Inotropes may not be effective because of persistent tissue hypoxia. In fact, they may further delay oxygen delivery *(59)*. Cardiac dysrhythmia can occur due to hypo- or hyperkalemia, acidosis, or cardiac irritation with a catheter. Progressive bradycardia is often a preterminal event.

6.9. Sepsis

Avoidance of sepsis is imperative in patients designated for liver transplant. Daily cultures of all available specimens, and heightened surveillance for emerging infection, is essential. Positive cultures are treated with appropriate antibiotics. The issue of whether to use prophylactic antibiotics has not been resolved. Controlled studies are in progress to assess the need for selective gut decontamination in these patients.

7. PROGNOSIS

The cause of liver failure is the most important variable in predicting survival. Survival is poor in non A, non B hepatitis, and idiosyncratic drug-induced FHF *(6)*. In acetaminophen overdose, a factor V level of less than 10% is considered a poor prognostic sign and an indication for transplantation *(60)*. As a general rule, in patients with acute liver failure, a prothrombin time greater than 30 s and grade 3 coma or cerebral edema with the need to intubate should precipitate active consideration for transplantation. Overall, because of improved intensive management of patients with FHF, survival has improved from 20% in 1973 to 50% in 1988 *(49)*.

8. LIVER TRANSPLANTATION

Liver transplantation is the definitive solution to the loss of hepatic function. As previously mentioned, the development of encephalopathy and associated progressive coagulopathy are the two most commonly used criteria to assess the need for transplantation. Liver transplantation is indicated in patients felt to have less than a 20% chance of survival without it. Although 1- and 5-yr survival in patients transplanted for acute liver failure is good, it is not as good as for relatively stable cirrhotics *(61,62)*. Prior to transplantation, it is necessary to consider whether the function of other organs, specifically the brain, is preserved, whether the patient is actively infected, and whether the disease will recur in the graft. Unfortunately, because of considerations such as inadequate insurance, geographic location of the patient, and lack of donor supply, only approx 10% of patients with this condition are transplanted.

9. INDICATIONS FOR CONSULTING THE SUBSPECIALIST

In the early stages of acute liver failure, patients will often come to the attention of their primary care physician with nonspecific complaints as described above. As the situation is recognized, namely that the patient undergoes rapid, and progressive hepatic decompensation, the patient should be referred to a specialist with access to a tertiary care facility that possesses the full range of intensive care technology.

10. CONCLUSIONS

FHF is a true medical emergency similar to cardiogenic shock and acute renal failure. Unfortunately, unlike renal failure, there is no currently available artificial device to perform essential hepatic function for the patient. Ultimate survival of these patients often depends on aggressive supportive care until either the patient's native liver recovers or a donor liver can be found. A rapid search for etiology is important, because, occasionally, a specific antidote can be used to reverse the deteriorating hepatic function.

Early consideration for transplantation and aggressive intensive care directed at specific problems associated with liver failure, including cerebral edema, bleeding, infection and renal failure, improve prognosis.

SUMMARY

Fulminant hepatic failure represents a medical emergency caused by rapid onset of severe hepatocellular dysfunction.

Identification of etiology is critical in determining prognosis and if an "antidote" is available.

Recent improvement in survival of patients with fulminant hepatic failure is a result of better critical care management and liver transplantation.

Effective monitoring and management of patients with fulminant hepatic failure involves the use of an epidural catheter to measure intracerebral pressure.

Current research efforts are aimed at finding a way to keep patients with fulminant hepatic failure alive until either their liver recovers or a graft liver can be found.

Timing of liver transplantation is a critical issue and involves assessment of liver function using prothrombin time and stage of encephalopathy.

REFERENCES

1. Martin P, Pappas SC. FHF. Dig Dis 1980;8:138–151.
2. Trey C, Davidson CS. The management of FHF. In: Popper H, Schaffer F, eds. Progress in liver disease, 3rd ed. Grune and Stratton, New York, 1970, pp. 282–298.
3. Bernuau J, Rueff B, Benhamou JP. Fulminant and subfulminant failure, definition and causes. Semin Liv Dis 1986;6:97–106.
4. O'Grady JG, Schalm SW, Williams R. Acute liver failure;redefining the syndrome. Lancet 1993;342:273–275.
5. O'Grady JG, Gimson AES, O'Brien CJ, et. al. Controlled trials of charcoal hemoperfusion and prognostic factors in FHF. Gastroenterology 1988;94:1186–1192.
6. O'Grady J, Alexander G, Hayallar K, et. al. Early indicators of the prognosis in FHF. Gastroenterology 1989;97:439–445.
7. Brenuau J, Goudeau A, Poynard T, et al. Multivariate analysis of the prognostic factors in fulminant hepatitis B. Hepatology 1986;6:648–651.
8. Omela M, Ehale T. Mutations in the precore region of the HBV DNA in patients with FHF and severe hepatitis. N Engl J Med 1991;324:699–704.

9. Liang TJ, Haregawa K, Wanda JR, et al. Characterization of an HBV variant associated with an epidemic of fulminant hepatitis. Hepatology 1990;12:869.

10. Hoofnagle JH, Dushenko GM, Schaffer DF. Reaction to chronic hepatitis B virus infection by cancer chemotherapy. Ann Int Med 1982;96:447–449.

11. Hansen CA, Sutherland DE, Snover DC. FHF in HBs Ag carrier renal transplant patient followed by cessation of immunosuppressive therapy. Transplantation 1985;39:311,312.

12. Liang TJ, Jeffers L, Reddy RK, et al. Fulminant or subfulminant non A non B viral hepatitis, the role of hepatitis C or E viruses. Gastroenterology 1993;104:556–562.

13. Smedile A, Veeme G, Cargnel A, et al. Influence of delta infection on the severity of hepatitis. Lancet 1982;2:945–947.

14. Asher LVS, Innis BL, Shesthra MP, et al. Virus like particles in liver of patients with fulminant hepatitis and antibody to hepatitis E virus. J Med Vir 1990;31:228.

15. Sobue R, Mijazaki H, Okamoto M, et al. Fulminant hepatitis in primary human herpes virus infection. N Engl J Med 1991;324:1290.

16. Smilkstein MJ, Knapp GL, Kulig KW, Rumack BH. Efficacy of oral N acetylcysteine in the treatment of acetaminophen overdose. N Engl J Med 1988;319:1557–1562.

17. Seeff LB, Cuccherine BA, Zimmerman HJ, Adlee E, Benjamin SB. Acetaminophen hepatotoxicity in alcoholics, a therapeutic misadventure. Ann Int Med 1986;104:399–404.

18. Speilberg SP, Gordon GB, Blake DA, et al. Predisposition to phenytoin hepatotoxicity assessed in vitro. N Engl J Med 1981;305:722–727.

19. Brunt EM, White H, Marsh JW, Holtmann B, Peters HG. FHF after repeated exposure to isoflurane anesthesia, a case report. Hepatology 1991;13:1017–1021.

20. Walton B, Simpson BR, Strunin L, et al. Unexplained hepatitis following halothane. Br Med J 1976;1:1171–1176.

21. Rehdev K, Forbes J, Alter H, et al. Halothane biotransformation in man, a quantitative study. Anesthesiology 1967;28:711–715.

22. Chase RE, Holaday DA, Fiserova-Bergerova V, et al. The biotransformation of ethrane in man. Anesthesiology 1971;35:262–267.

23. Holaday DA, Fiserova-Bergerova V, Latto IP, et al. Resistance to isoflurane biotransformation in man. Anesthesiology 1975;43:325–332.

24. Kenna JG, Satoh H, Christ DD, et al. Metabolic basis for a drug hypersensitivity, antibodies in sera from patients with halothane hepatitis recognize liver neoantigens that contain the trifuroacetyl group derived from halothane. J Pharmacol Exp Ther 1988;245:1103–1109.

25. Sandle GI, Layton M, Record CO, Cowan WK. Fulminant hepatic failure due to Budd-Chiari syndrome. Lancet 1980;1:1199.

26. Klein AS, Hart J, Bernes JJ, Goldstein L, Lewin K, Busuttill RW. Amanita poisoning;treatment and the role of liver transplantation. Am J Med 1989;86:187–193.

27. Goodwin JE, Coleman AA, Sahn SA. Miliary tuberculosis presenting as hepatic and renal failure. Chest 1991;99:752–754.

28. Rab SM, Alam N, Hoda AN, Yee A. Amoebic liver abscess;some unique presentations. Am J Med 1967;43:811–816.

29. Sherlock S. Fulminant hepatic failure;diseases of the liver and the biliary system. 9th ed. Oxford: Blackwell Scientific Publications, 1993:102–113.

30. Williams R, Alexander AES. Intensive liver care and management of acute hepatic failure. Dig Dis Sci 1991;36:820–826.

31. Traber PG, Dal Canto M, Ganges DR, Blei AT. Electron microscopic evaluation of brain edema in rabbits with galactosamine induced FHF, ultrastructure and integrity of the BBB. Hepatology 1987;7:1272–1277.

32. O'Brien CJ, Wise RJS, O'Grady JG, Williams R. Neurologic sequlae in patients recovered from FHF. Gut 1987;28:93–95.

33. Gimson AES, Brande S, Mellon, et al. Earlier charcoal hemoperfusion in FHF. Lancet 1982;2:681.

34. O'Grady, Langley PG, Isole LM, Aledort LM, Williams R. Coagulopathy of FHF. Sem Liv Dis 1986;6(2):159–163.

35. Rubin MH, Weston MJ, Bullock G. Abnormal platelet function and ultrastructure in FHF. Q J Med 1977;46:339.

36. Robert HR, Cederbaum AL. The liver and blood coagulation, physiology and pathology. Gastroenterology 1972;63:297.

37. Stanley NN, Salisbury BG, McHenry C. Effect of liver failure in the response of ventilation and cerebral circulation to carbon dioxide in man and in the goat. Clin Sci, Mol Med 1975;49:157.

38. Wilkinson SP, Arroya VA, Moodie H. Abnormalities of sodium excretion and other disorders of renal function in FHF. Gut 1976;17:500.

39. Hoyumpa AM, Desmond AV, Avant GR. Hepatic encephalopathy. Gastroenterology 1979;76:184.

40. Munoz SJ, Maddrey WC. Major complications of acute and chronic liver disease. Gastroenter Clin North Am 1988;17:265–287.

41. Sanson RI, Trey C, Jimmne AH. Fulminant Hepatitis with recurrent hypoglycemia and hemorrhage. Gastroenterology 1967;53:291.

42. Weston M, Talbot I, Howorth P, et. al. Frequency of cardiac arrhythmias and other cardiac abnormalities in FHF. Br Heart J 1976;38:1179–1188.

43. Rolando N, Harvey F, Brahm J, et al. Prospective study of bacterial infection in acute liver failure. Hepatology 1990;11:49–53.

44. Canaalese J, Gove CD, Gimson AES. Reticuloendothelial system and hepatic failure. Gut 1982;23:265–269.

45. Fagan EA, Williams R. Fulminant viral hepatitis. Br Med Bull 1990;46:462–480.

46. Wyke RJ, Canalese JC, Gimson AES, Williams R. Bacteremia in patients with FHF. Liver 1982;2:45–52.

47. Metselaar HJ, Hesselink EJ, DeRave S, et al. Recovery of failing liver after auxiliary heterotropic liver transplantation. Lancet 1990;334:1156,1157.

48. Boudjemak K, Jaeck D, et al. Auxiliary liver transplantation for fulminant and subfulminant hepatic failure. Transplantation 1995;59:218–223.

49. Hughes RD, Wendon RD, Gimson AES. Acute liver failure. Gut 1991;Supplement:586–589.

50. Munoz S. Management problems in FHF. Sem Liv Dis. Vol 13. 1993;14:395–413.

51. Harrison PM, Keays R, Bray GP, Alexander GJM, Williams R. Improved outcome of paracetamol induced FHF by the late administration of acetylcysteine. Lancet 1990;334:1572,573.

52. Ede RJ, Gimson AES, Bihari D, Williams R. Controlled hyperventilation in the prevention of cerebral edema in FHF. J Hepatol 1986;2:43–51.

53. O'Grady J, Portmann B, Williams R. FHF. In: Schiff L, Schiff E, eds. Diseases of the liver. 7th ed. Philadelphia: JB Lippincott Company, 1993:1077–1090.

54. Forbes A, Alexander GJM, O'Grady J, et al. Thiopental infusion in the treatment of intracranial hypertension complicating FHF. Hepatology 1989;10:306–310.

55. Canalese J, Gimson AES, Davis C. Controlled trial of dexamethasone and mannitol for cerebral edema of FHF. Gut 1982;23:625–629.

56. Lidofksy SD, Bass NM, Prager MC, et al. Intracranial pressure monitoring and liver transplantation for FHF. Hepatology 1992;16:161–167.

57. Munoz S, Robinson M, Northup B, et al. Elevated intracranial pressure and CT of the brain in FHF. Hepatology 1991;13:209–212.

58. Preston FE. Hemorrhagic diasthesis and control. In: Williams R, Hughes RD, eds. Acute liver failure, improved understanding and better therapy. Miter, London, UK, 1991, pp. 36–39.

59. Bihari D, Wendon J. Tissue hypoxia in FHF. In: Williams R, Hughes RD, eds. Acute liver failure, improved understanding and better therapy. Miter, London, UK, 1991, pp. 42–44.

60. Pereira L, Langley P, Hayllar K, Tredger JM, Williams R. Coagulation factors V and VIII/V ratio as predictors of outcome in paracetamol induced FHF and the relation to other prognostic factors. Gut 1992;33:98–102.

61. Bismuth H, Samuel D, Gugenham J, et al. Emergency liver transplantation for fulminant hepatitis. Ann Int Med 1989;107:337–341.

62. Devictor D, Desplanques L, Debray D, et al. Emergency liver transplantation for liver failure in infants and children. Hepatology 1992;16:1156–1162.

INDEX

ABOUT THE EDITORS

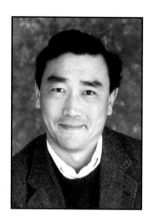

Dr. George Y. Wu received his M.D. and Ph.D. in Biochemistry from the Albert Einstein College of Medicine in 1976 and went on to Internal Medicine training at Harlem Hospital. He moved to the University of Connecticut in 1983 where he is now Professor of Medicine, Chief of the Division of Gastroenterology-Hepatology, and Herman Lopata Chair in Hepatitis Research. He received a number of awards and honors including an American Liver Foundation Research Prize and was elected to membership in two of the most prestigious national medical societies: the American Society of Clinical Investigation and the Association of American Physicians.

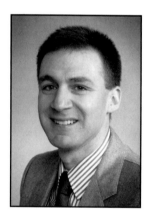

Dr. Jonathan Israel is a clinical assistant professor of medicine at the University of Connecticut. After graduating summa cum laude from Rensselaer Polytechnic Institute he attended Albany Medical College where he graduated with distinction in research. Dr. Israel did his internal medicine training at Johns Hopkins Hospital. He did his gastroenterology and hepatology fellowship at the University of Pennsylvania where he was awarded an American Liver Foundation Postdoctoral Research fellowship award. He is a member of the American Gastroenterologic Society, American College of Gastroenterology, and the American Association for the Study of Liver Diseases.